Comprehensive
Nursing Manual

Comprehensive Nursing Manual

Cecy Correia
Nursing Tutor
Uday General School of Nursing
Cardinal Gracias Memorial Hospital
Sandor, Bangli, Vasai (W)
Thane, Maharashtra, India

Forewords

SA Pinto
Pranita S Pereira

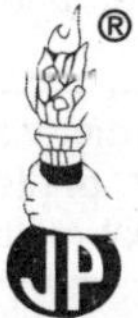

JAYPEE BROTHERS MEDICAL PUBLISHERS (P) LTD

Mumbai • St Louis (USA) • Panama City (Panama) • London (UK) • New Delhi • Ahmedabad
Bengaluru • Chennai • Hyderabad • Kochi • Kolkata • Lucknow • Nagpur

Published by
Jitendar P Vij
Jaypee Brothers Medical Publishers (P) Ltd

Corporate Office
4838/24 Ansari Road, Daryaganj, **New Delhi** - 110002, India, Phone: +91-11-43574357, Fax: +91-11-43574314

Registered Office
B-3 EMCA House, 23/23B Ansari Road, Daryaganj, **New Delhi** - 110 002, India
Phones: +91-11-23272143, +91-11-23272703, +91-11-23282021
+91-11-23245672, Rel: +91-11-32558559, Fax: +91-11-23276490, +91-11-23245683
e-mail: jaypee@jaypeebrothers.com, Website: www.jaypeebrothers.com

Offices in India

- **Ahmedabad**, Phone: Rel: +91-79-32988717, e-mail: ahmedabad@jaypeebrothers.com
- **Bengaluru**, Phone: Rel: +91-80-32714073, e-mail: bangalore@jaypeebrothers.com
- **Chennai**, Phone: Rel: +91-44-32972089, e-mail: chennai@jaypeebrothers.com
- **Hyderabad**, Phone: Rel:+91-40-32940929, e-mail: hyderabad@jaypeebrothers.com
- **Kochi**, Phone: +91-484-2395740, e-mail: kochi@jaypeebrothers.com
- **Kolkata**, Phone: +91-33-22276415, e-mail: kolkata@jaypeebrothers.com
- **Lucknow**, Phone: +91-522-3040554, e-mail: lucknow@jaypeebrothers.com
- **Mumbai**, Phone: Rel: +91-22-32926896, e-mail: mumbai@jaypeebrothers.com
- **Nagpur**, Phone: Rel: +91-712-3245220, e-mail: nagpur@jaypeebrothers.com

Overseas Offices

- **North America Office, USA,** Ph: 001-636-6279734, e-mail: jaypee@jaypeebrothers.com, anjulav@jaypeebrothers.com
- **Central America Office, Panama City, Panama,** Ph: 001-507-317-0160, e-mail: cservice@jphmedical.com, Website: www.jphmedical.com
- **Europe Office, UK,** Ph: +44 (0) 2031708910, e-mail: info@jpmedpub.com

Comprehensive Nursing Manual

© 2011, Jaypee Brothers Medical Publishers

First Edition: **2011**

ISBN 978-93-5025-173-7

Typeset at JPBMP typesetting unit

Printed at Rajkamal Electric Press, Plot No. 2, Phase-IV, Kundli, Haryana.

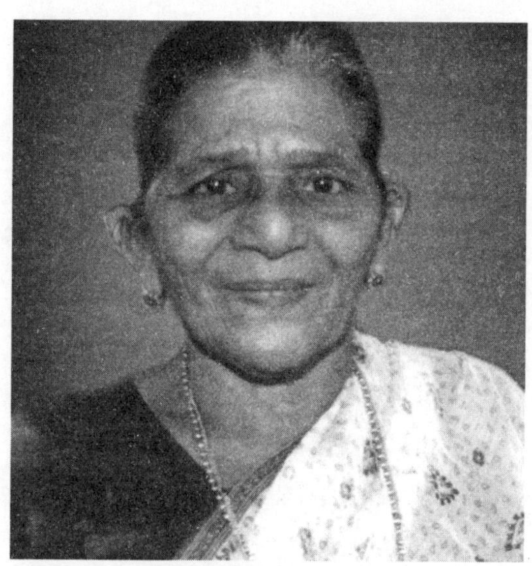

This book is humbly dedicated
to my Mother **Santan Correia.**
She is my teacher and first guru whom I salute.
May this book bring blessing to one and all.

Foreword

It is a great honor to introduce a book titled *Comprehensive Nursing Manual* by Cecy Correia. I am impressed by the content, which is challenging in today's nursing field. Let me congratulate Cecy Correia for having prepared such a wonderful book in time.

The aim of this book is to provide a well-illustrated, up-to-date text for the nurses. I am sure the response of this book will be no less and will use it as a textbook for the further studies.

As a person associated with nursing education for a few decades, I have come to realize more and more the vital importance of such knowledge in the changing scenario of modern nursing profession.

I hope, together with students, the trained nurses as well will find it a useful book of reference.

People today have to deal with a good number of clients and health care professionals whether working in one's country or abroad, associating a great deal of proficiency in nursing care.

I have no doubt that Cecy Correia's book *Comprehensive Nursing Manual* is just the ideal tool to achieve these objectives. She is a renowned author and lecturer, so let me once again congratulate her in well advance. I am confident that nurses can develop critical thinking skills that provide the high quality care that is expected by the 21st century.

I am sure that the authorities of nursing schools and colleges will browse through the pages of this highly recommended work and value it. This book is available to all the nurses to guide in their quest for knowledge, skill and excellence. The book will make a valuable contribution to the nursing literature.

It is my great privilege to be asked to write the foreword to *Comprehensive Nursing Manual* published by well-known publisher Jaypee Brothers Medical Publishers (P) Ltd, New Delhi. The publishers have responded magnificently with format, page layout, etc. This book will sharpen nurses' perception in several ways.

SA Pinto
Principal
Uday General School of Nursing
Cardinal Gracias Memorial Hospital
Sandor, Bangli, Vasai (W)
Thane, Maharashtra, India

Foreword

The content of the book *Comprehensive Nursing Manual* gives in nutshell, under one roof, information for nursing students, staff nurses, graduates and postgraduates. This book is also a useful guide to nurses who are preparing for interviews and planning to go abroad.

Due to lack of availability of continuous medical education in every hospital, many of the staff nurses feel lack of confidence to work in hospital equipped with latest technology. This book updates their knowledge to latest technologies.

The author has taken immense effort to give in nutshell all the information required by the nursing faculty. This book is written in a simple manner to understand all categories of people.

Today with high-tech and scientific revolution, the world has developed with latest technologies. This book gives complete information to present-day nurse to enrich her professional skills.

The initial chapters deal with nursing care. They describe the basic procedures starting from hand washing, back care to sophisticated procedure like hemodialysis, biopsies, etc.

More focus is given on adolescence and sex education in detail.

There are two chapters dealing with nurse and counseling also is the need of the hour to deal with illness giving psychological support in sickness.

Another chapter 'Medical Nursing, Doctor and Patient Relationship' is also explained well on human relationship.

Last chapter 'Health and Internet' 'Research—Nurses' Role with Eye on the Future' talks about nursing information and research.

Pranita S Pereira
Casualty Medical Officer
Cardinal Gracias Memorial Hospital
Sandor, Bangli, Vasai (W)
Thane, Maharashtra, India

Preface

More than two decades of my Nursing career, I always felt a dying need to acquire more knowledge but could not get due to the inadequate materials around. This gave me the inspiration to write this book on this content which all the nurses who are under training and all who are working as a staff and all graduates and postgraduates need to know and always may not find the right materials.

Moreover, in all the hospitals, the staff are not privileged to have 'continuous medical education' and so they feel outdated without up-to-date knowledge and thus feel lack of confidence to work in hospitals equipped with latest technologies. This concern for such lack of knowledge has been shared with me by a number of nurses. Hence, I have made my humble attempt to give all that is missing for them who will find every thing in one book and thus it will boost their self-esteem and confidence.

As one advances in Nursing Practice, some of the details with the daily practice becomes the second nature automatically. But there are certain things the nurses will always like to know and revise in nutshell reading, under one roof, which will be handy and useful tool for rest of life and their career as it is based on nursing principles and scientific principles.

The content and the very title of the book that is "Comprehensive Nursing Manual", which will be very useful to all the nurses to acquire all-round development as there are lots of things for each of you. It can be used in multipurpose ways for the nurses and many other graduates in medical field.

It will provide in-service education, nursing guide for senior nurses, a guide to nurses who are preparing for interview and plan to go abroad, challenges of nursing field, to walk towards a nurse of 21st century, where today there are new and divers approaches to nursing profession.

This book will provide unique content and right choice for the nurses who will be looking for it. The book has something new, valuable, unique, precious to one's work and written in a simple manner to understand all the categories of people. It gives new ways of perceiving knowledge and skill to a nurse looking towards 21st century who has diverse roles and responsibilities to play and the issues challenging her profession.

This book helps nurses to wake up and equipped well to face competitive modern nursing world. Change with changing times and keep abreast with things that are evolving; otherwise get ready to grow in darkness. Be a new way of becoming a nurse. Improve your professionalism; today, you have many opportunities to be creative and innovative, so get trained in skills. Be future orientated and make effort for excellence. Today, the world has become small, within a fraction of a second, you can reach any corner of the world and contact. Today, with high tech and scientific revolution, the world has developed with latest technology one can ever imagine a few years before. Today, man is living in rocket/robot age which has opened the wider horizons in professional nursing too.

Today's era is such that we must keep learning and enriching our knowledge capital with new viewed technology adding milestone in the pursuits of excellence. Today, you have to be smart. Your mind should be far more developed than a few decades before. With internet, satellites, website and email, and computer which in older times people could never think of.

Today, computer is taking over human mind. Advanced equipment like digital monitors and microscopes help to grasp nursing concept better than before, computer presentation, advanced technological aids, facilities like laser projector, laptops, online education courses and knowledge-oriented technology in the midst of all advances, where are you? Where has Nursing Profession reached? Do you feel outdated / or lost? Or do you feel confident enough?

The workload connected with human beings is never constant. Human needs are varied at various stressful situations. Nurses are with the patients round the clock. Nursing plays a vital role in safeguarding the health of the people. Nursing needs to develop in its potentialities as millions are in need of expert care by nurses. There is always a shortage of nurses for high quality care. The ability, intelligence, aptitude , initiative, and particular knowledge are considered in favors in promotion. A technical knowledge in their field enables the task be dynamic, creative and innovative.

Certain details are avoided in order that topics may not become cumbersome, which will help in smooth reading. Health is the greatest gift and contentment, the greatest wealth and believe that health is the condition of wisdom and sign of cheerfulness.

The best six doctors anywhere and no one can deny it are—sunshine, water, rest, air, exercise and diet—they will mend you and change you to stay well.

So, here is the book for you to enhance your confidence. I am sure it will deepen your knowledge and enrich your professional skills. It will enhance nurses to keep an eye on the future.

Cecy Correia

Acknowledgments

Teachers are those who use themselves as bridges, over which they invite their students to cross. Then having facilitated their crossing, joyfully collapse, encouraging them to create bridges of their own.

"What we do for ourselves dies with us, what we do for others remains immortality".

"The world of tomorrow belongs to the person who has the vision today".

"A child's life is like a piece of paper on which every person leaves a mark".

Inspired by such words and the almighty God whose grace, blessings and constant accompaniment was felt all through working on this book.

I express my profound attitude of gratitude to my husband *Alois Macwan*, for his constant support and encouragement which sustained me to complete this book.

I extend my gratitude to my Principal, Dr Pranita (MO), nursing colleagues, students and hospitals and clinical fields who motivated me towards this book.

I am highly privileged to get 'Jaypee Brothers' as the 'pioneer medical publishers' which has link to the world through and is committed to the cause of medicine. They are distinct and have a finest quality work.

I was impressed by the prompt response and constant touch with the writers that make them distinct in their approach and attitude.

I wish to give a special recognition to M/s Jaypee Brothers Medical Publishers and their production team who has directed me to make this book a reality. I humbly express my million thanks to Mr Tarun Duneja, Director-Publishing, Mr K Ramesh, Mumbai branch, because of their constant guidance, phone calls, emails, and their leadership has been praiseworthy. My reviewer, proofreader and all who worked behind this book unassumingly I wish to acknowledge. Without whom the edition would not have been possible.

To write a book is not a small fear, I hope it meets the standard for our readers.

Gratitude is attitude of life, which flows from my heart; I extend my sincere thanks to every well-wisher for completing this book.

Contents

Section II : Nurse Connecting Herself to Institution and Community or Transferring Technology from Hospital to Rural Field

**Section I I I : Nurse and Nursing Art as Science and
Nurse in Clinical Field with Procedures**

Section I V : Nurse and Her Psychological, Emotional Aspect with Client and School Health Education—Adolescence and Counseling

Marching and Moving Ahead with Her Career in 21st Century

Heart Attack and Nursing Interventions

WHAT IS SILENT HEART ATTACK?

Most people enormously assume that all heart attacks are always preceded by a series of symptoms such as chest pain, pain in the left arm etc. however; a heart attack can also be asymptomatic as is the case with a silent heart attack. Through it comes without warning signs; it is still life threatening, often goes undetermined clinically. This increases the chances of underlining heart diseases becoming more serious heart attack and there fore the first and only symptom of a silent heart attack could be sudden death. Here section of heart does not receive blood. This lack of blood flow can cause the heart tissues to scar and even die.

Heart attack? When? Blood pressure and diabetes are not the only silent killers. Heart attack too may occur without any warning signals. Silent heart attack, offers no warning signs and no symptoms. In fact, you may have suffered one without being aware in the least. Scary? It can be scarier, if you are ignorant about it.

Certain atypical signs such as sweating, dizziness and nausea, headache, pallor, nervousness and anxiety may accompany silent heart attack. A feeling of fullness in the center of the chest, mild pain in the arms, breathlessness while doing routine physical activities such as walking to the bus stop. Usually such symptoms are mild and subside within a short span of time.

How can it be **detected?** It can be detected by talking ECG, talking medical history, testing blood for cardiac enzymes, a stress test, echocardiogram, coronary angiography.

Since clients have not experienced symptoms, they tend to take it lightly, or think that doctors are making a big deal.

The high **risk group**—You are likely to have silent heart attack if you are above 65 years, are diabetic, high blood pressure, have high elevated serum cholesterol level, are obese, lead a sedentary lifestyle, smoke regularly, had a history of strok, lack of exercise, type of personality.

Treatment—A heart attack is a medical emergency. Delaying treatment can mean lasting damage to your heart or even death. The sooner the treatment begins the better your chances of recovering almost completely.

Thrombolytic drugs or clot busters are used to dissolve blood clots that are blocking blood flow to the heart. When given soon after a heart attack begins, these drugs can limit or prevent permanent damage to the heart. The drugs to be administered within one hour of silent heart attack. Treatment measures also involve angioplasty to unclog the blocked arteries or a coronary bypass surgery where, in arteries or veins from other areas in your body are used to bypass the blocked arteries.

How to prevent it? Tobacco and passive smokers can damage heart health. Stress levels, which are extremely high in metros, avoid food high in saturated fats, switch to food rich in fibers. Do regular exercise. After age of 35 have yearly checkups and ECG, stress test, lipid profile, sugar is tested.

Angina pectoris is pain in the chest that is caused by *hypoxia of the cardiac muscle*. It is a sign of *myocardial ischemia*. Angiana pain comes during activities. Tab. *Nitroglycerine* placed under the tongue three minutes before activity and repeats the dose in 5 minutes if pain occurs. The two coronary arteries are the 1st branches of the aorta and carry blood with high oxygen content to the myocardium. Coronary occlusion is caused by ischemia of the heart muscles. After cardiac catheterization check pulse distal to the insertion site.

Complication of MI is cardiac dysrhythmia; Catheter in pulmonary artery to provide information of Left Ventricular heart failure. Lab, MI, LDH, CK-MB, is enzymes released into the blood from cardiac muscle cells when myocardium is damaged.

Apical pulse less then 60 and more than 120 contraindicated when talking drugs digoxin at home. Patient receiving anticoagulant drug observe for epitaxis and hemorrhage —INR test anticoagulant cardiac shock is failure of circulatory pump, always drop BP. Adrenaline is used to treat the shock because it increases cardiac output. Atropine blocks vagal stimulation of the SA node, resulting in increased heart rate.

The SA node is the hearts natural pacemaker. Instruct patient to take daily pulse and keep accurate records, pulse remain at least equal to the pacemaker; Lidocaine decreases the irritability of ventricles; Asystole refers to absence of arterial and ventricular contraction. Which causes death? During cardiac arrest time, the patient is anoxic, irreversible brain damage will occur if patient is anoxic for more than 4 minutes.

Patient found unconscious, unresponsive, initiate a code, help must be obtained immediately; Edema comes during the day and disappears night is Right ventricular heart failure; Edema can be classified on a four point scale from 1+ to 4+. Check the degree of edema; Right ventricular heart failed patient complains of dyspoea, edema and fatigue. Elevation of plasma hydrostatic pressure at the venous end of the capillary bed, increases pressure within circulatory system causing ascities- with air conditioning the heart is relived of the strain of pumping blood through many miles of the blood vessels in the skin. Pulmonary edema associated with mitral stenosis. 6L oxygen via nasal cannula, patient in an orthopric position; cardiac catheterization check patients pedal pulses if complains of numbness. After cerebral angiogram procedure asses symmetry of the radial pulses.

Cardiorespiratory failure—The heart consumes more oxygen per minute than any other organ in the body, because it is constantly beating. Consequentently, when the lung stop working, the heart fails occurs. Conversely, the ventilation of the lungs fails soon after the heart stops. Due to this medulla oblongata cannot function without the continuous supply of oxygen that is normally transported to it by cardiovascular system.

It is marked by sudden fail in the arterial oxygen tension and rise in the arterial carbon dioxide content. Due to it, the oxygen content in blood fails. Tissues of the body too are affected due to that. Brain is less tolerant of hypoxia then the heart. Brain tissues begin to deteriorate and irreversible changes take place in the brain tissues. Chest pain that is angina pectoris produced due to hypoxia. Clinical death occurs with the cessation of blood flow and the respiratory arrest. If the cardiac arrest is identified quickly and cardiopulmonary resuscitation is started immediately, we will be able to bring back the patient to life from clinical death. However, 5 to 6 minutes of cerebral ischemia results in biologic death and no revival is then possible.

Causes of cardiac arrest airway obstruction, Myocardial Infarction, anesthetic depression, hypotension, retention of carbon dioxide, drowning, electric shock, poisoning, drug reaction, pulmonary embolism, extensive hemorrhage, brain injuries, and hypothermia.

The three *cardinal signs* are *apnea, absence of carotid and femoral pulse and dilated pupils.*

Sequence of *cardiopulmonary resuscitation* is *A- Airway; B-Breathing; C-Circulation.*

Because of an emergency, no time is lost for this procedure. The success of the CPR depends on the speed with basic life supporting measures are effectively initiated. Noting the cardinal signs and symptoms, get quickly help.

Clean airway to restore respiration and circulation. Keep the heart and neck in a hyper-extended position to prevent tongue falling back and obstructing airway. Place ore-pharyngeal airway if breathing is not restored start artificial ventilation. Pinch the nostrils closed, using an index finger and thumb of the hand near the patients face. Take a deep breath, place your mouth into the rescuers mouth ensures airtight seal. The expansion of the chest ensures ventilation of the lungs.

HOW TO SURVIVE A HEART ATTACK WHEN ALONE

Let us say it is 7:10 PM and you are driving home alone, after an unusually hard day on the job. You are really tired, upset and frustrated.

Suddenly you start experiencing severe pain in your chest that starts to radiate out into your arm and up into your jaw. You are only about five kms from the hospital nearest your home.

Unfortunately, you do not know if you will be able to make it that far. You have been trained in CPR, but the person that taught the course did not tell you how to perform it on yourself.

Since many people are alone when they suffer a heart attack, without help, the person whose heart is beating improperly and who begins to feel faint, has only about 10 seconds left before losing consciousness. However, these victims can help themselves by coughing repeatedly and very vigorously.

A deep breath should be taken before each cough, and the cough must be deep and prolonged, as when producing sputum from deep inside the chest.

A breath and a cough must be repeated about every two seconds without letup until help arrives, or until the heart is felt to be beating normally again.

Deep breaths get oxygen into the lungs and coughing movements squeeze the heart and keep the blood circulating. The squeezing pressure on the heart also helps it regain normal rhythm.

In this way, heart attack victims can get to a hospital. It could save their lives!

Follow the above mentioned tips to lead a healthy and a happy life.

ALWAYS LISTEN TO YOUR FAMILY DOCTOR

What is the Cardiopulmonary Resuscitation (CPR) ?

Heart attack is of an emergency, do not waste valuable time.

Keep following things ready

Oxygen administration sets

IV infusion sets and cut down sets

Ambu bag and mask devices

Endotracheal tubes of different sizes

Oropharyngeal and nasal airways

Laryngoscope of different sizes

Tracheotomy sets

Suction apparatus

Cardiac monitor and defibrillator

Mechanical respiratory aids

Emergency drugs such as epinephrine, sodium bicarbonate, cardiac and respiratory stimulants

Clean rag pieces or gauze pieces of container

No valuable time is lost in explaining the procedure to the patient/relatives.

Procedure

Clean the airway of obvious foreign matter, e.g. Vomitus, secretions.

Hyperextend the head and neck of the patient by tilting it backward as far as possible

Pull the victim's jaw forward by placing the fingers behind the angle of the jaw and is lifted forward until the teeth on the upper jaw and the lower jaw is approximated

If breathing is restored, place on oropharyngeal airway

If breathing is not restored start artificial ventilation

To initiate breathing can be given [mouth to mouth]

Pinch the patient's nostrils closed, using an index finger and thumb of the hand near the patient's face. Take a deep breath, place your widely opened mouth over the patient's mouth and blow forcefully enough to make the patient's chest rise. Turn the face towards the patient's chest to observe its expansion.

After each inflation move, your mouth ensures airtight seal. The expansion of the chest ensures ventilation of the lungs. In children [the rescuer's mouth is placed over the mouth and nose], less volume of air is introduced, but they are given about 20-30 times per minute.

If cardiac massage is to be given, the artificial breathing should be carried at a rate of 5% or 15 : 2, i.e. one inflation after every 15 cardiac massage when there is only one rescuer.

To maintain circulation begin external cardiac compression immediately following initial four rapid breaths.

Position the patient on his back on a flat, firm surface.

Kneel on bed at the side of patient.

CR cardiac compression at rate of 60-80/Minutes; Assess the vital signs.

Lung inflations and cardiac compressions must be followed until patient starts spontaneous respirations and pulse.

Keep patient under observation 48 to 72 hrs.

Watch pupils, pulse, movements of chest wall no retraction of muscles, blood pressure, temperature, pulse and respirations, watch for convulsions, insert Foley's catheter. Start IV infusion

Record each thing with observation

Basic CPR – follow the ABCD → *that is* Average Breathing Circulation Defibrillation

Advanced → Drug, ECG

CPCR → Cardiac Pulmonary Cerebral Resuscitation

Congenital heart block can be treated but city needs to make surgeries more easily available to kids. Medical science has progressed to a point where doctors can detect a slew of problems in the fetal stage itself, can detect chromosomal abnormalities, congenital neoplasm a abnormalities that is tumors, skeletal abnormalities, renal cystic disease, congenital infections as well as neurological abnormalities.

The non-invasive test- done between 11 and 13 weeks are:

The Test Detects

Downs syndrome and neural tube defects

Low levels of Pregnancy Associated Plasma Protein A (PAPP-A) in maternal serum during the first three months of pregnancy may be associated with fetal chromosomal anomalies that indicate genetic abnormality. Low PAPP-A levels in the first trimester may also predict that the outcome could be different pregnancy.

Triple AAA marker done between 16 and 18 weeks. This includes tests that can detect neural defects. Congenital malformation and genetic disease conditions like tiresome, Ed wards and Downs syndrome.

Nuchal cord translucent C test-done 9 and 13 weeks, it can detect neural defects such as DS, Turners or spina Bifida in which a part of the spinal cord is not formed, leads to a life long disabilities in some

3D or 4D anomaly scan at 10 weeks. This is a detailed 3D/4D scan. Every single angel and every minor and major physical anomaly ranging from an eye problem to defects in the heart to cleft lip.

Fetal echocardiography done in 20 and 24 weeks.

It gives the complete picture of the heart and any malformation is detected.

The invasive tests are done only when any of the screening tests turn positive. Also recommended if there is a family history of genetic diseases or the parents are old.

Amniocenteses done at 16 and 18 weeks– a needle is passed into the amniotic cavity inside the uterus. The amniotic fluids contain fetal cells, which can be grown in culture from chromosome analysis biochemical analysis and molecular analysis/it shows genetic abnormality.

Chorionic villus sampling done in 9 and 12 week.

A catheter is passed through the cervix and into the uterus to the placenta under ultrasound guidance. This allows sampling of cells for chromosome analysis for genetic abnormality.

Fetoscopy—An endoscope is introduced into the amniotic sac to get a visualization of the fetus. This helps in getting fetal blood sample, skin biopsy and liver biopsy.

USG based fetal blood sampling. This uses sonography probe/catheter to get sample of fetal blood.

We have to understand that 90% of children born with heart defects are normal after an operation. We cannot change the incident of heart defect, but we need public trust hospitals and government to come together to ensure that such operations are made easily available to children.

Abortion of such a child has adverse moral, ethical, and inhuman consequences. Know the trauma parents who have such child with disability go through. A baby with malfunctioning organs cause unlimited and cannot be explained the tribulation. We have to react when technologies is alerting us. If do not follow why technology at all. Who will be responsible for child's agony? Parents will have to watch child's agony helplessly. Which can be unbearable? Parents are not able to afford to give child latest treatment thus putting child in distress. Life will be hell for such a child. Child will lead a terrible life and will not have normal childhood.

Adding with life long medical expenses

The law is clear no person has the right to kill an unborn child.

The almighty deciding the fate of human beings

Destiny is playing its role people will misuse the law. May use as a pretext for terminating perfectly healthy child. As this issue was discussed few days back and appeared in newspapers remains unanswered.

Beating heart bypass surgery—Coronary artery disease caused by atherosclererotic narrowing of coronary arteries. If it is not treated, it can cause chest pain on exertion, when multiple coronary arteries are narrowed the treatment of choice is coronary artery bypass grafting (CABG). It requires anastomosis of grafts taken from the patients own body. A new technique of operation done without the use of heart-lung machine. It is a new technique and the result of surgery is very satisfying. Old and sick patients too fare well after surgery.

Ventilation is the movement of air in and out of the lungs. The primary function of the lungs is gas exchange. The physical structure and the airway allow air to be warmer, filtered and humidified as it enters the body. In the alveolar sacs, oz is exchanged for coz. The mechanics of breathing are coordinated by the ribs, diaphragm, pleural space, elastic recoil of the lungs and nervous system provides one form of acid base balance. When there process of structure and function are altered, various disorders can occur.

During inspiration, air flows from the environment into the trachea, bronchi, bronchioles and alveoli. During expiration, alveolar gas travels the same route in reverse.

Physical factors that govern air flow in and out of the lungs are collectively referred to as the mechanics of ventilation and include air pressure variances, resistance to air flow and lung compliance.

Air flows from a region of higher pressure to a region of lower pressure. During inspiration, movement of the diaphragm and other muscles of respiration enlarge the thoracic cavity and there by lowers the pressure inside the thorax to a level below that of atmospheric pressure. Therefore, air is drawn through the trachea and bronchi into the alveoli.

During normal expiration, the diaphragm relaxes and the lungs recoil, resulting in a decrease in the size of the thoracic cavity. The alveolar pressure then exceeds atmospheric pressure and air flows from the lungs into the atmosphere.

Airway resistance is determined chiefly by the size of the airway through which the air is flowing. Any process that changes the bronchial diameter and alters the rate of air flow for a given pressure gradient during respiration. With increased resistance greater than normal respiratory effect is required by the patient to achieve normal levels of ventilation.

When pressure changes are applied in the normal lung, there is a proportional changes in the lung volume. A measure of the elasticity, expandability and dispensability of the lungs and thoracic structure is called compliance. Factors that determine lung compliance are surface tension of the alveoli and the connective tissue of the lungs. Normal compliance is (1.0 L/cm H_2O) increased compliance occurs when the lungs have lost their elasticity and thorax is over distended. When lungs and thorax are stiff there is decreased compliance. Conditions associated with this pneumothorax, hemothorax, pleural effusion, pulmonary edema, atelectasis etc.

Lung function, which reflects the mechanic of ventilation. It is categorized as tidal volume, inspiratory reserve volume expiratory reserve volume and residual volume.

Tidal volume (TV) is the volume of air inhaled and exhaled with each breath 500 ml which may not vary, even with sever diseases.

Inspiratory reserve volume (IRV) is the maximum volume of air that can be inhaled after a normal inhalation 300 ml.

Expiratory reserve volume (ERV) is the maximum volume of air that can be exhaled forcing after normal exhalation 1100 ml, it is decreased in obesity, ascities and pregnancy.

Residual volume (RV) 1200 ml, it increases in obstructive diseases.

Vital capacity (VC) 4600 ml and inspiratory capacity 3500 ml total lung capacity 5800 ml functional residual volume of air remaining in the lung a normal expiration, coz is waste product of tissue metabolism.

Ventilation air flow and perfusion/blood flow determines the efficiency of gas exchange. The primary function of lung is gas exchange.

The rhythm of breathing is controlled by respiratory centers in the brain. The inspiration and expiratory centers in the medulla oblongata and pons control the rate and depth of ventilation to meet the body's metabolic demands.

Ventilation is the flow of gas in and out of the lungs and perfusion is the filling of pulmonary capillaries with blood.

Ventilation—Perfusion ratio in different areas of lung, the ratio may vary. Alteration in perfusion may occur with a change in the pulmonary artery pressure, alveolar pressure and gravity. Airway blockage, local changes in compliance and gravity may alter ventilation.

Imbalance occurs from inadequate ventilation. Ventilation and perfusion imbalance causes shunting of blood, resulting in hypoxia. Oxygen can eliminate hypoxia. Once the air enters the trachea, It becomes fully saturated with water vapour, which displays some of the gases so that the air pressure within the lung remains equal to the air pressure outside.

Low ventilation perfusion states may be called shunt producing disorders. When effusion exceeds ventilation, a shunt exists. Blood by passes, the alveoli without gas exchange occurs. Oxygen and carbon dioxide are carried simultaneously by virtue of there abilities to dissolve in blood. Oxygen is carried in the blood in two forms. First as physically dissolved oxygen in the plasma, second in combination with the hemoglobin in RBC.

High Ventilation—Perfusion Ratio Dead Space Results

The normal value of paoz is 80 to 100 mm Hg (95% to 98% saturation)

Paoz partial pressure of alveolar coz

Normal levels paoz above 70 mm Hg

Dangerous levels below 40 mm Hg

Nursing management of the client on *mechanical ventilation* indicated when the patient is unable to maintain safe levels of oz or coz by spontaneous breathing even with the assistance of other oz delivery devices. Mechanical ventilation helps to minimize the work of breathing while effectively promoting gas exchange oxygenation and ventilation. It requires the establishment of an artificial airway (usually by ET intubations initially) and use of positive pressure ventilator.

Endotracheal tube is a longer, slender hallow tube usually made of polyvinyl, chloride that is inserted into the trachea via the mouth or nose. Oral intubations is usually used for short term airway management nasal intubations is more secure and believed to be more comfortable and does not move as much in the airway. However many instillations are not using nasal intubations because of risk of sinusition if prolonged intubations required ET tube will be replaced with a tracheotomy.

Inserting the tube the client is positioned supine with all dental bridge work plates remove the head of hyperextended the lower except of the neck flexed and the mouth opened this position bring the mouth, pharynx and larynx into a straight line oxygen saturation adequate checked.

Checking tube placemen immediately after on ET tube has been inserted

Tube placement is verified by auscultation and chest X-ray to ensure to see the position of tube and if the tube is slips can correct reestablishing quickly. Secure the ET tube immediately after intubations with adhesive tape specially designed. ET tube holds.

Seal the tube against the tracheal wall to facilitate positive pressure ventilation

Protects the respiratory tract from the aspiration of foreign the amount of air required to seal on ET tube cuff I to replace by the cuff pressure which usually maintained at less than 20 mm Hg. Low cuff pressure is necessary to prevent drainage to the tracheal mucosa arterial pressure in he tracheal wall are approximately 20 to 25 mm Hg while venous pressure is

20 mm Hg therefore cuff pressure greater than mucosa and necrosis may develop cuff pressure should be every 8 hour.

Care of the cuff- suction and hyperventilate before and after procedure

Clean the area for secretion by suctioning gently deep into the oropharyx, advance the suction catheter to the end of ET tube, deflate the cuff while applying suction to suction catheter, so that any secretion lying above the cuff will be removed. Repeat pharyngeal suctioning.

Managing cuff leaks can be a major problem. It may be because by a rupture or tear in the cuff or pilot system or by the ET tube.

The pilot balloon not filing when air is injected

The client's ability to talk when the cuff inflated

Air heard leaking during positive pressure breathing that the client is at high risk of aspiration while the cuff is leaking during positive pressure breathing.

Suctioning—ET tube improve the clients ability to cough while stimulating increases secretion formation in the lower tracheobronchial tree. It is usually required to help maintain a patient airway. It should perform only when it is needed excessive suctioning if used can lead to airway trauma, and other problems.

Sign and symptoms indicate the need for suctioning is noisy breathing restlessness; increase respiration mucus bubbling into the ET tube can identify by auscultation and increase in peak airway pressure during continuous mechanical ventilation.

Communication—Due to ET tube passes trough the vocal cords therefore the client can not laugh effectively or speak. So help the client develop a means of communication by keeping paper and pencil, pad or a picture board readily available.

Provide oral hygiene—Careful oral hygiene is essential every few hours for a client with an ET tube secretion frequent oral suctioning above the cuff is highly recommended. The client's teeth should be brushed on a oral mucosa moistened and dry mucus membranes apply lubrication to decrease the risk of necrosis of the mouth and pharynx from pressure the ET tube should be rotated from one corner of the mouth to the other at least every 24 hours.

Turn patient from side-to-side every two hours. Lateral turn of 120 degree is desirable, from right semiprone to left semiprone. Position and make patient sit in upright at regular intervals if possible. Upright posture increases lung compliance. Carry out passive range exercises of all extremities for patients unable to do so. Asses for need of suctioning at least every 2 hours. Patient with MI are unable to clear secretions on their own. Suctioning may help to clear secretion and stimulate the cough reflex.

Asses breath sounds every two hours. Listen with stethoscope to the chest for bottom to top on both sides. To confirm airway patency and placement of ET. Determine breath sounds weather normal or abnormal.

Humidifier must change every 24 hours

Assess airway pressure at frequent intervals

Monitor for pulmonary infection. This helps for earlier detection of infection

Measure abdominal girth to asses' degree of distension daily

Test all stool and gastric drainage for occult blood. Abdominal distention occurs frequently with respiratory failure and further hindrance respiration by elevation of the diaphragm.

Establish means of assign effectiveness and progress of treatment.

Continuous Mechanical Ventilation

Maintain adequate ventilation

Deliver precise concentration of froze

Deliver adequate tidal volume is obtains on adequate minute ventilator and oxygenation

Lessen the work of breathing in those clients who cannot suction adequate ventilation on their own.

Types of Ventilators

Pressure cycled ventilators deliver a volume of gas to the airway using positive pressure during inspiration. This positive pressure is delivered until the preselecled pressure has been reached when the preset pressure is reached the machine cycles into exhalation pressure cycled ventilators are used in only a small portion of clients who require continuous mechanical ventilation.

Volume—Cycled ventilators deliver a present tidal volume or inspired gas. The tidal volume that has been preselecled is delivered to the client regardless of the pressure required to client. This volume a pressure limit can beset to prevent the occumence of dangerously high airway pressures.

Mode of Ventilation

Control ventilation—delivers gas at present rate and tidal volume or pressure regardless of patient's inspiratory effects.

Assist control ventilation—Delivers gas at present tidal volume or pressure in response to clients inspiratory effects and will intake breathe if client fails to do so with in present time.

Synchronous intermittent mandatory ventilation—Delivers gas at present tidal volume or pressure and rate while allowing client to breathe spontaneously. Ventilator breaths are synchronized to clients respiratory effect.

Positive end expiratory pressure—Positive pressure applied at the end of expiration of ventilator breaths.

Constant positive airway pressure—Positive pressure applied during spontaneous breaths.

Pressure support ventilation—Preset positive pressure used inspiratory efforts, client controls rate in spiratory flow and tidal volume.

Volume—Assured pressure support ventilation-tidal volume is set to ensure client receiving minimum tidal volume with each pressure support breath.

Independent lung ventilation—Each lung is ventilated separately.

High frequency positive pressure ventilation delivers 60-100 breaths/min.

High frequency jet ventilation delivers 100-600 cycles/min.

High frequency oscillation delivers 900-300 cycles/min.

Inverse ratio ventilation proportion of inspiratory to expiratory time is greater than 1.1 can be initiated using pressure.

Nursing responsibility—Altered respiratory function, ineffective airway clearance auscultate lung sounds and respiratory rate and pattern every one to two hours as needs,

Check ventilation setting drams and connect at lest hourly and after any removal of ventilator from client

Suction as needed provide pre- and post-hyper inflating nebulizer every 2 hours

Secure the ET tube properly

Use block or oral airway

Monitor arterial blood gas values and arterial oximetry

Anxiety related to dependency while on mechanical ventilator—develops means of communication. Place a nurse call device within the clients reach. Be available and visible. Provide distraction, explain all procedure, provide privacy, and provide a calm environment. Medicate as necessary for anxiety.

High risk for complications—assess for acute rising or severe dyspoea, agitation, panic, absence breath sounds localized hyperresonence ring breathing effort tracheal deviation abnormal findings.

Asses for acute or gradual fall in blood pressure tachey cardia, dysrthias, weak peripherals pulses, and acute reduction pulmonary copilot's pressure.

Monitor for signs of adverse estuation vocalization low pressure alarm, bilateral decrease in upper lobe airway sounds, gastric distension clinical manifestation of, inadequate ventilation, keep on incubation tray readily available.

Risk for infection related to impaired defense, wash hands thoroughly, use sterile technique for suctioning. Monitor client for increase breathing effort localized changes in auscultation and change in paoz, provide oral care every two hour. Drain water from ventilator tubing and do not drain water back into humidify. Monitor sputum for changes in colour, consistency, amount and odour. Monitor laboratory values, blood cell count etc.

Continuous mechanical ventilation is used for many different reasons. Ventilation support may be needed for short term care like severe pneumonia or long term stroke, in some emergency cases, ventilator support is to stabilize a patient's condition. Positive benefit is the continuous ventilator allows the lungs to rest so that healing may take place.

Continuous Mechanical Ventilator Artificially Prolong Death

Alteration in nutrition provides adequate nutrition, begin tube feeding as soon as it is evident that the client will remain on continuous mechanical ventilator for a length of time. Avoid excessive carbohydrate loads. Weight the client daily. Monitor intake and out put, monitor bowel sound. Asses for complication of tube feeding, aspiration, constipation; Use feeding or between bolus feeding obtain.

Conclusions—You could save a life if you identify stroke or an attack. Sometimes symptoms of a stroke are difficult to identify. Unfortunately, lack of awareness spells disaster. The stroke victim may suffer severe brain damage. If one can get stroke victim within 3 hours he can totally reverse the effects of a stroke.

10 leading causes of death—Heart disease, cancer, stroke, unintentional injuries, COPD, pneumonia, influenza, DM, suicide, chronic liver diseases and cirrhosis etc. Remember that men over age 60 years; one who has family history of high blood pressure, heart attack and diabetes, pressure 200/110 mm of Hg, IDDM uncontrolled, eight 50% or more over weight, cholesterol level over 280, serum triglycerides, fasting 400 to 1000, percentage of fat in diet over 50%, no activity, sedentary occupation, cigarette smoking over a 40 a day, stress at work and home extremely high, women who takes oral contraceptives, high air pollution, one who has only 4 to 6 hours of sleep at night. Also his social problem can affect his well being such as job being more important than family, excessive competitiveness in all areas of life, divorce, dissatisfaction with job, the primary gratification is money etc.

Choose a diet low in fat, saturated fat and cholesterol, use salt and sodium on moderation, eat a variety of foods, maintain healthy weight, choose diet with plenty of vegetables, fruits and grain products, use sugar only in moderation, fats and sweets use sparingly.

Evaluate what things in your life are important to you and help you want to live each day, e.g. health, respect for others happiness, loving relationship, time spend with loved ones, friendship, religious beliefs, financial security, having job/work to do.

How important is your health to you? What do you hope to accomplish in your life time? For example, rare children successfully, become rich and famous, have satisfying career? Have you accomplished what you set out to do in your life? Are you satisfied/dissatisfied/have any of your beliefs and values challenged you? What do you wish you could change about yourself? Describe how you feel when you become ill? Have a balance perspective of life experience, persist despite adversity and discouragement, and believe in oneself and one capability. Realization that life has purpose, realization that each persons life path is unique, some of which must be walked alone.

Responsibility of Nurse in Drug Administration

Primitive men looking for food soon learned that eating parts of some plants caused diarrhea or other discomforting effect. Knowledge about drugs gained by this kind of practical experience through trial and error handed down from generation to generation. For example, Opium, cannabis, belladonna are drug of ancient origin. Most of today's drugs are synthetic chemicals that found a place in modern treatment only after undergoing extensive trials in several species of animals and in human volunteers and patients. The process, by which new drugs are discovered, developed and tested for efficacy and toxicity, are long and difficult.

Chemicals are constantly being screened to determine whether they are worth trying in the treatment of cancer, bacterial infections or other diseases. No drug has only a single action. Drugs usually has a variety of names, is often a cause of confusion, when the drug is offered in combination with other agents; the mixture has still another trade name.

We need to understand some of the general principles that apply to the actions and clinical uses of all drugs. The factors that influence the actions of all drugs in the human body. In addition, the prevention and treatment of drug over dosage and other types of toxicity.

The nurse is legally responsible for being fully informed about any investigational drug that she is administering to a patient consult patients physician, do observation and chart recording of it. When a drug enters a living system, its millions and millions of molecules immediately begin to react with those of the body's cells.

How body cells *respond to the presence of drugs* that are capable of altering their functioning. How the body handles drugs in order to detoxify and remove them. How various factors influence both the responsiveness of the reacting target tissues to drugs and the ways in which drugs are eliminated and their actions are terminated? Knowledge of the drug exact sites of action has practical value in various ways.

How the *drug metabolism* takes place. Drugs absorbed into the body fluids from the site of it are entering into the body. Transported or distributed to distant points in the body. Detoxified or inactivated/transformed into breakdown products. Excreted or eliminated from the body via various routs. Factors such as body weight, age, disease states, tolerance, physiology, environment, immunologic factors influencing the effects of drugs.

Individual *variation* in responsiveness different to the same dose of drugs, elderly, young children age affects his body ability to metabolize and eliminate potent drugs. Patient has history of other illness, besides the disorder receiving drugs. Patient's personality, mental and emotional state can influence his response to drugs. Diet and alcoholic intake, time, appropriate scheduled dose affects.

Be *alert* for drug interaction, whenever new drugs are added to patient's medication regimen or when one of several drugs is being discontinued following prolonged administration. All drugs are potentially harmful. The nurse to be aware that every drug that is used in therapy is capable of causing adverse effects in some patients. Nurses especially alert to avoid any error in administering dosage with greatest efficacy and safety. Acquire fundamental knowledge about the medication such as therapeutic use, side effects, potential toxicity, usual dosage range and route of administration. Check the patient's drug history to see how he responds to drug therapy during an earlier episode.

The root cause of ill health in India is malnutrition, lack of clean water and sanitation and unemployment. Major portion of our population living in abject poverty, can barely afford a square meal a day, and let alone having the means to spend on costly medicines. More and more drugs flood in our market every year whereas resources for the purchase of drugs is scare.

Therefore, WHO has in this view formed *essential drug policy* of minimum rational drugs that will satisfy the health care needs of the majority of the people. Which is affordable price and easily available. Which will improve the quality of drug management and reduce the cost of the consumer, which will ensure rational use of drug and reduce the risk of irrational and hazardous drug? It will be economically beneficial and will respond the real health needs of people.

Essential drugs will make *quality control* easier because of the limited number of drugs involved. The WHOs action programmed on essential drugs recommends about 350 drugs to meet most of the health care needs of the people. This recommendation has been ignored by the govt. of India only two states have taken the initiative and implemented the essential drug concept in India they are Delhi and Tamil Nadu.

There are over 100,000 *formulations* in the country. It is common practice of doctor to use brand names when, prescribing is often influenced by the marketing practice. Quality drugs are cheaper when purchased under their generic names rather than their brand names, which are valuable aid to memory, as it is easier to remember. Rs 9000 crores of drugs are consumed every year in India. There are certain criteria for withdrawal of irrational and hazardous drugs. The combination of an antibiotic with other antibiotic, or antibiotics with corticosteroid or other active substances will be prohibited.

Drug is any substance used for the purpose of diagnosis, prevention, relief or cure of a disease for the benefit of the recipient.

Once the drug goes into body it absorbs, distributes, binders, localizes, stores, bio-transforms and excretion of the drug by the body.

Routes of drug administration are- through via *oral, which* is the common route. Both solid and liquid preparations can be given easily by oral route. It is slower onset of action. In *sublingual drug* is put under the tongue where it can be rapidly soluble. *Rectal drug* is placed inside rectum as suppositories or enema. Some times this route is used when oral ingestion is not possible due to some reason like frequent vomiting.

Inhalation drugs are in the form of vapour and absorption of drugs occurs through respiratory tract mucosa. *Cutaneous drug* is applied locally over the skin or mucus membrane in the form of lotions, ointments, creams, liniments or transdermal patch. *Parenteral drug* is injected with the help of an injection directly into the blood.

Intravenous drug injected in one of the superficial veins. A large volume of drug can be infused through this route. This route also provides rapid onset of action. *Intramuscular drug* is injected directly in the muscles. Moreover, *subcutaneous drug* is injected directly in the loose subcutaneous tissue. Only small amount of drug can be injected through this route. Intradermal injected into the skin.

Infants, children and elderly require smaller amount of dose as compared to adults. Children find it difficult to swallow tablets so liquid preparations or crushed tablets are preferable. They are flavored to colored to encourage the child to take the medicine. A nurse should confirm the dose before administrating a drug to children.

Age, sex, weight factors affect the drug response. Many drugs are metabolized in liver and excreted through kidney. When drug is given orally, it is absorbed from the gastrointestinal tract and reaches the liver before reaching the general circulation. Prolonged administration of some drugs requires increasing dosage for producing same response. Drugs, which are eliminated slowly from the body, may accumulate in the body and may produce toxicity.

Adverse drug reactions are undesired effects and it is important for the nurse to know and be aware of the possibility of its reactions, so that appropriate steps can be taken. Over dosage may result in drug poisoning. Drug allergies or hypersensitivity and some drugs cause sensitization of the skin to ultraviolet radiation that is photosensitivity. There are drug dependency and withdrawal reactions to be noted.

Always check prescription for name of the client, name of the drug, dose of the drug, route of administration, and date. Always check the label for date of manufacture, expiry date, dose and amount of drug, any instructions mentioned on the label or any warning. Record the administration in the file or register.

Check ward stock regularly, drugs of emergency life savings should be kept on the emergency trolley. Drugs requiring low temperature for storage must be stored in refrigerators. Ask always about previous drug reactions before giving a drug. Certain drugs should not be used during pregnancy, lactation and childhood.

Avoid mixing drugs in the same syringe. Maintain a high fluid and good urinary flow during sulfonamide therapy. Alkalinization of urine also minimizes crystallization and precipitation of sulfonamides in urinary tract. Avoid direct exposure of client to sunlight during sulfonamide therapy.

Antiviral drugs are not much effective, support natural defense mechanism of client, encourage intake of food rich in immune stimulating nutrients. Dependency can occur with long-term use of all sedative-hypnotics. Use the minimum dose for the minimum period. Avoid engaging in hazardous activity like driving, swimming. Client should be advised to avoid irritating foods and alcohol and stop smoking.

Client's education and understanding about the disease is very important to manage their own disease. They should be taught to modify their lifestyle giving repeated instructions and helping them recognize the danger sings. Administer the diuretics in the morning so that the maximal effect will occur during the waking hours that are during the day. The best way to monitor the efficiency of a diuretic is to weigh the client regularly.

Over use of purgatives can inhibit normal bowel habits and induce dependency on it. This can lead to laxative abuse. They are usually given at bedtime to promote defecation in the morning. If treatment with steroid lasts more than 10 days, withdrawal must be gradual, as adrenal suppression will have occurred. Client must be taught not to stop taking steroids suddenly. Antihistaminic are best given in the evening since they cause drowsiness. Client advised not to drive. Intravenous fluids should be administered slowly, except where there is marked fluid and electrolyte deficit. Otherwise, fluid overload may precipitate pulmonary edema, in client with renal and cardiac failure.

Rationality of drugs- means the use of drug, which are efficient, safe, low-cost and easy to administer. For this practitioner to have adequate knowledge and appropriate skill for correct diagnosis and treatment. Lack of scientific knowledge when doctors have not kept abreast of currant developments in medicine and inaccurate diagnosis occurs due to lack of time, over crowed OPD, inadequate health personnel and lack of diagnostic aids. Ordering right medicine for the right patient at the right time and in the right amount with due consideration of costs.

Prescribe drug only when indicated, choose drug, which is effective, and relatively safe, and has cheaper alternatives. Eliminate new drug, which are expensive and use essential drug list. Be aware of banned drugs and follow the ethics of drug; use your clinical judgment. Most clients especially from rural areas will not be able easily to come back to you, see how you can make your client well in one trip and if possible with few drugs. Remember getting ill and getting well are socioeconomic processes.

Fixed dose combination of drugs needed out by the drug controller of India, e.g. fixed dose combination of vitamins with analgesic; but still they are sold in Indian market, let these drugs be separately available for their appropriate use. More expensive does not necessarily mean better. India has one of the best-developed pharmaceutical with over 20,000 units producing between 60,000 to one lakh formulations and turnover of more then Rs, 15,000 cores. Yet such large scale production has not had any significant improvement in the availability of drugs to meet the country's needs, because most of the formulations produced are unnecessary, being therapeutically ineffective, irrational and even dangerous.

Today essential drugs are in short supply. Quality of drug, should act for what it is prescribed for. All drugs have a declared shelf life between 18 months to 5 years. Drug promotion done by unethical method such as heavy advertising, free sample drugs, bribes like diaries, posters, calendars, pen gifts, medical conferences held in five star hotels with lavish meals, sponsoring television program.

Medical information is exploding and along with the internet revolution. A lot more information is now easily available. Still internet is inaccessible to most people in the third world. The explosion of medical information seldom caters to ordinary literate lay persons. We need to fill this gap. Those who are not doctors have little or no access to information about the use and effect of medicines, and doctors have very little time to inform their client about the correct use of the medicine they prescribe. The widespread crisis in medicine created by drug policies, which go against the safe interest of all people.

Drugs are chemical substances, which affect living organism. They are used to cure diseases, relieve symptoms and remove pain. Pharmaceutical companies through chemical processes produce most drugs. They are marketed only after testing for safety and efficacy. Testing is done on animals and human volunteers and marketed with approval of the food and drug administration.

They are dispensed in the human body in various forms, which are designed to ensure correct dosage. Each drug has three names. First is the generic, the other is the brand name chosen by the manufacturer so that it can be easily recognized and remembered. Finally, there is the chemical name of a drug, which describes it technically. Drugs are classified in different ways. According to their chemicals, of their use, biological effect, legal status. some drug have multiple use. One must recognize the class of the drug, one is taking.

Non-prescription drugs are called over the counter drugs. Drugs available on prescription and are to be used under medical supervision. Generic products are usually cheaper than brand product. Over the counter drugs do not need prescription, and which are widely available at provision stores as well as at chemist shops. These medicines are usually used for self-treatment; like all medicines, they can be harmful, if misused. Over the counter preparation have no legal recognition and are better referred to as non-prescription drugs or household remedies. What is not prohibited is permitted. Other dues to be sold by retail on the prescription of the registered medical practitioner only. Caution- it is dangerous to use this preparation except under medical supervision.

Drugs once enters the human body, it acts on various parts of the body, sometimes curing the disease while sometimes just relieving the symptoms. Although different drugs act different ways, their mechanism of action against micro-organisms such as virus, bacteria, protozoa and fungi that attack the body or abnormal cell body, causing infectious diseases. Some drugs can kill these micro-organisms or stop their multiplication in the body and thus cure the disease. Certain diseases such as cancer are caused due to abnormal cells. Some drugs treat such diseases by killing the abnormal cells.

Human body needs certain vitamins and minerals to function properly. It obtains from a balanced diet. If for any reason, the body does not get the essential vitamins/minerals. Various deficiency diseases may occur. Such diseases can be cured by replacing the deficient vitamin or minerals. Similarly, deficiency diseases also occur when there is a lack of hormones. Such diseases are treated with drugs that replace the hormones. Certain drugs alter the way in which a cell acts, that is, they either increase or decrease the cell activity to produce the desirable response. This is achieved in different ways by different drugs. Certain hormones act on the cells to produce undesirable effects. Some drugs either block the action or treat undesirable conditions. Some drugs alter the transmission of the messages from one part to another part.

If the dose is too low, it may not have any effect at all, if it is too high, it may not produce any additional benefits but may produce adverse effects. This means that the dose should be in optimum range that is called therapeutic range varies for different drugs. Hence their dose has to be calculated accurately to achieve the desired beneficial effect. The dose dependent on factors such as age, weight and general health of patient. Children weight lesser than adults so they required lesser amount. Besides their metabolic activity is not as developed as the adults are, so it is given from mg of drug/kg body weight of a child. As children of the same age may have difference in their weights.

Dose for older people have also to be adjusted. Elderly people are more prone to adverse effects because their liver and kidneys are not as efficient as those of the normal adult are. The adult dose for most of the drugs can be generalized and hence the same dose is recommended for all adults irrespective of their age.

Liver is that organ in the human body in which breaks down the drug into simpler substances. If the liver is not functioning properly, the break down process is affected and the drug gets accumulated in the body. Accumulation of certain drugs leads to dangerous effects. A person with liver problems is prescribed fewer drugs and in lower doses. Besides drugs that cause liver damage.

People with poor kidney function are also at a greater risk from drug side effects. Kidney excretes the drug in urine. When kidney not working properly, a lesser amount of drug is excreted while a major portion remains in the body causing harmful effects. Certain drugs bind to protein leading to harmful effects. So care to be taken that kidney damage as an adverse effect should not be given to people with kidney problems.

Some drugs produce a very rapid effect while some drugs effect after a long period causing anxiety to the patient. Similarly, the effect of certain drugs lasts for a very short time while certain drugs exert their effect for a longer period.

For oral medicines, it is very important to follow the instructions regarding the intake of food, to get maximum effect of the drug. Certain drugs to be taken on empty stomach one or two hours before the food, so that they get into the blood more quickly while others are to be taken with the meal so that they do not cause stomach irritation. Instructions regarding avoiding certain foods, which may impair drugs action. Tablets should be swallowed completely in upright sitting position/standing position with at least half glass of water. This helps medicine to act faster. Liquid medicines should be always taken, after shaking the bottle properly. The doses should be measured carefully.

The frequency of doses will depend on how long the action of the drug will last. Do not miss a dose as woman taking oral contraceptives forgets a pill, she may become pregnant, missed dose may produce return of symptoms to alter the effects of drugs are insulin, anti-epileptics etc.

The way one ends a drug treatment is very important in the case of drugs to be taken regularly for a long time. Usually people tend to stop drug treatment on their own once they begin to feel better or they experience adverse effect of the drug; this should not be done without doctor's advice. The full course of treatment should always to be completed, specially drugs like antibiotics which are used for treatment of infection. The occurrence of side effect does not imply that the drug treatment should be stopped. One should check with the doctor.

Many times people have false beliefs that if, they take an additional amount of drug than what is prescribed, they will feel better faster. Some times elderly people take dose twice, forgetting that they had already taken a dose before. One should always be conscious enough to notice any unusual symptoms, report to the doctor immediately. Over dose may create lot of unwanted effect and may lead to dangerous consequences. Also people with impaired liver or kidney functions should be extra careful not to exceed a prescribed drug as there breakdown process is not efficient as in normal patient, and this may cause accumulation of drug in the body leading to dangerous side effects.

It is important to give relevant information to the doctor to prescribe the drug rationally and reduces the chances of adverse effect of the drug. Tell your doctor about any other drugs you are talking already. Tell your doctor if you are pregnant, breast feeding, past you had any specific health problem, if you have undergone any kind of surgery, any kind of special diet, have any allergic reaction to any past treatment.

Many drugs are known to cross the placenta and cause adverse effects on the foetus. Hence, it is always better to let your doctor decide whether you should take a particular drug or not. If pregnant woman is suffering from chronic condition such as epilepsy, high BP, diabetes, it is necessary to give her drug treatment. The doctor then, balances the possible benefits and risks of the drug and decide if it should be taken or not.

Most drugs can pass from the mother's blood stream into the mother's milk just like the way they pass from the mother's blood stream into the baby's blood stream. A baby who is being breast-fed will thus receive small amount of drug that the mother is receiving.

Nutritious food, cleanliness and vaccinations are three important bodyguards that protect children against many diseases. The way child's body deals with drugs in completely different from that of an adult body. Thus, avoid unnecessary drugs, as certain drugs are harmful. A drug needs invariably calculation based on weight. Older people are at more risk to the adverse effects of drugs than normal adults are, drugs must be used with caution.

Possible adverse effect whenever drug is consumed. As drugs once taken, it is distributed all throughout the body and not restricted to just one particular organ in the body. Thus, a drug produces the desirable effect in one particular organ for which it is taken and undesirable effects in all other organs where it also acts simultaneously. For example, anti cholinergic drugs are taken to relieve spasm in the wall of the intestine, but they also affect the eyes causing blurred vision, the mouth causing dryness and the urinary bladder causing retention of urine. All the effects caused in organs other than the intestine are undesirable and will be called side effect of anti cholinergic drugs. Such side effects disappear slowly as the body gets used to the drug. One must consult the doctor persist for a longer time. The doctor may change the drug or the dosage regimen to reduce the side effect.

Sometimes a patient may have to tolerate the side effects of certain drugs, which are the only available drug for the treatment of disease which itself may be very serious and could prove fetal if left untreated, e.g. a disease like cancer. Such cases regular and careful observation/ monitoring by the doctor throughout the treatment is necessary.

Adverse effects are unexpected, unusual and unpredictable reactions of the drug. They may be caused when person is allergic to the drug or due to some genetic deficiency in the person such as the lack of an enzyme, which inactivates the drug, may lead to accumulation of the drug causing adverse reactions. They may also occur due to interactions with other drugs.

Adverse effects may be either mild or serious in nature, which determines the steps one should take if they occur. One should be alert to significant changes that occur in ones body while talking drugs. Inform doctor regarding your medical history in detail to prescribe a correct drug. Even the mildest drugs can produce adverse effects if misused or abused. Just because a drug can produce, certain side effects one should not hesitate to use it. It is necessary to read the warnings on the labels of drugs, which you are talking. Certain drugs interact if taken along with alcohol, which has toxic effect on intestinal lining which alters secretion of digestive enzymes. It reduces absorption of vitamin B_1, folic acid, reduces blood levels of vitamin B_{12}.

Antifungal increased urinary excretion and reduces blood levels of magnesium and potassium. Antidepressants weight gain, altered blood glucose and increases excretion of calcium. Drug nutrient interactions and dietary recommendations like antacid has effect on nutritional status such as bloating, constipation, nausea, loss of appetite. Dietary recommendations are taking between meals, increase intake of vitamin A, iron, and folic acid.

Many disorders require long-term drug treatment either to control the symptoms or to prevent them occurring again. Certain drugs cause adverse effect, especially on long-term use. One must never stop using the drug without consulting the doctor. Doing so may cause worsening of the symptoms, which can sometimes prove more dangerous than the adverse effects of the drug. To take the drug at the same time every day to avoid the chance of missing any dose.

For effective drug use know the name and the correct spelling of the drug you are talking with brand name and its generic name. Check the label before purchase to ensure expiry date is valid at the time of consumption of the drug. Read the inserts and get familiars with the content of product. Follow dosage instructions correctly. Shake all the liquids suspensions of drugs thoroughly. Follow doctor's instructions on dietary and other treatment measures. Keep written drugs taken and the drugs you have allergy, discard outdated drugs and keep them away from children, heat, light in dry container.

Do not pressurize doctor to prescribe unnecessary drugs. Do not take the drugs on the advice of friends who have had similar symptoms. Do not take drug when you are pregnant or breast feeding unless prescribed by your doctor who is aware of your condition. Do not take drug in dark, identity carefully in the light.

How some drug works- analgesics/painkillers- pain is unpleasant symptom and not a disease. Pain suggests some disturbance in the body. It is important to determine the cause of pain in all cases; it is always not easy, so pain killer play an important role in providing immediate relief until the cause is found and treated.

Each *antibiotic* is different used in the treatment of specific organisms. They are not effective against virus they are anti bacteria's. Bacterias are present all around us in the air we breath, our natural immunity protects us form them. However, when our immunity breaks down infectious diseases set in. bacteria multiply rapidly, destroying tissues, releasing toxins and threatening to spread via the blood stream to such a vital organs as the heart, brain, lung and kidneys. The exact infection can be detected by client's blood, sputum, urine, stool or pus tests confirming the nature of bacteria. Antibiotics come in the form of tablets, capsules, liquids, dry syrups or injectable. There are also antibiotics used for topical skin, eye and ear infection. Antibiotics must be used with caution.

Steroids are an important and potent group of drugs. They are found in the body naturally as hormones, being secreted by the adrenal glands. They have many different actions in the body, involving the immune response, water and mineral metabolism, and anti-inflammatory action. They may be given orally or by injections, or used locally in the form of ointment or creams. They should be used with precaution; they produce rapid relief of symptoms like fever, body ach so it is most common type of misuse.

HOW TO DEAL WITH AN ANAPHYLACTIC SHOCK?

Anaphylactic shock occurs as the result of a severe allergic reaction to a drug. It usually occurs within minutes of taking the drug. In anaphylactic shock, the blood pressure falls drastically and the airways may become narrowed. The main symptoms include pallor, tightness in the chest, breathing difficulty, rash, facial swelling, and collapse. Give artificial respiration immediately. Once the victim is breathing normally, lay him down; face upward with legs raised above the level of the heart to ensure adequate circulation of the blood. Use a footstool to support the feet. Cover the victim with the blanket while waiting for medical help. Do not give anything by mouth to the victim.

If anyone takes on overdose of medicines such as aspirin, heparin, insulin, colloquies, dioxin etc immediate medical attention must be sought.

Individual consumer action may be taken by having basic knowledge of medicines and how they work. Knowing which drugs are hazardous, banned or need to be avoided. Avoid irrational drugs. Ask your doctor to prescribe the drugs by their generic names and avoid OTC wherever possible.

Nurses play a very significant role in the use of drugs. It is they who are responsible for administration of drugs, observation of client's acceptance and untoward reaction of the drug. It is essential for them to know the actions, uses and contraindications of the drug dispensed.

80 years of penicillin—Penicillin is one of the earliest discovered and most widely used antibiotic agents in treatment of bacterial infection.

History—In 1875, first published reference in London. In 1928, rediscovered by Alexander Fleming; In 1939, Dr. Howard Floury showed penicillin's ability to kill infectious bacteria; In 1941, Andrew J Mayer increases yields of penicillin by Ten, first patient treated; In 1942, mass production of penicillin starts; In 1945, Flaming, Florey and Ernest Chain awarded Nobel prize for discovery of penicillin.

How it works—As by competitively inhibiting the Transpeptidase enzyme, leaving the new bacteria without a strong net for a cell wall. Penicillin inhibits growth of bacteria by destroying its cells walls, bacteria grows, cannot multiply, bacteria bursts.

Resistance—Some organism produce an enzyme, penicillin's, that destroys the antibiotic, other bacteria have altered cell wall structure that penicillin cannot destroy

Side effects—Diarrhea, hypersensitivity, nausea, rash, fever and vomiting, can cause allergic sensitivity (skin reaction, allergic shock).

Nurses responsibility—Read physicians orders and copy correctly, compare the label, expiry date, measure calculated dose. Do not touch with hands. Pour liquids from side of bottle. Do not mix medicines. Identity patient with medicine card, call patient by name, verify identification, stay with patient until he has taken the medicines. Record medicine amount, time, dose, rout etc. always make sure of routes of giving medicines, safety measures, abbreviation, medication effects, and precaution to be taken. Dangerous drugs are given by special orders. All poisonous drugs kept separately and medicines for external use kept separate cupboard from medicines for internal use. No drug should be kept without label. Emergency drugs kept in a place where they are readily obtainable for emergency use.

Medicines are substance used to promote health, to prevent, to diagnose, to alleviate or cure disease.

No medicines are given without doctors written orders. Give drug at correct time and do not leave with patient.

Drugs contraindication and precautions- most drugs are contraindicated in pregnancy to lactation. High alert medications needs extra care and safeguards such as insulin, opiates and narcotics, heparin, injectable potassium chloride and sodium chloride.

Dose miscalculations, incorrect drug administration, handwriting is a major source of error, telephone and verbal orders are prone to misinterpretation. Drugs with similar sounding or similar looking names frequently confuse, Latin abbreviations are confused with other units of measurement. When medication, dose adjustment of renal or hepatic impairment, children, elderly, serious underlying illness are at greatest risk. Nurse needs to clarify abbreviations, recalculate formulas and confirm the dosage with the prescribed. Have another nurse to check the original order. Do not start a patient a new medication by borrowing from another patient. Be sure fully understand any drug administration device before using it. This includes infusion pumps, inhalers and transdermal patches. Educate patient about the medication they take. Install a computer physician order entry system. Implement bar code technology to ensure right drug reaches the right patient. Whenever there is a negative change in a patients condition when an new drug has introduced, nurse must recognize and be familiar with most commonly encountered adverse reaction from escalating into a serious health problem. Stop the drug and monitor patients status for improvements, every patient is an individual with specific drug handling capabilities. Patient should know generic and brand names of the medication, purpose, dosage, what to do if a dose is missed, duration of therapy, minor side effects/serious side effects and what to do if they occur, and which medications to avoid, foods to avoid, how to store and follow up are. Provide written instructions in a simple and easy to read format.

Each drug has indication, action, contraindication, precautions, adverse reactions and side effects, route and dosage, availability, generic available, nursing implications, implementations, patient, family teaching, evaluation; that is effectiveness of therapy.

Each disease has pathophysiology and etiology, clinical manifestations, diagnostic evaluation, management, complications, nursing assessment, nursing diagnosis, nursing intervention, patient education health maintenance , outcome based on evaluation.

CHAPTER 3

Investigation and the Nurse

NURSE'S RESPONSIBILITY IN COLLECTION OF SPECIMEN FOR DIAGNOSTIC/ LABORATORY TEST

Nurse herself should have thorough working knowledge of the diagnostic test, which will help her to prepare the patient with compassion and clarity. She has to make sure that patient understands it correctly.

Factors to consider would be what pathologic process underlines the patient's manifestations? Are there laboratory results you would want to check? What other precautions should you institute based on the patients other manifestation and the laboratory data? What other data are significant to collect at this time? What laboratory results would be appropriate to evaluate? What teaching should be considered with the patient? What additional assessment would you need to make? What interventions should you anticipate at this time?

The nurse must carefully explain the diagnostic tests to patients and prepare them adequately for the examinations. She also provides emotional support to complete the diagnostic process so that appropriate treatment may be initiated. Nurses need to assess the effectiveness of their teaching, nurses should closely monitor and report, so that patient can adapt to the changes in their lives. Sometimes problems can be life threatening and the nurse must help to ensure patient to receive prompt treatment.

Nursing investigations are designed to help to maintain health, cope with long term illness and comply medication regimen and achieve and maintain maximum health. She must have clear understanding of herself, of the structure and functions of the body to provide apt knowledge and work with other professional team members for positive outcome. In order to provide effective interventions. Once she has a thorough knowledge of it, she must understand the diagnostic assessment, findings, and specific indications. Explain the importance of procedure and ask if they have questions. You are an important resource person and patient requires help and education, as patient is particularly vulnerable during this period of illness. A high level nursing surveillance can mean that patient recovers successfully. Keep in mind that the degree of nursing interventions is directly related to the severity of the illness and patients over all condition. She must have knowledge of bacteriology, there mode of transmission, effect on the body and different methods used in eliminate them, practice nursing principle and safety and has therapeutic effective broad knowledge of infection, prevention and control. If lapse it may further aggravate the problem and pose severe threat to health of patient. Her responsibility is to provide safety, consistency and effective care. Using scientific principle to relieve anxiety and encourage adjustment and meet all the needs of patient.

Instruct, patient to wash genitals with soap and water. No antiseptic should be present in the collection bottle it should be clean and dry.

For cultural specimen use sterile containers and get the midstream. Avoid collecting specimen during menstruation.

Do not contaminate inside the bottle and keep specimen at room temperature. To avoid decomposition and multiplication of undesirable pathogenic bacteria, she should follow certain principles, which are:

- Specimen should be fresh and sent as soon as it is collected. Motility of the organism can be noted only when they are fresh.
- Sometimes preservatives should be added to prevent decomposition of urine.
- For diabetic patient several times specimens are collected. The accuracy and reliability of findings depends upon the correct method of collection, transportation of specimen to the laboratory and documentation/recording of reports.
- Inaccurate results may mistake the physician in the diagnosis and treatment of patient.
- Label each specimen as soon as it is received with necessary data, nature of test to be done.
- Specimens serve as a media for transmission of disease producing organism of the person who handle them incorrectly.
- Carry specimen in tray rather than in hands.
- Wash hands thoroughly after handling the specimen bottle.
- Container should have a wide mouth to prevent spilling; proper containers are used according to the nature of specimen.
- The containers once used are cleansed and autoclaved before re-used.
- Wax lined disposable paper cups are used for the collection of sputum and stool because they can safely dispose after use.
- There should be no cracks in the specimen bottles it may leak.
- The nurse typically reinforce the physicians explanation, confirms the patients comprehension and takes the written consent.
- Sent specimen within two hours of collection, if not refrigerate, urine become alkaline on standing.
- In 24 hours, its quantity is around 1,000–1,800 ml and its specific gravity 1.012–1.024.

Give supportive care, discard urine and note time, measure all urine in large specimen bottle, add preservative, store in cool place.

Specimen collection is a small quantity of a substance or object, which shows the kind and quality of the whole sample. Contaminated and improperly collected specimens will produce false results which will adversely affect in diagnosis and treatment.

- Adequate explanation to patient's relatives to collect specimen (what, how, and quantity).
- They should not be misplaced, send them to proper place. Record the reports immediately and accurately on the patients chart.
- Nurses must use gloves and other barriers as necessary before nurse is exposed to the patient's body fluid and take appropriate precautions.

The field of laboratory medicine has undergone many changes in the past two to three decades. The results of test vary with age, sex, season, race, diet, genetic constitution, the geographical area, laboratory to laboratory. Therefore, standard methods of collection, storage, and preparation of specimens are extremely important in assuming reliable results.

- The urine contaminated with blood, pus, vaginal discharges, seminal fluids etc. may give false reports. So that the nurse should instruct the patients how to collect the urine specimen for laboratory tests.

     For preparation of patient and method of procedure; see that request slip is completed and correctly prepared.

- Instruct patient's relatives to collect or save first urine voided in the morning, if possible have patient void directly into specimen container, send proper lab slip – chart collection-receive report and place chart where easily physician can see.

Bacterial infections are common in clinical practice, causing infections of various organs. Both gram-positive and gram-negative bacteria and cocci produce a variety of infections like bronchitis, tonsillitis, pneumonia, ear infection. Most infections need use of chemotherapeutic agents to control them, with the help of defence mechanism of the body. If infection is present in one part of urinary tract, it may travel to another part. To find out the cause of infection urinalysis is to be done is as follows:

Urinalysis

In physical urine examination, color, appearance, volume, reaction, specific gravity and odor is examined.

Urine *Volume* usually normal about 1200 to 2000 ml/day.

Its *color* pale yellow to deep amber color.

Appearance clears without any sediment.

Odor aromatic, fruity odour may be due to ketone, bodies as seen in diabetes mellitus.

Its *Specific gravity* 1.003 – 1.030. The specific gravity may be low in renal diseases and it may be high when the urine contains albumin, sugar, urea, phosphate etc.

Reaction pH 4.5 to 8. Get fresh urine specimens for reaction. On standing at room temperature, the urine becomes alkaline due to the formation of ammonia.

Albumin/protein is usually negative. It is found in nephritis, febrile conditions, poisoning, eclampsia, hypertension and some forms of cardio-vascular diseases.

Sugar found in the urine is in uncontrolled diabetes mellitus, pancreatic disorders and impaired tubular reabsorption. It may result also from eating a heavy meal or from emotional stress. I.V. infusion of glucose also may raise the blood glucose level above the renal threshold.

Acetones are found in the urine when the body fat is metabolized for energy, producing an excess of metabolic products. This occurs in uncontrolled diabetics, starvation, severe infection accompanied by vomiting and diarrhea, pregnancy and lactation.

Pregnancy test/chorionic gonadotrophin – collect concentrated morning specimens. Positive results are seen in pregnancy, chorionepithelioma and hydatidiform mole. Ultrasonic detection of pregnancy can be detected 10 days after the first missed period and the twin pregnancy as early as five and a half weeks of amenorrhea.

Bilirubin negative, bilirubinuria is usually indicative of biliary tract obstruction. Other causes include hepatitis, portal inflammation, and hepatocellular damage.

RBC in urine often indicates glomerulonephritis, tuberculosis of the kidney, renal calculi, sickle cell anemia, tumors of the kidney, systemic lupus erythematosus, anti-coagulation therapy, excessive use of analgesic etc. when collecting urine from a menstruating women, the nurse has to be careful to get the urine without contaminating it with blood. When a patient complains of haematuria, it is necessary to note whether the bleeding takes place at the beginning to at the end of each voiding.

The presence of *WBC/pus* cells in the urine designates an infectious process somewhere in the urinary tract.

Presence of *casts* indicates tubular/glomerular disease.

Hyaline casts are found normally after strenuous exercise, but there presence in people at rest may indicate acute glomerular-nephritis, malignant hypertension, acute pylonephritis, chronic renal diseases, congestive heart failure or diabetic nephropathy.

Red cell casts may denote bleeding within nephron because of glomerulonephritis.

The presence of crystals in the urine is an important predisposing factor in calculus formation.

Since urine is normally sterile, a bacterium represents infection within urinary tract. Some special tests are carried out in order to isolate microorganism for the diagnosis of tuberculosis of kidney, well's diseases etc.

Amylase is increased in acute pancreatitis. Calcium excretions are increased in Hyperparathyroidism, vitamin D intoxication etc. It is reduced in hypoparathyroidism and vitamin D deficiency.

Urine *chloride* levels very with excretion of sodium, potassium, ammonia and bicarbonate.

Creatinine increased levels are seen in typhoid fever, salmonella infections and tetanus. It is decreased in muscular atrophy, anemia, leukemia and advanced degeneration of kidneys.

Prophobilinogen positive results are seen in acute liver disease. Collect fresh urine for qualitative tests and protect the urine from direct light.

Urobilinogen increased levels are seen in liver diseases, biliary tract diseases and hemolytic anemia's. Reduced excretions are seen in complete obstruction, diarrhea, and renal insufficiency.

Uric acid increased in gout and reduced in nephritis.

Culture and Sensitivity—To determine presence of specific organism and their sensitivity to antibiotics abnormally high in infection in UTI, careful cleansing metus, clean catch by catheterization do not contaminate inside basin or specimen bottle.

Dilution and concentration test to measure the capacity of the kidneys to concentrate urine withhold food and all fluid after the evening meal or 12 hrs before start of test.

Insulin clearance test—Tests for glomerular filtration rate 0.3 gm/36 mg minute in urine.

Phenolsulfomethalein (PSP) excretion of dye indirect measure of tubular excretion and dye is injected, dye will temporarily affect urine color pink to red.

Gastrointestinal secretion—stool, gross, microscopic – presence of parasites, fat, bacteria (salmonella and shigella), ova, amebas, blood, infestation, malabsorption, GI hemorrhage, peptic ulcer, hemorrhoids .

Faeces—color light to dark brown. Melaena/tarry black stool indicate bleeding into upper GI tract, the blood being altered by the gastrointestinal juices or it may result from the administration of iron.

Clay colored stools indicate obstruction to the flow of bile into the intestinal canal.

Presence of blood in large amounts is suggestive of bleeding piles, destruction of a blood vessel in the large intestines by an ulceration process or contamination of the stool with menstrual blood.

Blood and mucus are found in amoebic dysentery.

Pus cells are seen in bacillary dysentery.

EH cyst is found in amoebic dysentery. *E. coli* are nonpathogenic and is commonly found in the colon.

Presence of ova indicates *roundworm,* pinworm or whipworm. The ova of each worm have its own characteristics. Segments of tapeworm are seen in tapeworm infestation.

Positive *occult blood* is seen in Melaena, Vibrio-cholera is seen by its motility in cases of cholera infection.

The stools should be freshly collected. It should be examined without any delay.

Sputum: Culture for bacteria and parasites, abnormally high in the presence of infection and malignant growth. Presence of sputum indicates respiratory infection and inflammation.

Polymorph nuclear cells are found in large numbers along with lymphocytes, in cases of lung diseases and tuberculosis.

Eosinophils are seen in conditions of asthma, allergic conditions etc.

AFB will be positive in cases of tuberculosis of the lungs.

Gastric Fluid Analysis

Fasting residual volume 2.0 – 0.6 m Eq/hr low in pernicious anemia, gastric carcinoma, pellagra and high in peptic ulcer, certain endocrine disorders. Delay breakfast, intubations is an unpleasant experience. To ease procedure, patient sits up, encourage to swallow as tube is advanced to help reduce gagging and nausea. Emergency drug tray and resuscitation equipment should be available.

Semen Analysis

Absence of sperm in the semen is associated with primary testicular disorders or complete obstruction of the seminal tract.

Lowered sperm density is often associated with decreased spermatogenesis. A sperm density of less than 20 million/ml is considered as infertile.

Decreased sperm mobility contributory factors in infertility.

Discharges from wounds or body cavities: Smear culture for bacteria and for cancer cells.

Serous Fluids spinal fluid—for bacteria specially meningococcal, pheumococus, streptococcus, tubercle bacillus, negative, 3–4 specimens of 2–4 ml each, surgical procedure.

Thoracic fluid (thoracocentesis) gross, microscopic and chemical exam for color and transparency, specific gravity, proteins, cell count, cytological study. Add anticoagulant to specimen.

PERITONEAL FLUID (ABDOMINAL PARACENTESIS)

Pericardial Aspirations

Synovial fluid—Straw colored, clear of cloudy viscous good mucin clot 200 – 600 WBC/cu mm. low viscosity in gout, rheumatoid arthritis, tuberculosis, septic arthritis, TB has low value.

Blood investigations—Let us understand the blood components and functions of blood before understanding its investigations.

Blood components are red blood cells, platelets, white blood cells, granulocytes, neutrophils, Eosinophils, besophils, lymphocytes, monocytes, plasma water, proteins albumin, globulins, and fibrinogen.

A significant deficiency or alteration in the procedure during an individuals life time will have grave consequences. Several of the more serious diseases affecting humen are derived from or are related to pathologic change in the blood forming system.

Blood mediate the exchange of oxygen and carbon dioxide between lungs and tissue. Form platelet plug to arrest bleeding, promote thrombin production. Protection from bacteria and other foreign substances. White cells containing granular structures, broken down into three subcategories, phagocytosis, allergic and inflammatory reactions. Prevention of clotting in microcirculation. Allergic reaction, formation of immunoglobins, cellular immunity, phagocytosis. Liquid in which cells circulate, maintains colloidal osmotic pressure, contains antibodies for body's defence, blood coagulation.

Blood may be collected as whole blood or clotted blood. Blood films are made for the cell counts.

Whole blood collected only by venipuncture under strict aseptic technique. A syringe of proper size, needles tight fitting. Whole blood is collected in a test tube or bottle with suitable anticoagulant EDTA (ethylene diamine tetra acetic acid) used.

The containers should be clean. Transfer the blood fron syringe to the container as soon as it is collected. Remove the needle from the syringe before putting blood into container. To prevent clotting blood mixed thoroughly.

Do not keep blood for long at room temperature, send to the lab immediately, and keep it in a refrigerator at 4 to 6° C.

All specimens labeled with patient's identification data. Reports are to be entered in chart.

Nurses responsibility and understanding on possible manifestations of a transfusion reactions—fever, chills, muscle aches, pain, back and chest pain, headache, heat at the sight of infusion, apprehension, tingling, numbness, changing respiration rate, nausea, vomiting, abdominal cramping, shock, hypo or hypertension, cyanosis, facial flushing, edema, temperature, changes in urine volume, rashes, itching, diaphoresis.

In acute reaction-allergic due to sensitivity to foreign proteins in plasma which could be prevented by prophylactically with antihistamines. Febrile non hemolytic caused by sensitization to donor WBC, platelets or plasma proteins. Acute hemolytic due to infusion of ABO incompatible RBC. Anaphylactic, circulatory overload when infusion of blood at a rate too rapid for size, place patient in upright position and adjust transfusion volume and flow rate on the basis of patient size and clinical status. If slow transfusion will exceed 4 hours. Septicemia transfusion of component contaminated with micro-organism—treat symptoms and administer antibiotics. Obtain blood culture.

Hematologic diseases are complex disorders that requires the nurse to understand the hemato-system. The nurse involved in the administration of blood and blood products for the treatment of wide variety of disorders. It is vital that the nurse understand blood transfusion procedure and use proper technique of administration so the patient will receive safe and effective care.

Blood Hematology—Hemogram

RBC, low value in anemia, aplastic anemia, bone marrow depression 5 – 20 ml for complete blood exam, tourniquet or lancet for skin puncture.
WBC 4.500 – 10.500/cu mm. Low values in leukemia— bone marrow depression.
Differential count WBC – bacterial infection, virus infection, Allergic reaction, Hodgkin's disease.
Hematocrit (HCT) packed cell volume – for anemia.

Platelet count—145,000 – 375,000/cu mm. Thrombocytopenic purpura, aplastic anemia, septicemia.

Reticulocyte—Determines bone marrow activity.

Coagulation time—Time takes for blood to clot after removal from a vein., lack of vit K, liver disease, hemophilia atibrinogemenia. Record time.

Bleeding time—Measures of blood vessel retract ability. Note time of puncture.

Sedimentation rate—Time for solid materials in blood to settle, low value in CCF and high value in inflammation, cell destruction, toxemia.
Arterial Blood gas analysis gives an indication of the efficiency of the lungs in the exchange of oxygen and carbon dioxide. It generally includes arterial PH— purpose acidity or alkalinity of arterial blood, low acidosis, high value respiratory alkalosis, drawn only by specially trained personnel, careful pressure 5 minutes applied following puncture.

PCO_2—Plasma carbon dioxide pressure of arterial blood/venous blood— For male – 34-45 mm Hg and for female – 31-42 mm Hg. Low alkalosis high acidosis.
Total CO_2 content—For male is 24-30 and for female is 21–27 mEq/liter.

PO_2 – Plasma oxygen pressure of arterial blood 80–90 mm Hg. Low value in respiratory insufficiency, shock syndrome acidosis. Supplementary O_2 is needed with low values.

Oxygen Saturation (96–97%)

The procedure may be performed for the assessment of acid-base balance, which may be disturbed due to metabolic or respiratory disorders, especially when mechanical ventilation of the lungs is used.

Bromsulphalein (BSP)—To determine amount of dye in blood stream at end of 45 minutes. O.4 mg BSP/100 ml blood.

Lactic acid dehydrogenates LDH—Serum transaminase level 25 – 120 units. High in MI, acute hepatitis obstructive jaundice.

Non-protein nitrogen NPN—Low in severe liver disease, high in kidney disease/urinary obstruction/dehydration.

Phosphates acid—Metastatic carcinoma of prostate.

RA test—Rheumatoid arthritis test- Negative.
Serologic tests for syphilis STS— Negative
Triglycerides 140 mg/100 ml (arteriosclerosis)
Urea nitrogen (BUN) 8–25 mg/100 ml low in hepatic failure, nephrosis high in renal insufficient nephritis, UTI, acute nephritis.
Uric acid 2–7.5 mg /100 ml high in gout, toxemia of pregnancy, leukemia, polycythemia renal insufficiency.
Blood cultures—To determine specific organism.
Bone marrow examination— To examine cells being produced by bone marrow 10,000 – 50,000 nucleated cells per cu mm.

Prothrombin time (PT)— To indicate ability of blood to form intravascular clots 15 – 30 seconds high in liver disease, vitamin K deficiency, frequent evaluation necessary to determine dosage of anticoagulant.

Central Venous Pressure Measurement (CVPM) – 5-8 cm H_2O high value insufficient cardiac output above 15–17 cm, fluid overload. Catheter is inserted percutaneously or by cut down usually through external jugular or subclavin vein into the midsuperior vena cava, low blood volume need for fluid replacement
ECG — Electric impulses of heart contraction
EEG — Electric impulses of brain
Electromyogram — Electric impulses of muscular mass
Gallbladder series — Filling and emptying gallbladder, dye administration, delay breakfast, fat free supper, nil by mouth after mid-night, dye given after supper 12 hrs prior to exam.
IVP intravenous pylelogram—Outline of urinary tract, dye excretion by kidneys, NPO by midnight, Laxative/enema every before
Pneumoencephalogram—Outline of ventricles of brain – painful for patient – support.

Angiograms—Often lengthy and fatiguing procedure, site observed for shock.

Mammograms—Soft tissues of breast visualized. Films taken of breasts.

Scans–bone, brain, liver – tumor mass, obstruction.

CSF and other cavity fluids- the fluid collected in three sterile test tubes which should be numbered. 6 to 8 ml of fluid is collected at a time. Sent to the lab. To be examined within 30 minutes of its collection. Handle the specimens very carefully as repetition of lumber puncture is no simple matter. Specimens should be collected before antibiotics. Specimens obtained for isolation of virus should be frozen immediately.

Pulmonary function test is a method of assessing pulmonary volume, lung capacities and flow rates by the use of spirometry. It is used to screen high-risk patients such as cigarette smokers, industrial workers who are exposed to dust, diagnosis of pulmonary diseases.

Diagnostic Aids

- *Endoscopes* are a direct visual examination of the internal body parts by means of an endoscope passed along the interior of hollow organs or cavities.
- *Pandoscopy* is a term used for the visualization of more than one organ with the same endoscope. The endoscope is usually inserted into a natural body orifice such as mouth, anus or urethra. From head to foot, nearly every area of the body can be visualized with it. It's Size and shapes varies according to usage all have similar working elements. It must be handled carefully; it is delicate and expensive instrument, cleaned immediately after use, using large quantity of water to flush out blood, pus and other deposits. Never keep it moist, which gives rise to fungus. It is non-autoclave. They are hanged until next use.
- *A biopsy* is the removal and examination of tissue for diagnostic purpose.
- *Open-biopsy* is an surgical excision at the time of exploratory surgery; it depends upon the size of the tumor, if the suspicious tumor is small, the entire tumor is excised for examination e.g. lump in the breast; if the tumor is large, only a part of the tumor is removed. This is called subtotal incision biopsy.
- *The needle biopsy*: The needle fitted with a syringe is inserted into the suspicious site of the organ and a small sample of cells are aspirated for microscopic examination. This type of biopsy is done for lungs, liver, etc. a probe needle is inserted to the specific area of the organ, after the needle is positioned, the probe is removed and the slitted biopsy needle is inserted and rotated. Small pieces of tissues trapped in the needle. The chances of complications such as hemorrhage, pain, shock and collapse, perforation of the adjacent organs. Needle biopsy trough special needle and endoscope biopsy by means of endoscope.
- *Aspiration* of the body cavities is done by introducing a needle for the purpose of removing blood, serous fluid, pus from cavities. It is done for diagnostic or therapeutic purpose, e.g. in chronic nephritis, congestive cardiac failure.
- *In bone marrow biopsy,* specimen of bone marrow taken from the sternum, iliac crest, posterior superior iliac spine, spine of the vertebrae to tibia by means of thick needle. Purpose is in

aplastic anemia, leukemia, and thrombocytopenia etc. bone marrow depression or destruction, metastatic neoplasms.

- *Closed renal biopsy* is the retrograde renal and urethral brush. Procedure done as a cystoscopy, a ureteric catheter is passed and its position is confirmed by fluoroscopy. A biopsy brush is then passed through the catheter and the lesion is brushed over several time. The brush is then removed and any tissue adhering taken and send to lab test. If no tissue is found on the brush, 24 to 48 hour urine specimens may be collected to catch any cells that may be disloged by the bristles. Patient placed in prone position for procedure with a firm pillow under the abdomen. Under local, asked patient to take deep breath and hold it, then a probe needle is inserted through the skin and positioned inside the renal capsule. After confirming the position, a biopsy is taken, after removing needle, firm pressure is applied.
- The contraindications are single functioning kidney, infection, tumors, hydronephrosis, severe hypertension, coagulation disorders, history of renal failure, pregnancy and un-cooperative patient.
- *Cervical biopsy* is the removal of a small piece of the cervix for the histopathological examination. It can be done as a punch biopsy or cervical conization. In punch biopsy, one or more small pieces of tissues are removed from the cervix with a punch biopsy forceps. The cervical conization is done by talking a cone shaped section of the cervix with a scalpel or by diathermy conization. Done in OPD basis does not have pain as cervix does not contain nerve ending for pain. Instruction such as report bleeding, 24 hours no strenuous activity, abstain sexual activities, use clean pads.
- *Endometrial biopsy* is done by scraping the lining of the uterine cavity with a curette. D&C done for diagnostic purpose. It is done to control dysfunctional uterine bleeding, in complete and incomplete abortion, to relieve dysmenorrheal, remove polyps, diagnose uterine malignancy, diagnose sterility, etc.
- In *needle biopsy*, diagnosis is done by using a Vim Silverman's needle or a Menghini's needle with a cannula with a stitted probe. It is introduced into the liver substance and rotated to get a biopsy. Hemorrhage and biliary peritonitis are the complications.
- The *site of the puncture* in the hypochondriac region in the eighth or ninth intercostal space. It can be determined by X-ray and by scanning. Patient lies in supine position with his right side as close to the edge of the bed as possible. A pillow is placed under the left side turning face away from procedure.
- *Liver aspiration* is an introduction of a needle into the liver substance to drain the abscess. Instead of liver biopsy needle, long aspiration needle with wide bore are introduced into the liver to remove the thick pus.
- *Open renal biopsy* requires surgical procedure involving an incision through the flank. The procedure is costly and has prolonged recuperation period for the patient.
- *Thoracocentesis* is to puncture by needle through the chest wall into the pleural space for removing pleural fluid, blood, serous fluid, pus etc. and *air* that is *pneumothorax*. In diagnostic purpose, usually 20-30 ml fluid removed and in therapeutic purpose larger amount of fluid drawn to relieve the pressure caused by accumulation of fluid in the pleural cavity. The purpose to study the chemical, bacteriological and cellular composition of the plural

fluid. Effusion occurs in patients with tuberculosis, lymphoma, carcinoma etc. to instill medications into thoracic cavity.

Complications that may occur during procedure is sudden rise of sharp pin in the chest, persistent cough, shortness of breath, fall in blood pressure, rapid pulse, anxiety, restlessness, profuse sweating, pallor and cyanosis, decrease or absence of lung sounds on the affected side, due to collapse of lungs. Cessation of normal chest movements on the affected side.

- In *pericardial aspiration* removal of fluid from the pericardial sac, there is a possibility of puncturing the heart or injuring the coronary vessels. ECG monitoring is essential during the procedure.
- *Abdominal paracentesis* is the removal of fluid from the peritoneal cavity. In healthy body, the fluid formed in the peritoneal cavity is absorbed into the lymph circulation, but in disease processes, fluid accumulates within this cavity and cause ascites. Purpose is to relieve pressure on the abdominal and chest organs, if a transudate collects as a result of renal, cardiac or liver diseases.
- *Complications*—Hypovolemia leading to shock and collapse, infection, injury to the blood vessels and other abdominal organs, renal failure due to reduced systemic circulation, hypoproteinemia as a result of repeated tapping.
- *Lumbar puncture* is the insertion of a needle into the lumbar region of the spine, in such a manner that the needle enters the lumbar arachnoid space of the spinal canal below the level of the spinal cord, so that the CSF can be withdrawn or a substance can be therapeutically or diagnostically injected. The CSF is formed through the choroids villi, in each of the four ventricles of the brain and it circulates freely through the ventricles, the subarachnoid space and the central canal of the spinal cord. Purpose is to administer spinal anesthesia before surgery in the lower half of the body. To administer medications into the spinal canal as in the case of meningitis. To remove blood, pus, CSF contained in the subarachnoid space, thereby reduce the intracranial pressure, if it is dangerously high. Diagnosis purpose, to measure the CSF pressure and, to remove CSF and to replace it with air, oxygen or radio opaque substances for diagnostic X-rays in order to locate tumors or other brain disorder.
- *Complications*—Injury to the spinal cord and spinal nerves, infection introduced into the spinal cavity which may give rise to meningitis. Leakage of CSF through the puncture site and lowering the intracranial pressure and may cause post puncture headaches. Damage to the intervertebral discs. Local pain, edema and hematoma at the puncture site. Temperature elevation, rapid reduction in the intracranial pressure caused by the removal of CSF can cause herniation of the brain structures into the foremen magnum. This in turn causes pressure on the vital centers in the medulla, causing respiratory failure and sudden death. Site on lumbar puncture in adult is usually between the second and third or fourth and fifth lumbar vertebra. In small children and infants, the site is still lower because the spinal cord extends up to the third lumbar vertebra. The patient is placed side lying position at the edge of the table or bed. The body of patient should be in 'C' shaped with full flexion of the spine. Draw both knees up towards the chin; keep the hands between the knees. Open Liver biopsy- a wedge of the liver is removed for study and the remaining edges are

sutured together. Surgical procedure and has major abdominal incision. It helps to visualize entire liver which allows to see altered tissue area.

Diagnostic Assessment/ Radiographic Examinations (X-rays of the skull and spine)

Plain X-rays of the skull and spine are used to determine the body fractures, curvatures, bone erosion, bone dislocation, possible calcification of soft tissue, which can damage the nervous system. Several views are taken, anteroposterior, lateral, oblique and when necessary special views of the cervical must be ruled out by radiography as one of the first priorities. During procedure client will have to remain, if the patient is in traction, nurse has to assist with positioning if portable X-ray unit is not available. Any patient cannot walk from a wheel chair to the X-ray table should go to the radiology department on a stretcher. The patient is positioned for each of the views desired and is asked to move just before each X-ray.

- *X-ray* is a form of electromagnetic energy of very short wave length. Due to this, they have ability to penetrate into matter and it is this characteristic that makes them useful in the study of tissues. X-ray examination may be commonly done by taking plain X-rays and contrast studies. Bone, chest, skull, sinus, abdomen plain X-rays taken. To study specific organ either air or opaque chemicals introduced into the body cavities. Chemical contras agents can be introduced into a hollow organ such as gastro intestinal tract that is barium meal and barium enema— the bronchial tree bronchography, spinal canal myelography, gall bladder and kidney cholecystogrphy, intravenous pylography, e.g. to study the functions of the gall bladder— a dye may be given either by mouth or intravenously.

  The dye is excreted selectively by the liver with the bile and is then concentrated by the gall bladder, which is seen in the X-ray. The commonly used contrast agents are hypaque, pantopaque, cardiographine, barium sulphate etc. Routine chest films are important as a part of any complete physical examination— they revels disorders involving the lung tissue, abnormalities in the heart position, size, disorders of bone of the chest wall, presence of large volume of fluid in the pleural space, abnormal changes in the pulmonary arteries and veins.

- *Angiography* is the roentgenographic visualization of the blood vessels any where in the body following the injection of a contrast medium. It is useful in evaluating the disorders of the brain, heart, lungs and other body segments.

- *Angiocardiography* is the study of the chambers of the heart and the large thoracic blood vessels done in conjunction with the cardiac catheterization. Immediately after the dye is injected— a series of X-ray films are taken which reveal the course of the dye as it circulates through the patient's heart, lungs, great vessels.

  The purpose to check the valves of the heart competence, to diagnose congenital septal defects. To reveal calcifications or occlusions of the coronary arteries. To study the structure and functions of the heart in detail prior to cardiac surgery.

- *Pulmonary angiography* is the roentgenogrsphic visualization of the blood vessels of the lungs. It is helpful in diagnosing such condition as pulmonary embolism, lung tumors, aneurysms, vascular changes associated with emphysema, congenital defects, it also involves the cardiac catheterization.

- *A cerebral angiography* allows X-ray visualization of the brain vascular system. The dye may be injected directly into the common carotid artery or with the insertion of a catheter into the brachial artery or femoral artery to the descending aorta and from there into the desired vessels of the heart. Once the appropriate vessel has been reached, the contrast material is injected and a series of films are rapidly taken.
- *Venography* is designed to identify and locate deep vein thrombosis and other structural abnormalities of the veins. A radio-opaque dye is injected into the venous system of the affected limb under fluoroscopy and X-ray films are taken.
- *Cardiac catheterization* is complex procedure involves the insertion of catheter into the heart and surrounding vessels to obtain detailed information abut the structure and functions of the heart, its valves and the circulatory system. This procedure can be used to study the entire heart confined to the right or left side exclusively.

Purpose

- To obtain a clear picture of cardiac structure and functions prior to heart surgery.
- To obtain the pressure within the heart chambers and the great vessels.
- To inject contrast medium directly into the heart chambers and the great vessels in order to obtain X-ray films of the heart and blood vessels.
- To diagnose the existence of congenital abnormalities.
- To confirm the diagnosis of the heart diseases and to determine the extent to which the disease has affected the structure and functions of the heart.
- To obtain the measurement of the cardiac output.
- To draw blood samples directly from the heart chambers and vessels in order to measure the oxygen content of the blood and the extent of oxygen saturation. This information indicates weather abnormal congenital shunts are present in the heart or not. To detect the pulmonary and mediastinal abnormalities, the displacement of vessels from their normal positions or reduced blood flow to an area caused by emboli, timorous obstruction, congenital defects etc.

A cardiac catheterization is usually done only in one side of the heart, although it is necessary to insert the catheter into both sides of the heart. For a right sided cardiac catheterization the physician first performs a cut down either on the antecubital vein or in the femoral vein and passes a sterile, radiopaque catheter of 100 to 125 cm long through the vein into the vena cava— then trough the right atrium and ventricle into the pulmonary artery. The ECG is constantly monitored during the procedure. Pressure within the atrium, ventricles and the pulmonary artery are measured.

The blood samples also are taken— the dye is injected into the right side of the heart and the films are taken. For the left sided cardiac catheterization, the catheter can be passed retrograde from the brachial or femoral artery into the left ventricle. Once the catheter is positioned, the left side of the heart can be studied by means of pressure readings, blood studies, dye injection or X-ray films. The coronary arteries may be studied during the left heart catheterization. The catheter is advanced under the fluoroscopic control, to the base of the aorta and the dye is injected into the opening of each coronary artery.

Preparation of the Patient

Prepare the patients psychologically for this procedure. Patient may fear the cardiac catheterization, since it is pertaining to their heart. Tell the patient that he will experience no pain, except certain sensations.

- Get the written consent for the procedure.
- Make sure that the patient has not suffered from allergies.
- The sensitivity test for iodine should be carried out.
- Make the patient to fast for 6 to 8 hours prior to the procedure.
- Antibiotics are administered prior to the procedure to prevent possible infections, especially if the patient has the history of the rheumatic heart diseases or congenital heart diseases.
- Record the pulse, respiration, temperature, BP etc prior to the procedure for reference in the post procedure period.
- Record the height and weight of the patient on the chart in order to asses the amount of dye to be injected.
- Pre medications are given to relax the patient.
- Mark the site of peripheral pulses with skin pencil, this will aid in locating the pulse during or after the procedure.
- Other preparations are as for a surgical procedure.
- Strict aseptic techniques are to be followed.
- Emergency equipment and drugs for resuscitation of the patient should be at hand to act immediately in emergency.
- A continuous cardiac monitoring using an electro-cardiogram should be done to detect cardiac arrhythmias.

Watch for early sings of complications during or after the procedure. The complications expected are cardiac arrhythmias, thrombophebitis, myocardial infarction, pneumothorax, pulmonary embolism, anaphylactic shock and even death.

After Care of the Patient

On completion of procedure, when the catheter is removed, a sterile sponge is placed on the site and firm pressure is applied to prevent bleeding from the punctured site and hematoma formation. Later on ice may be applied to minimize the swelling and discomfort.

The cardiac monitoring should be continued after the procedure also. After the procedure, the patient should be placed comfortably and safely. He should be advised to take complete bed rest for 12 to 24 hours.

The skin color, temperature and peripheral pulses etc should be carefully evaluated for the signs of complications. Warmth of the skin distal to the side of the catheter insertion must be assed for phlebitis. The affected extremity is kept straight, the arm may be immobilized on an arm board or the leg must be kept straight at the groin to prevent clot formation.

The patient should be carefully watched in the post procedure period also. The vital sings are checked every 10 to 15 minutes during the first hour, and then every 30 minutes for the next few hours or until stabilized. Any change should be reported to the physician immediately. The puncture site is checked for bleeding, swelling or hematoma and signs of thrombosis.

The temperature is checked frequently. It may be slightly elevated; the BP may be low due to the diuretic effect of the dye.

Check for the peripheral pulses in the extremity in which the catheter was inserted. Absence of pulse or weakening of the pulse could signify occlusion of the vessel.

Watch for allergic reactions following angiography. Be guard on such allergic symptoms as flushing, nausea, vomiting, numbness, tingling, chills, diaphoresis, faintness, urticaria, tachycardia are the danger signals of anaphylactic shock. Occasionally their may develop tissue sloughs due to leakage of the contrast medium into the area surrounding the vein and thus causing venous thrombosis. Sudden death may occur if the dye was injected rapidly.

- *Barium-X-ray*—Abdomen shows the shadows of the relative densities of the structures photographed. But the inside of the gastrointestinal tract cannot be visualized unless a contrast medium is ingested or instilled into it. Barium sulphate is a white chalky, radiopaque, non-toxic, non-absorbable and relatively cheap contrast media that can be used safely for the gastrointestinal tract studies.

- *Barium swallow* may be performed as a part of barium meal. Barium swallows study the filling and the emptying of the esophagus. The patient drinks the barium sulphate solution. As the patient swallowing mechanism studied and abnormality such as strictures, hiatus hernia, tumors detected.

- *Barium meal* is useful in diagnosing obstructions, ulcerations and growths within the esophagus, stomach and duodenum and to find out the structural and functional abnormalities of the small intestines. The first part of the barium meal is done as for a barium swallow. When the barium reaches the stomach, it outlines the walls of the stomach and fills the lumen of the stomach. The thickness of the gastric wall and the mucosal pattern are observed for evidence of spasms, ulcerations and filling defects that could be caused by tumors. The motility and the emptying time of the stomach are also observed. The patency of the pyloric valve and the anatomy of the duodenum observed, the intestinal loops are observed. Films of the stomach are taken at various intervals that is 3 hours after the first X-ray, 6 hours, 24 hours etc.

- *Barium enema* by which the large colon is studied with barium given per rectum. About 2-3 pints of barium sulphate is given to distend the bowel and the X-rays are taken. It will show any abnormalities in the structure of the colon. The bowels should be thoroughly empty before a barium enema is given. Any retained faecal will cause a filling defect to show on the X-ray and confuse the diagnosis.

- *Cholecystography* is the radiographic examination of the gall bladder after administration of opaque medium for detection of gall stones and to estimate its ability to fill, concentrate its contents, contract and empty in normal states. *X-ray KUB* is an X-ray of the kidney, ureter and bladder, is a simple film of the lower abdomen. This helps to identify size, shape, location and soft tissue masses, malformations, radiopaque calculi.

- *Intravenous pylography/excretory urogram* is visualization of the kidney, ureters and bladder by injecting a dye into the vascular system. Intravenous injection of a radio-opaque dye that is filtered and excreted through the kidneys into the urinary tract. It reveal the position, shape and the dimensions of the kidneys, anatomic peculiarities of the urinary system, such as horse-shoe kidney, polycystic kidneys, hydronephrosis, double ureters, displacement of the ureters, enlargement of the prostrate gland, tumors, renal calculi, abnormalities urinary bladder etc.

- *Hysterosalpingography* is an X-ray study of the uterus and fallopian tubes using contrast medium—in order to evaluate the uterine abnormalities and tubal patency in sterility problems. The patient is placed in a lithotomy position, with the cervix exposed and a canula is inserted into the cervix and a sterile, acqueous radio-opaque substance is injected into the uterine cavity and the tubes. This examination is not carried out for more than 7 days after the end of the menstrual period, since the ovulation would be taking place. The test may need the dilatation of the cervix, prepare patient for a D and C.

Electroencephalography [EEG]

The electroencephalogram may be compared with electrocardiogram, in that the electrodes are placed over the skull in many areas and the electric activity of the various segments of the brain is recorded. EEG is painless and a safe technique for evaluating the brain pathology such as brain tumors, brain abscess and epilepsy. EEG records the electrical activity of the cerebral hemispheres. Each graphic recording represents the voltage changes in various areas of the brain (determined by recording the difference between two electrodes) the test is performed to:

- Determine the general activity of the cerebral hemispheres.
- Determine the origin of seizure activity (epilepsy).
- Determine cerebral function in pathologic conditions such as tumors, abscesses, cerebrovasular disease, hematoma, injury, metabolic disease, and degenerative brain disease and drug intoxication.
- Differentiate between organic and hysterical or feigned blindness and deafness.
- Monitor cerebral activity during surgical anesthesia.
- Diagnose sleep disorders (all-night EEC).
- Determine brain death.
- *Patient Preparation*—The preparation of the patient for EEG is extremely important because it can directly affect the accuracy of the test results. He should be told that it is not a form of shock treatment or a way of hypnotizing the patient. The co-operation and a relaxation of patient is necessary. The patient should not be disturbed mentally before the test. Mental excitement and depression can alter the EEG tracing. The patient may be hospitalized during the test or OPD basis.

Instructions—Thoroughly explain the procedure if the order is for the patient to be 'sleep-deprived', tell the patient to awaken about 2 to 3 am and stay awake for the rest of the night. Avoid CNS depressants or stimulants; withhold anticonvulsants only if instructed by the physician. Not to drink caffeine containing fluids, coffee, and tea on the day of test, reassure patient that test, is not dangerous or uncomfortable. Ask patient to wash hair in the morning of test, hair need to wash again to remove the electrode glue.

MRI—Magnetic Resonance Imaging

Magnetic resonance is a new imaging modality based on the use of high powered magnets. It is a method of protons within the body, enabling very high quality anatomical images to be obtained. Resent advances in the development of needles, catheter and guided wires have lead to their increasing therapeutic use.

Radiology is rapidly changing. The wide spread acceptance of digitalization and subsequent computerization pioneered in CT is now making an impact on conventional radiograph.

MRI is one of the newest diagnostic tools for detecting neurological problems. With a large magnetic field and the introduction of a specific radio frequency, protons of the body absorb and emit energy. This energy is then converted to a picture or images are clear for all densities of tissue. MRI is particularly useful as a diagnostic tool for multiple sclerosis. It surpasses CT in clarity for many types of tissue and lesions such as meningiumas and acoustic neurmas as well as arteriovenous malformations and other cerebral anomalies. MRI does not involve exposure to radiation and is noninvasive.

PET   Position Emission Tomography
SPECT   Single Photon Emission Computed Tomography.

PET is a new diagnostic tool available only in larger medical centers at present. Its benefit over CT scan or MRI is that it provides information about the *function* of the *brain* and provide information about the *structure* of the *CNS*.

The physician injects the patient with the radioisotope doxyglucose. The isotope emits activity in the form of positrons, which are scanned and converted into an image by computer. The image is displayed in colors. The more active a given part of the brain, the greater the glucose uptake. This test is being used extensively for diagnosis and research on Alzheimer's disease and other dementias, epilepsy and movement disorders. The level of radiation is equivalent to five or six X-rays but much less than the exposure during CT. Because the radioisotope have a such a short life, there must be a cyclotron on the premises to prepare them. This limits the number of medical centers able to offer the test.

This limitations of PET may be overcome through the use of a single-photon emission (SPECT) gamma-emitting radionuclides have longer half lives, thus SPECT is less expensive than PET, the resolution of the images is limited. SPECT is particularly useful in studying cerebral blood flow and cerebral blood volume, among other things.

Patient Preparation

The nurse explains the test and avoid coffee, alcohol and tobacco before 25 hours of test, meal 3-4 hours before procedure, diabetic patient no insulin given before test. The nurse withholds any other drugs that alter glucose metabolism.

Procedure

The patient sits on a reclining chair in front of the scanner. An IV line is started on each hand / arm – one to inject the isotope and the other to obtain blood samples. The arm used for blood samples is warmed to get arterial (shunted) and venous blood. The patient may be blindfolded and have earplugs inserted for all or part of the test and must be still for 1 ½ hours. The patient is asked to perform certain mental functions, which activate different areas of the brain.

Follow-up care : The radioisotope is eliminated in the urine.

EMG—Electromyography

Electromyography records the electrical activity of peripheral nerves by testing muscle activity. EMG usually helps in the diagnosis of neuron and peripheral nerve disorders.

Preparation—Inform patient. EMG may cause temporary discomfort–specially patient is subjected to episodes of electrical current–pretest serum muscle enzyme determination with post-test levels 7–10 days after EMG–mild sedation is ordered.

Procedure—The test may be performed at the bedside–nerve conduction studies are done–it is usually tested first. Flat electrodes to the nerve and muscle innervated are used. If nerve conduction is accomplished– the muscle contracts.

For testing muscle potential, multiple needle electrodes varying from ½ -3" inserted. The patient may be asked to perform activities for measurement of muscle potential during minimal and maximal contraction. The degree of nerve and muscle activity is recorded on an *oscilloscope*, which provides the graphic readout for later interpretation.

Follow-up— a few medical complications are associated with EMG. The nurse provides comfort measures and inspects the needle sites for hematoma formation. Apply ice to prevent this complication. Patient may feel increased pain and anxiety after test.

ENG—Caloric Test or Electronystamography

Tests vestibular function. In caloric testing, the examiner instills cold water into the ear canals to elicit nystogmus. For this test electrodes placed near the eyes transmit eye movements, which are recorded on graph paper. The two tests can be done separately or together.

Preparation—Withhold food and fluids 6-8 hours before the caloric test in order to lessen vomiting. (ENG there are no such restrictions). The caloric test– the tympanic membranes must be intact with no perforations. Remove any make-up around the eyes.

Procedure—Patient positioned in a chair with a head titled forward 30 degree. Patient to maintain eye contact with a certain object, which enables examiner to observe eye movement during the test.

For caloric test—The examiner irrigates one ear with cold water, 7°C/144.6°F, below body temperature for 30 seconds. The normal result is slow movement of the eyes towards the side of irrigation followed by fast movement to the opposite side. After 5 minutes ear is irrigated with warm water, 7°C above body temperature. The normal results nystamus to the irrigated side. Same way done to the other ear. Instillation of fluids may cause nausea, vertigo, vomiting. Cerebellar assessment that is finger-to-nose touch or the Romberg test. Abnormal findings of no nystamus or nystamus in directions other than normal are elicited in meniere's disease, coma, certain brain tumors and pathogenic states of the brainstem.

For ENG, the patient is recumbent– electrodes are secured to the skin near the eyes and then attached to a machine that records the eye movements graphically. Patient must keep his eyes closed during the entire test and asked to change positions at various intervals. The examiner may instill a small amount of cold or warm water 2 ml into the ear canal as a stimulus.

Follow-up – for the caloric test, the patient is restricted to bed rest until abatement of any nausea or vertigo, ENG requires fly care.

Oculoplethysmography

It studies carotid artery blood flow by monitoring one of its branches– the ophthalmic artery. The systolic pressure of each this artery is measured by raising the intraocular pressure above systolic artery pressure. Instilled anesthetic eye drops, place suction cups that resemble contact lenses on the cornea, and applies pressure. The pressure is then released. The reappear range of pulsation is measured as the systolic pressure. The eyes are compared for circulatory assessment, check for corneal abrasion after the procedure.

Cerebral Blood Flow Determination

Withhold CNS depressant and stimulants, make sure hair is clean and hairpins removed. The technician attaches sensors/probes connected to a computer to the scalp. Radioactive isotope injected IV or inhales radioactive gas through a mouthpiece. The patient receives various stimulants during the test. Increases in local blood flow can be seen with any neuronal activity, such as reading, hand movement, seizures and temperature evaluation. Local blood flow decreases with degenerative disease, comas of metabolic origin increase ICP and subarachnoid.

Brain Scan

It is a radionuclide imaging study-dye is injected to detect certain pathologic conditions. Test useful for evaluating vascular abnormalities, locating tumors, hematoma, and abscesses.

The dye is injected—there is a delay in the test up to 2 hrs while isotope is absorbed by the brain. Patient remains still on table. Test takes 1–2 hrs, depending on the number of scanning used.

Carotid Phonoangiography and Carotid Doppler Flow Analysis

Tests determine narrowing/occlusion of the carotid arteries. The lumen size of the carotid arteries can be measured through the use of amplified sound, which is then converted to a graphic picture. An electronic microphone is placed over patients carotid arteries a direct canal Doppler probe is used in the flow analysis.

Arthroscopy

It is a tube inserted into a joint for direct visualization, the knee and shoulder are most commonly tested. Moreover, synovial biopsy and surgical procedures to repair traumatic injury can be accomplished with arthroscope.

ROM—Range of motion exercises are taught.

Procedure—Patient given light general epidural of spinal anesthesia. In some hospitals, a large pneumatic tourniquet is used around the thigh to minimize bleeding during the procedure. Knee is flexed to 40 degree and saline/RL used to irrigate the knee. Arthroscope is inserted through a small incision 0.6 cm long. Multiple incision may be required for variety of angles. After procedure elastic bandage is required. Encourage exercise taught before examination. For increased joint pain, thrombophlebitis, infection, severe joint or leg pain contact physician.

Bone Scan

It is a radionuclide test – dye injected for visualization of the entire skeleton. Used to detect – tumors, arthritis, osteomylitis, osteoporosis, vertebral compressions, unexplained bone pain.

Patient placed on the scanning table—for accurate image patient must be able to lie still 30-60 minutes during scanning, elderly, restless patient is given mild sedation. The examiner looks for areas of bone in which there is an increased uptake or concentration of isotope. These hot lesions indicate abnormal bone metabolism, a sign of bone disease, cold lesions in which there is a decreased uptake, indicate poor blood flow to bone—as in severe arteriosclerosis. The substance excreted in urine, stool.

HBO—Hyperbaric Oxygen Treatments

It is the administration of oxygen at greater than atmospheric pressure. Oxygen is greatly increased in the tissues and neovascularizations– fibroblast activity, collagen synthesis and phagocytes are increased to speed wound healing.

An air-flotation—Low air loss support surface that provides pressure relief used in care of patients who are at high risk for skin breakdown. A fluid air bed- these beds feel like waterbeds but are composed of air-fluidized silicone beds. Used in care of patients who cannot tolerate turning nor have only one turning surface.

Cerebral Angiography—(Arteriography)

Illuminates the cerebral circulation. Contrast medium is injected into an artery usually the femoral and X-rays are taken sequentially as the contrast medium flows with the blood for visualizing carotid, vertebral and cerebral circulation. The test is used for diagnosis of vascular aneurysms, malformations, displacements and, occluded or leaking blood vessels.

Contrast Media Method

Client preparation— The nurse ascertains that the patient has no allergies to iodine. Written consent to be obtained, it is necessary to immobilize the head of the patient. The expectation of burning or heat sensation, which lasts just a few seconds and is often noted behind eyes or in the face. Patient is told to keep 6 to 8 hrs nil by mouth before the test. Remove patients hairpins, jewelery, hearing aids, and dentures. Records vitals, empty bladder – administer the pre-angiography hypnotic, sedative or analgesic as ordered by physician.

Procedure

The patient is placed within a headrest device or immobilized with tape. The radiologist locates the artery to be used cut and inserts a catheter into a artery–patency of the catheter is maintained with IV fluid–injects 40-50 ml contrast medium and X-rays are automatically taken – after the catheter is removed, pressure is maintained over the puncture site for 5 minutes to prevent arterial bleeding. Follow-up care — patient restricted to bed rest for 6 to 24 hours. The extremity into which the contrast medium was injected is kept straight and immobilized for approximately the length of the bed rest. The nurse checks the extremity for adequate circulation, which is demonstrated by *skin color* and temperature, pulses distal to the *injection site, capillary refill.*

A pressure dressing, sandbag, ice bag or maintained 6-12 hours to prevent bleeding swelling or hematoma formation.

Digital Subtraction Angiography (DSA)

It is used to evaluate the carotid and other cerebral arteries–food taken is restricted for 2 hrs before the test, but fluids are not.

Procedure—Because DSA is done through the IV route, it has the advantage of causing less risk of bleeding or spasm. DSA is OPD procedure. The radiologist threads a large angiocatheter into the brachial vein and position it in the superior vena cava near the right atrium. IV fluid is given via catheter. An initial X-ray is taken, the image is placed in a computer to be used as a reference for the subsequent images. The radiologist then injects the contrast medium. As subsequent images appear on a screen and are transferred to the computer, the original reference image is subtracted from the later images. This produces a heightened image.

Myelography

To perform myelography a contrast medium, or dye, is inserted into the subarachnoid space of the spine. A lumbar puncture is the usual insertion site. Myelography enables the vertebral column, intervertebral disks, spinal nerve roots, and blood vessels to be visualized. Now CT and MRI is popular and replace this diagnostic techniques.

Client preparation—Increase oral and IV fluids and liquid breakfast on the day of test. Adequate hydration. Promotes the manufacture of CSF, prevents dehydration, which could result from post-test vomiting. Increases the rate at which the water-soluble contrast medium is used–is excreted by the kidneys.

CNS depressants and stimulants are not administered for 48 hours before the myelogram. They decrease the seizure threshold and thus increase the risk of a seizure. Take history of allergies to iodine, seafood, renal, liver dysfunction. Most of the media are iodine based and may cause allergic reactions ranging from rashes to anaphylaxis. Metabolism and excretion of the water soluble contrast medium depend on proper functioning of the liver and kidneys.

Health education before and after procedure is important patient may fear discomfort or possible paralysis from having a needle inserted close to the spinal cord.

Procedure—Special procedure room in the radiology department or in OT and patient is carefully monitored. Three types of contrast media are available. Iophendylate metrizamide is water based iodine solution. A prone position with a pillow under the abdomen, a sitting position flexed at the waist, a side–lying, knee-chest position. After that physician inserts a large-gauge spinal needle into III rd or IV the lumbar interspace. Approximately 6-15 ml of CSF is removed to allow room for the contrast medium. Physician then slowly injects contrast medium equal to amount of CSF removed while observing for allergic reaction. By fluoroscopy the cervical and thoracic regions are visualized. Serial radiographs are taken during this procedure, patient is not allowed to move so as not to dislodge needle and must maintain neck hyperextension to the solution from entering the cranium. If Iophendylate is used, solution is withdrawn after the films are obtained. As a water soluble medium, metrizamide mixes with the CSF and cannot be removed.

Follow-up—For preventing leakage of CSF place patient flat in supine position for at least 8 hours. To prevent the contrast medium from ascending into the brain, patient who received metrizamide is placed in a sitting position at a 15 to 45 degree angle for 8-16 hours. This may be followed by an 8 hrs in flat lying position. Patient neurologic status monitored for 24 hrs after myelography. Assess vital signs at frequent intervals, patient's ability to move the lower extremities, unusual sensation, such as tingling in the feet and legs, complains of radiating pain and discomfort in the lower back or extremities, changes in motor or sensory status, inspect injection site for leakage of blood or hematoma formation is reported immediately. A large loss of fluid can result in a spinal headache, causing severe pain often not relieved by medication. If headache lasts for a week or more, a 'blood patch' performed in which 10 ml patients blood inserted into the injection site for clotting and sealing the leak, not common, is performed by anesthesiologist.

Nausea with vomiting common 3-8 hrs after the test 20-25% undergone myelography have at least one complication–observe carefully then can be treated and possibly reversed.

CT Scanning: Computed Tomography

CT Scanning has been a significant tool in advancing neurological diagnose with the aid of computer, pictures are taken at many horizontal levels, or slice of the brain or spinal cord. A contrast medium may be used to enhance the image. CT scans distinguish bone and soft tissue such as brain, the vascular system and the ventricular system. Tumors, infarctions hemorrhage, hydrocephalus, and bone malformation can be identified.

Patient Preparation—Explain procedure, instruct patient to remove hair-pins, hair pieces or wigs. If contrast medium is used, food is withheld for 4-6 hours before the test. Note patient unduly anxious, fearful or unable to cooperate.

Procedure—The patient is placed on a movable table. The patient's head in a holding device, which is then secured. The angles for the desired pictures are determined by the X-ray technician. The patient must be completely still during the test which may be difficult. The table is then positioned within the machine, a large cylinder type structure. Some patients are fearful of the machine or of being confined in a small space. A non-contrast series of pictures taken first. Contrast media enhance the visualization of the vascular system and are frequently used. Except for the IV injection of contrast media, the procedure is noninvasive. The entire procedure takes 10 minutes or less with the newer machines and 40 minutes with older machines or the use of contrast media. Flu observe delay allergic response.

What is the ultravist in CT—Progress in X-ray diagnostic has also been archived by the introduction of safer contrast media. It fulfills all requirements for a modern diagnostic agent like client comfort, very good safety profile as well as an excellent imaging quality. Monomeric X-ray contrast with low osmolality reduces the risk of adverse reactions such as pain or heat sensation. It has high tolerance for the client as well as its reliability and easy usage for the radiologist and cardiologist doctor. With low viscosity, it allows good contrast enhancement and facilitates rapid administration of large volumes and high concentrations. Due to minimal histamine, release side effects such as urticaria and anaphylactic reactions are less likely to occur. This reduces the potential for toxicity and minimizing the retention of ultravist within the body when used in CT (computed tomography) procedures thus improves diagnostic efficacy. Good image quality in CT; and its minimal disturbance of the blood brain barrier make it a convenient contrast medium for cranial CT, thoracic and abdominal CT. It facilitates the rapid delivery of high concentration of the site of investigation.

CHAPTER 4

Medical Nursing

Medical nursing is a vast subject. Therefore revision of the most important points that every nurse must know while she is dealing with patients with their precious lives.

What is a Celiac Disease?

Celiac disease is an immune to gluten causing impaired absorption and digestion of nutrients through the small bowel. Affect adult and children and characterized by inability to digest and use sugar, starches and fats (Gluten free diet).

What are Esophageal Varices?

It is a life threatening hemorrhage from torturous dilated, thin walled veins in submucosa of lower esophagus.

What is a Diaphragmatic Hiatal Hernia?

It is a protrusion of part of stomach through diaphragm and into thoracic cavity (rolling).

What is a Gastroesophageal Reflux Disease?

It is an inappropriate relaxation of the lower esophageal sphincter in response to unknown stimulus.

What is a Dumping Syndrome?

It is a hypoglycemic type — episodes occurs postoperatively after gastric resection, when food and fluid that are more hyperosmolar than the jejunal secretions–pass quickly into jejunum, producing fluid shifts from blood stream to jejunum, discomfort may occur during a meal or 30 minutes after meal and lasts 20–60 minutes. The reaction is greatest after the ingestion of sugar.

What is Total Parenteral Nutrition [TPN]?

Provides nutrition through a central venous line to patients who are in a catabolic state, malnourished and cannot tolerate food by mouth is in negative nitrogen balance.

What is Nonketotic Hyperglycemic Hyperosmolar Coma?

It is seen in non-insulin dependent diabetes, brought by infection or illness. This condition may lead to impaired consciousness and seizures, critically ill.

What is Diverticulosis?

It is a small pouch/sac composed of mucous membrane that has produced through the muscular wall of the intestine, specially sigmoid colon.

What is Crohn's Disease?

It is a chronic inflammatory disease causing ulceration in the small and large intestines – Crohn's colitis, when only large intestine–Crohn's enteritis, terminal ileitis – lower part of small intestine called inflammation bowed disease.

What is Lithotripsy?

It is an extracorporeal shock wave used to break up renal calculi.

What is Aphasia?

It is an impaired ability to understand or use commonly accepted words or symbols interferes with ability to speak, write or read; articulate words.

What is Meniereis Disease?

It is a chronic recurrent disorders of inner ear–attacks of vertigo, tinnitus and vestibular dysfunctions lasts for 30 minutes to full day, no pain or loss of consciousness.

What is Otosclerosis?

It is a disease of the bone of optic capsule, insidious, progressive deafness.

What is Stapedectomy?

It is removal of the stapes and replacing it with a prosthesis; steel wire, teflon piston or polyethylene, treatment for deafness due to otosclerosis, which fixes the stapes, preventing it from oscillating and transmitting vibrations to the fluids in the inner ear.

What is Glaucoma?

It is an increased intraocular pressure.

What are Transient Ischemic Attacks/TIAS?

It is a temporary complete or relatively complete cessation of cerebral blood flow to a localize area of brain producing symptoms – carotid endarterectomy – cranial nerve damage, causes vocal cord paralysis or difficulty managing saliva and tongue deviation.

What is an Ischemic Stroke?

It is a brain lesion resulting from damage to blood vessels supplying brain.

What is Compartment Syndrome?

It is an accumulation of fluid in the muscle compartment, resulting in an increase in pressure that reduces blood flow to the tissues – can lead to neuromuscular deficit, amputation and death.

What is Herniated/Ruptured Disk?

It is a strain or injury to a weakened cartilage between vertebrae can result in this causing pressure on nerve roots in spinal canal, pain and disability.

What is Spinal Shock?

It is a temporary flaccid paralysis and are flexia following a severe injury to the spinal cord.

What is Autonomic Dysreflexia?

It is a group of symptoms in which many spinal cord autonomic responses are activated simultaneously. This may occur when cord lesions are above the 6th thoracic vertebra; it is most commonly seen with cervical and high thoracic cord injuries may occur up to 6 years after injury.

Cushing's disease is an endogenous overproduction of adrenocorticotropic hormone that can caused by pituitary hyperpigmentation.

Adrenalectomy is a surgical removal of adrenal glands because of tumors, also bilateral adrenalectomy performed to control metastatic breast/prostate steroid therapy given.

Addison's disease is a hormonal endocrine disorder destruction of adrenal gland unable to produce adrenal hormone / cortisol necessary for normal body function.

Multiple sclerosis: Neurological disease – brain and spinal cord leading to be generative neurological function (visual problem, weak extremities).

Cystic fibrosis is a generalized dysfunction of the exocrine glands that produces multi system involvement. Although the disorder is inherited as an Autosomal recessive defect, its probable cause is an alteration in a protein or an enzyme e.g. pancreatic enzyme deficiency. The basic problem is one of thick sticky tenacious mucous secretions that obstruct the ducts of exocrine gland.

Down syndrome is a chromosomal abnormality involving an extra chromosome 47 chromosome. As consequences the child usually has varying degree of mental retardation, characteristic facial and physical features and other congenital abnormalities. (Small round head).

Reye syndrome is a multi system disorder primarily affecting children between 6-12 years of age. It is Characterized by acute metabolic encephalopathy and fatty degeneration of the visceral organs, particularly liver. Earlier diagnosis by more sophisticated monitoring equipment and more aggressive treatment have improved survival rate in children elevating ALT, SGOT, SGPT, hypoglycemia bleeding.

Autoimmune disorders are streptococcus infection/sequelae – cause illness in children and is highly contagious, e.g. step throat, otitis impetigo, scarlet fever, carditis, rheumatic fever, acute glomerulonephritis.

Apnea of infancy is the unexplained cessation of breathing for 20 sec or long. Bradycardia, acute post-streptococcal glomeneloneph is a bilateral infection of the glomeruli of kidney, common noninfection renal disease of childhood.

Kawasaki disease is a mucocutaneous lymph node syndrome – affecting skin, mucus membrane of respiratory tract, lymph nodes and heart – children.

Hirschsprung's disease is a congenital ganglionic Negacolon of lower GI tract, absence of peristalsis noted with Down's syndrome.

Wilms tumor-nephroblastoma – a malignant tumor of the kidney – common renal cancer in children – nephrectomy and adrenalectomy followed by chemotherapy and radiation.

Febrile seizures are transient neurological disorder of childhood.

What is Cleft Lip and Cleft Palate?

These are congenital facial malformations resulting from faulty embryonic development. Mutant genes chromosomal abnormalities treatogenic agents.

What is Hypospadias?

It is a congenital anatomical defect of the male genito urinary tract, defected at birth. Urethral opening is located on the ventral surface of the penile shaft. This makes voiding in the standing position virtually impossible.

Epiglottis is a swelling in the throat that can lead to total airway obstruction if not treated promptly.

Constipation is considered the classic sign of Hirschsprung's disease.

Sypipecac is cardio toxic – is an emetic.

What is Neutrogena?

It is an abnormal decrease in the number of neutrophils (the specific type of WBC) responsible for phagocytosis and bacterial destruction in patient of leukemia.

Patient who receives digoxin and lasix develop hypokalemia.

When there is an Injury to the *head* of the frontal lobe of the *brain* the nurse needs to keep instructions simple and brief because the patient will have difficulty concentrating. Orient the patient to the person, place and time because of memory problem arises. Due to the damage to the *frontal lobe* it affects personality, memory, reasoning, concentration and motor control of speech. Disorientation and restlessness in level of consciousness is the first sign indicative of early increasing *intracranial pressure (ICP)* in most critical injuries. Patient knows what he wants to say but cannot verbalize the appropriate word that is known as *"Expressive aphasia"*. Nurse should show the pictures of common objects and needs to give him an opportunity to indicate what he would like.

Pressure on the heel and Achilles tendon could lead to nerve injury and foot drop. It is important that the appliance be set up to avoid complications. During *rheumatic fever* provide rest to prevent cardiac complications. Osteoarthritis affects the hips and knees because they are weight bearing and undergo the most stress. Steroids reduce inflammation of joint in arthritis. Bony ankylosis of the joints is irreversible and causes immobility. Rheumatoid arthritic patient has pain, tingling in the morning on awakening. Regular diet with vitamins and minerals; medicine Aspirin 0.6 gm qut; Encourage motion of the joint within limits of pain, Heat and cold application reduce infection and discomfort. Diet; a variety of meals, fruits, vegetables, milk, cereal grains. Required total hip replacement; do manual stretching exercise during break to avoid carpal tunnel syndrome.

When suctioning a patient with a *tracheotomy* tube assemble the proper equipment, to decrease patient's anxiety and increase trust in procedure.

When the Neonates born with *esophageal artesia* there is a sign of fluid from the blind pouch is aspirated into the trachea, causing cyanosis, coughing and choking.

In early signs of *asthma* there is a respiratory distress increased pulse rate, and a decrease in oxygen content of the blood.

Sore throat, fever and sudden onset of other flu like symptoms are sings of *agranulocytosis*, the condition is caused by lack of sufficient number of granulocytes a type of WBC, which causes the individual to be susceptible to infection. Thus such Patients WBC weekly to count throughout the treatment.

Patient with Emphysema

Needs the nurse to teach diaphragmatic pursed-lip breathing. Administer low flow oxygen. Encourage alternating activity with rest periods. Teach use of postural drainage and chest physiotherapy. In Pulmonary embolism is a potentially life threatening complication of deep vein thrombosis.

In Detached Retina

Nurse should approach the patient from unaffected side. Discourage bending down, deep breathing, hard coughing and sneezing that can increase intraocular pressure. Orient the patient. to the environment to reduce the risk of injury. Administer a stool softener to avoid straining during defecation. Lie on unaffected side or on back.

Hyperthyroidism

The conjunctivae should be moistened often with isotonic eye drops. Provide several small, well-balanced meals. Provide rest periods. Weigh the patient daily because metabolism is increased, heat intolerance and excitability result. Therefore, provide a cool and quit environment to promote patient comfort.

Hiatus Hernia

Abdominal pain and sternal pain after eating. Pain makes him difficult to sleep. Avoid constrictive clothing. Decrease intake of caffeine and spicy foods. Remain upright two hours after eating, to reduce gastric reflux, instructs the patient to sleep with his upper body elevated. Sleep in semi-fowler's position, and maintain a normal body weight.

Tumors of the Pituitary Gland

Take daily weight. Assess urine specific gravity. Monitor intake and output. Tumors can lead to diabetes insipidus due to deficiency of ADH which reduces the ability of the kidney to concentrate urine, resulting in excessive urination, thirst.

Reproductive System

LH is released by the anterior pituitary, simulating ovulation and the development of the corpus luteum preparing the endometrium for implant Fertilized ovum. With bilateral salpingo-oophorectomy for uterine cancer, allow patient. to verbalize her feelings. Assess for hemorrhage, infection, and thrombophebitis, May be given hormone replacement therapy (HRT).

Why Foly Catheter?

It will allow you to heal by keeping your bladder decompressed. An expanded bladder may interfere with wound healing by pressing on the wound. Catheter is usually removed when patient begins ambulating.

What is Cystic Fibrosis?

It is the most common inherited disease in children; it is inherited as Autosomal recessive trait, meaning that the child inherits the defective gene from both parents. The chances are one in four for each of the couple pregnancies.

With a hypertonic uterus, the placenta is not well perfused between contractions and the fetus is subjected to increasing periods of hypoxia, prepare for *cesarean section*. One of the earliest *maternal role* tasks is to accept the biologic fact of pregnancy and to incorporate the idea of a child into her body image.

Gonorrhea

Men complain of urethritis and epididymitis, women are frequently asymptomatic, diagnosed by culture of discharge from cervix or urethra. Treatment is ceftriaxone IM and doxycycline for seven days by mouth. Instruct patient how to prevent STD. Gonorrhea causes PID, which is one of the most common causes of sterility, it is treated with antibiotics. *STDs* are communicable diseases that must be reported, to the appropriate public health agency and maintain patients confidentiality.

Spermatogenesis occurs at the time of puberty. The testes are suspended in the scrotum to protect the sperm from high abdominal temperature, sperm cells are very fragile and can be destroyed by heat, resulting insterility.

Term condylomata acuminate refers to venereal warts. Syphilis treated with penicillin. Gonorrhea can produce sterility–Salpingitis result of gonorrhea.*Trichomonas vaginalis* is a protozoan that favors an alkaline environment.

When decreased blood supply occurs can result in gangrene and irreversible damage occurs after several hours. Syphilis incubation is about 3 – 6 weeks, clinical symptom appear 9 day or 3 months after exposure. The tertiary stage is noncontiguous. Gonorrhea is highly contagious getting sexual intercourse – Doxycycline with ceftriaxone specific – cures the infection.

Cervical Cancer

Patient who has poor appetite.—Provide small, frequent feedings.

Radioactive Cobalt Implantation

Patient on bed rest while implant is in place. Visitors should limited; less time spent in the patient's room, do not stand close or in line with radioactive source. Patient will have indwelling *Foley catheters* and tap water enema to prevent displacement of the implant. If the bladder or the bowel is distended, the chance that the *implant* will be dislodged is increased, keeping the bladder from overfilling decreases the chance of implant displacement, a Foley catheter will remain in place and the patient will be kept on a low residue diet, it is important to remember to decrease the time and increase the distance when dealing with a patient with a radium implant, rotating the staff members will prevent excessive harmful *exposure to radiation*. Radioactive implant *interferes* with ovarian function, which stops the menstrual cycle.

Heavy menstrual flow patient that needs extra iron—eat chicken liver which is an excellent concentration source of iron 12-15 mg/day.

BBT Method

At the time of ovulation, the basal body temperature increases about 1 to 2, this slight rise is important for patients who rely on methods of childbirth planning that depend upon knowledge of the ovulation.

Infertility

It is inability to conceive after at least one year of unprotected intercourse.

In a regulate *menstrual cycle* of 28 days, the time of ovulation is usually around the *14th day*, if the patient has intercourse 2 or 3 days before this time or 2-3 days after, it is possible that she will become pregnant, since the sperm live for 48 hours.

The use of *mild analgesics*, restriction of caffeine, and moderate exercise have all been shown to be effective in relief of the weight gain, irritability and muscle cramping of a menstrual period.

Diaphragm Birth Control Method

It is necessary to remain in place for at least 6 hours to be effective in preventing pregnancy, can be inserted up to 6 hours prior to intercourse, but spermicide must be inserted into vagina with every intercourse.

The Billing Method

It is also called cervical mucus/ovulation method depends on the characteristics changes in the cervical mucus.

Pap Smear

It is a specimen of cells used to identity abnormal cells, and hormonal changes. A routine procedure to identify infectious processes.

Colposcopy

Is to visualize the bladder. Examination of vagina and cervix using a colposcope, identifies precancerous lesions of the cervix by magnifying tissue for examination, instruct patient that some bleeding may occur, can use vaginal tampons, patient should report heavy bleeding.

Fibrocystic Disease of the Breast

It involves benign cysts of the breast, present as soft, tender, freely moving cyst that become enlarged during menstruation.

In a modified radical *Mastectomy*, the breast, axillary nodes, and superior apical nodes are removed, but the major and minor pectoral muscles are preserved. Postoperatively, encourage prescribed exercises and elevation of the extremity on the affected side to prevent *lymphedema*.

Breast Biopsy

Legation of an artery or vein is the greatest risk; *observe for bleeding* and pallor, cold, clammy skin, increase pulse, decreases blood pressure.

Vulvectomy

Patient to take size bath and keep the area clean and dry, both of these measures can be done to increase circulation to a vascular region such as the vulva, helping to promote healing.

Increase body temperature resulting from occupations or infections can contribute to *low sperm* counts caused by decreased sperm production. Heat can destroy sperm. Varicocele an abnormal dilatation of the veins in the spermatic cord is as associated cause for low sperm count. The varicosity increases the temperature within the testes, inhibiting sperm production. Frequent hot tubs may lead to a low sperm count. The temperature of the scrotum becomes elevated, possible inhibiting sperm production. Endocrine imbalance.

Childbearing – Antenatal Care

It is during the first trimester, or the first three months, that all the major systems of the fetus are developed, exposure of mother to noxious environment agents can interfere with proper development of fetus.

Additional nutrients required during pregnancy- two eggs and 8 oz of milk contains protein, calcium and calories, + 300 calories second and third trimester.

More calories but the same amount of protein, calcium and fluids are needed during *lactation*.

Fifth month auscultating fetal heart tones, visualization of the fetus by ultrasound /Doppler or x-ray, or fetal movement palpated by the examiner are all positive signs of pregnancy.

The advantages of breast-feeding include the nutrients are easier for the infant to absorb, it contains immune factors, it provides protection against allergies, and antibody responses to parenteral and oral vaccines are greater.

She should *exercise during pregnancy* at least three times per week, most important to determine regular exercise regimen before recommending and exercise program.

Warning signs of pregnancy swelling of face or fingers may indicate hypertensive condition, other danger signs include gush of fluid or bleeding from vagina, regular uterine contraction, severe headaches, visual disturbances, abdominal pain, persistent vomiting, fever or chills. Prenatal/antepartum teaching- *chills and fever* indicate infection, report immediately to the health care provider.

Toxoplasmosis/protozoan infection caused by eating infected uncooked meat or after handling infected kitty litter, infection can cross placenta and infect the fetus, pregnant woman should not clean animals and if she must, wear latex gloves and wash hands well afterward.

Fetal movement remains unchanged during *true labor*.

14-lb/pounds weight gain during first 5 months of pregnancy is appropriate. Eat frequent small meal. Discourage overeating large meals and gas-producing or fatty foods.

Breasts at 5th month are sensitive and sore apply cold compresses and wear a well-fitting supportive bra. *Breast soreness* due to hormonal changes.

Progesterone increases smooth muscle relaxation, thereby decreasing peristalsis. This slowed movement of contents through the GI system can lead to firmer stools and constipation.

BPP- biophysical profile is an ultrasound assessment of fetus well-being that includes fetal tone, fetal breathing movements and amniotic fluid volume.

In early pregnancy, amniocentesis can identify chromosomal defects and neural tube defects, sex of the fetus. It can be used to evaluate fetal lung maturity during last trimester.

Abruptio placenta—Evaluate vital sings, fetal heart tones, vaginal bleeding, intake and output, prompt cesarean delivery indicated if the fetus is in distress.

Hyperemesis gravidarum differs from the nausea and vomiting that normally occur during pregnancy. It is characterized by excessive vomiting that can lead to dehydration and starvation. Without treatment, metabolic changes can lead to severe complications, even death of the fetus or mother.

Headache, blurred vision, epigastric pain and severe nausea and vomiting can indicate worsening maternal disease.

Premature rupture membranes/PROM –fernlike pattern when vaginal fluid is placed on a glass slide and allowed to dry. Presence of amniotic fluid in the vagina, alkaline pH of fluid when tested with nitrazine paper.

Variable decelerations are transient drops in the fetal heart rate that can occur before, during or after a contraction. The *left lateral position* is the ideal position for any pregnant patient, as it prevents maternal hypotension caused by inferior vena cava compression which reduces placenta perfusion.

29 weeks pregnant having contractions every 8 minutes and is 3 cm dilated, administer terbutaline/brethine, betamethasone, IV fluids.

Adverse reactions to Oxytocin in the mother include hypertension, fluid overload and uterine tetany.

Early deceleration is a decrease in the FHR below the baseline. It result from head compression during normal labor and do not include fetal distress.

Glucose monitoring of the infant born to a mother with diabetes is essential because he is at risk for developing hypoglycemia after birth.

Mastitis is an infection frequently associated with break in the skin surface of the nipple, measures to prevent cracked and fissured, wash the nipples with soap and water, expose the nipple to the air for part of each day, wash hands before handling the breast and breast feeding, release the baby's grasp on the nipple before removing the baby from the breast.

Taking-in- phase is a normal first phase for a mother when she is feeling overwhelmed by the responsibilities of newborn care, while still fatigued from delivery. Taking hold is the next phase, when the mother has rested and she can think and learn mothering skills with confidence.

Taking cooing and cuddling with her son are positive signs that the mother is adapting to her new role as mother.

A postpartum woman should be suspected psychosis if she exhibits symptoms include delusions and hallucinations, the disorder rarely occurs without psychiatric history.

Sudden dyspnea with diaphoresis and confusion are classic signs and symptoms of dislodgment of a thrombus from a varicose vein becoming an embolus that loges itself into the pulmonary circulation.

Labor and Delivery

Membrane rupture—Serves for a prolapsed cord or meconium stained fluid, signs of possible life-threatening complications to the fetus that may require emergency delivery. No dry labor-because amniotic fluid does not function as lubrication for the labor process, helps maintain constant body temperature, provides oral fluids, cushions fetus.

Monitor fetal heart rate patterns to assure that the fetus is receiving adequate amounts of oxygen during labor.

Monitor for maternal complications that is changes in blood pressure and pulse elevated indicate hemorrhage.

Late decelerations—Fall in fetal heart rate after the peak of the contraction indicates fetal hypoxia, position patient on her left side, administer oxygen by mask, start IV or increase flow rate, stop oxytocin if appropriate.

The FHR slowing *Early fetal deceleration* occurs when the FHR falls below baseline for 15 seconds or more followed by a return, early deceleration occurs before the peak of the contraction and is a reassuring fetal heart pattern. Which is a normal finding?

Bradycardia below 60 beats/minutes indicates fetal distress; persistent Bradycardia may indicate cord compression or separation of placenta.

Active labor coach the patient in proper breathing and relaxation techniques, assist patient to cope with transition phase of labor, stay with patient, provide constant reassurance, help patient to reestablish breathing patterns, provide comfort.

8 cm dilatation encourage patient to *pant with pursed lips* to prevent pushing.

The opening of the cervix is 4 cm wide and the cervical canal is 60% shorter than normal. *Dilatation* is stretching of the external is from an opening a few mm in size to an opening large enough to allow the passage of the infant that is 0-10 cm, effacement is the thinning and shortening or literation of the cervix, occurs in late pregnancy or during labor.

From the beginning of labor until the cervix is completely dilated is the *first stage*, divided into phase 1 (latent 0-3 cm) phase 2 (active, 4-7 cm) phase 3 (transition, 8-10 cm).

Correct technique of *palpation uterine* contractions-place one hand on the abdomen over the fundus and, with the fingertips press gently.

Immediately after delivery *Oxytocin* purpose is to allow firm contraction of the uterus, stimulate smooth muscles of uterus to contract– used to treat postpartum.

The standard measurement for *uterine contractions* is from the beginning of one contraction to the beginning of the next contraction.

A short period of pace and an increase in blood show occur immediately before the baby is born at the beginning of the *second stage of labor.*

Third stage of labour fundus should be firm and globular and should rise.

After *normal vaginal* delivery check the lochial flow, directly check for hemorrhage.

Postpartum

Seventeen year old who delivered her age may interfere with positive mothering because the patient is still experiencing the dependency of childhood. The egocentric and concrete thinking of an adolescent may interfere with her ability to parent, adolescent may have unmet developmental needs and tasks that become as issue as she leaves the dependency of childhood and moves toward being an independent young adult.

Twelve hours after delivery, chart the results in the patient's chart, the fundus is about 1cm above the umbilicus within 12 hours of the birth, after this time, should descend 1-2 cm each day.

The *lochia pooled in the patient's vagina* when she lying in bed. Flow of lochia increases during ambulation and breastfeeding.

Twenty four hours after delivery, patient voiding large amounts of urine-*Diaphoresis* occurs for first 2-3 days postpartum in order to decrease the retained fluids from the pregnancy.

Notify the physician- *excessive bleeding indicates* perineal pad soaked, administer oxygen, tilt woman on side, elevate legs to at least 30, start IV with lactated Ringers or normal saline.

Severely *sore nipples* due to poor *infant positioning* or incorrect latch-on, make sure that baby is positioned at the level of the breast and the baby's mouth is directly in front of the nipple, asses the position of the infant during feeding.

The Neonate

Mothers drink *alcohol* has a CNS depressant effect on the baby.

Delivery room drops in *newborn's eyes* protect against infections that could lead to blindness, instill erythromycin or tetracycline.

Moros startle reflex, disappears at 3-4 months.

Newborn circumcision-observe for bleeding hourly during the first 12 hours, observe that infant is voiding, wash penis gently with water and apply petroleum around gland, yellow exudates should not be removed.

Care of cord- clean cord and surrounding area with alcohol or erythromycin solution, report redness, drainage, or foul odor.

Neonate can loose up to *10% of birth weight* due to low levels of intake and excretion of fluid through lungs, bladder and bowels, should regain weight by 10-14 days old.

First stool passed is meconium. It is passed in the first 24-48 hours of life. It usual appearance is green and sticky.

The infant has regained the initial weight loss; well-hydrated infants should have *6-8 wet diapers* per day, record results in the patient's record.

Two days old infant—shows tendency to bleed—cause is an absence of intestinal bacteria needed for the production of vitamin K. Newborn given vitamin K at birth, able to produce it by day 8.

Posterior fontanel: Triangular in shape, 0.5-1cm, it normally closes by the eighth to twelfth week.

Apical pulse on a 8lb, 4oz –place the bell of the stethoscope between the 2nd and 3rd intercostal spaces, the midclavicular line.

Change that takes place in the newborn circulation system after birth—The infant begins pulmonary ventilation. Lung inflation causes pressure in right atrium to decline, pressure is increased in the left atrium and the foramen ovale closes, ductus arteriosus occludes and becomes a ligament.

The baby's anterior *fontanel should close* after about a year and a half that is 18 months.

Childbearing – Maternal Complications

Due to hormonal interference in glucose metabolism, *insulin requirements* increase during pregnancy, however, immediately after delivery, the requirements usually decrease.

Lower level of narcotic given to prevent respiratory depression in the infant and drowsiness at birth, reversal of narcotics can be achieved by administering Naecan to the mother 15 minutes before delivery.

During labor induction with *oxytocin–stop* infusion if contraction occur at 2 min intervals and last more than 90 seconds.

After *cesarean section* monitor for hemorrhage and shock, incisional dressing, airway, amount of lochia.

Gestational diabetes diet- cheese and fresh fruit.

Painless vaginal bleeding indicates *placenta previa*, placenta abnormally implanted in the lower uterine segment; patient will be treated with bed rest. Immediate cesarean section will be done if patient is at term and in labor or bleeding persistently.

Meconium-stained amniotic fluid alert the possibility of fetal distress and hyperbilirubinemia possibly indicates hypoxia induced peristalsis and sphincter relaxation.

Gestational woman–It is important that she take prescribed *insulin* even though may not be eating regularly because insulin needs are increased during illness.

Preeclampsia – edema of the face and hands noted, 3+ proteins in the urine, high BP- bed rest lying on left side, maintain adequate intake of fluids and protein.

Magnesium sulfate IV- patients deep tendon reflexes are decreased-discontinue IV infusion. Is a sign of magnesium toxicity which may cause respiratory or cardiac arrest, keep calcium gluconate at bed side.

Neonatal Complication

Fetus produces increased *insulin* due to maternal hyperglycemia and continues to have increased insulin levels after birth, until infant's pancreas adjusts to extra uterine life with a lower glucose level, the high insulin output may result in a very low glucose level in first few days.

The baby's large size is due to the amount of *sugar* that she received in utero–infant has round face, chubby body, and a flushed complexion–child is at risk for hypoglycemia, hypocalcemia, and hyperbilirubinemia.

Infant has *mottling of the skin*, lab values indicate metabolic and respiratory acidosis-cold stress.

Red wrinkled skin, due to lack of subcutaneous fat that accumulates during third trimester, lanugo is downy fine hair found on shoulders, forehead and cheeks and is more noticeable in preterm infants, floppy, poor head control, and limp extremities indicate hypotonia.

Important to promote positive *parent child relationships*, both parents and child have emotional needs that must be met, he needs to develop a sense of trust and security and holding him promotes this.

Explain to parents that the child will set his own pace in achieving certain developmental tasks such as walking; many children don't walk until later on, whereas others walk earlier, there is no need for concern.

Separation anxiety—keep the child's toys from home near him, provide a familiar environment that will help to comfort the child.

Infant double *birth weight* at 5 months.

Otitis media—Eustachian tubes of children are shorter, wider, and straighter than those of adults. Infection travels from the pharynx via the eustachian tube to the middle ear.

Mother *addicted to narcotics*- narcotic withdrawal in newborn within 24-72 hours after birth, infant will be jittery and hyperactive, high pitched cry, disphoresis, tachypnea.

Phototherapy to a newborn with *jaundice*- check the infants temperature every hour, cover infants eyes to protect from fluorescent lights, remove during feeding so that eyes can be checked .

Physiologic jaundice results from the breakdown of excessive fetal red blood cells coupled with immature liver metabolism of bilirubin, declines in 5-7 days, normal bilirubin levels are 0.2-1.4 mg/dl.

Low birth weight infant is at greatest risk for developing respiratory distress syndrome.

Risk of developing infant *respiratory distress syndrome*-related to developmental delay in lung maturation due to underdeveloped lungs and the lack of surfactant, signs include labored respiration, grunting, nasal flaring, retractions, tachypnea, maintain body temp, IV fluid, TPN, maintain patient airway.

Pediatric Nursing

The inability to maintain eye contact is a characteristic of *autism–Establish* trust.

Having *imaginary friends* is a normal and common occurrence in children between the ages of 4-6, after that they outgrow the imagenary friends.

Children at 5 years of age are involved in imitative play, will play house, and play doctor.

Up to 9 month Babinskins reflexes present, 12 months it disappears–stroking the outer sole of the foot upward from the heel across the ball of the foot causes the big toe to dorsiflex and the hyperextend.

Infant with *pyloric stenosis* will present with projectile vomiting and abdominal distention, other symptoms include weight loss, constipation, dehydration, visible peristaltic waves.

Scoliosis—Lateral curvature of a portion of the spine, if patient wears Milwaukee brace, good skin care under pressure areas is necessary, brace is worn 23 hours per day.

Lead poisoning—Homes with lead paint should be cleansed weekly by wet cleansing and do not dry sweep.

18-month-old children drink some drain cleanser- Intubaton tray should be immediately available so that the airway may be protected.

Seizures can occur without warning, it is dangerous to have a thermometer in the mouth because the child may start seizing.

At 24 months child has steady gait and can use short sentences, goes up and down stairs alone, runs well with wide stance, builds tower of six to seven blocks, has vocabulary of about 300 words.

Discuss with *the parents* any problems or fears about childbearing that they may have. Important is that parents become active listener, become actively involved in children's education, and look at things from child's point of view.

Develop a structured routine for activities of daily living bathing, sleeping and playing.

Attention deficit disorder—may display impulsive, aggressive, and hostile behaviour- hug your child after a task is correctly performed. Child responds to positive reinforcement.

Kindergarten class child walks down stairs using alternative feet by age 4, indicates a delay.

It is not until 25 months that the child is physiologically and psychologically prepared to maintain daytime toilet training; at that time the child will not be able to achieve nighttime toilet training.

Cerebral palsy—Place toy out of the immediate reach of the child. Spastic cerebral palsy –fixed posture, clenched fists, and flexed forearms. The infant has poor head control after 3 months. Delayed gross motor development, signs stiff or rigid arms or legs, arching back, floppy or limp body posture.

It takes soft spot/ anterior *fontanel* 12-18 months /1.5 years to close.

Hemophiliac trait is an X-linked trait found primarily in males. This trait very rarely shows itself in females because their second sex chromosome is also X, they would need to have the trait linked to both chromosomes to show the disease, because males second sex chromosome is Y, they will show the disease, a female who has the trait linked to one X chromosome and not the other is considered a carrier.

A 7-year-old, 2.5 lb in one year is not an adequate weight gain. A 7-year-old girl may become shy at times because she experiences a conflict regarding her independence from her mother, this shyness period should be tolerated.

Developmental dysplasia of the hip is suspected – limited ability to abduct affected limb, a clunk heard on abduction.

Congenital hip dysplasia is pavlik harness, is applied to hold the hips in wide abduction, if the treatment does not achieve the correction in a few months, then surgery is indicated and a postoperative Spica hip bandage or body cast is applied.

Correct a scoliosis deformity emphasize that the brace should be worm 23 hours a day. Assess home environment for safety hazards, teach child how to prevent falls by using handrails and avoiding slippery surface.

Should be concerned- the infants *head lags* when pulled from a lying to a sitting position.

Cystic fibrosis is an altered viscosity of mucus. Is an Autosomal recessive trait. *Cystic fibrosis*- the child takes the pancreatic enzymes 1 hour after eating. Obstruction of the bile duct, absence of digestive enzymes, excessive salt loss through the skin, detected by the diagnostic sweat test.

Percussion accomplished by placing child in postural drainage position and striking chest wall with cupped hand's–vibration moves secretions during exhalation; chest physiotherapy is performed twice daily; administer bronchodilator medication before performing percussion and vibration.

Provide a safe play area, be aware of danger of aspiring foreign objects, *poisoning*, burns, and falls from infant seats, high chairs, walkers, and swings.

Mucomyst medication is given as an antidote after an Tylenol overdose/poisoning.

Cyanotic type of *congenital heart defect* is associated with clubbing of the fingers. Other symptoms include costal retractions and failure to thrive. It leads to polycythemia, chronic hypoxia, the body tries to compensate by producing more red blood cells to carry the limited amount of oxygen available to the tissues. They have difficulty eating and breathing at the same time, by providing small, frequent feeing and elevating the child's head after eating, the nurse can ensure better nutrition and decrease the possibility of aspiration. Surgical repair of it—postoperative care plan; elevate the head of the bed assists with respiratory effort and is essential.

Diagnosis of *idiopathic hypopituitarism*–observe characteristically have fine skin and delicate features; also have increased insulin sensitivity and premature aging common later in life. Will be given growth hormone–promotes growth of bone and soft tissues, affects linear growth, and conserves carbohydrate utilization.

According to Erickson, there is an overlap of *late adolescence and early adulthood* in which the indivual tries to develop intimate relationships/ sense of identity and intimacy.

To assess the pulse rate of an infant during cardiopulmonary resuscitation- the *brachial artery* near the axilla in the infant, infants arteries are naturally small–femoral, carotid and apical pulses may be difficult to palpate.

Turners syndrome- 45 chromosomes genetic abnormality resulting from a female having only one X chromosome, clinical manifestations include short stature, webbed neck, low posterior hairline, and shield shaped chest.

Vitamin E is given to infant to prevent oxidation of red blood cells.

Burns—Push the child to the ground and make her roll, smother flames, do not run because it will fan the flames.

Help parents to increase self esteem by making them feel accepted, empathize with parents about the *difficulty of childbearing..*

Rubeola— running nose, sneezing, and coughing that occur before the rash, it is communicable during prodromal phase.

Incubation period for *chickenpox/ varicella zoster* is about 10-12 days, approximately 2-3 weeks. About one week after onset of disease; also communicable 2 days before rash appears. Child can return to school when the lesions are crusted,

DPT vaccine–6 months second DPT vaccination is given. The side effects—baby crying continuously, convulsions, high fever, loss of consciousness.

In children younger than 3 years of age–straighten the *ear* canal by *pulling the pinna* down and straight back, children older than 3 years of age–pull the pinna up and back.

Myelomeningocele—place neonate in prone position. Neural tube fails to close and fuse during development, sac usually encased in fine membrane that is prone to tearing, which causes leaking of C.S.F, prone position helps prevent pressure on the fat like protrusion on the back, pressure on the area may result in increased intracranial pressure and may also cause a rupture of the sac, leading to infection. Infection may cause meningitis and damage the brain, the CNS is very delicate; asepsis is extremely important.

Five year old should have vocabulary of 2,100-3,000 words and use complete sentences containing 5-7 words.

At 9 months, the infant is able to pull himself up and assume a sitting position as well as say words such as dada and mama.

Second stage of separation is despair, at this time the crying stops and the child becomes depressed, apathetic and withdrawn.

Soyabeans are used as the protein source in formulas for children with allergies to cow's milk; this protein is less likely to induce allergies in infants.

Newborns have rapid respiration rate than adult which is 30-50 breaths/minute. Six month old infant likely to cause an *allergy with eggs and meat proteins.*

Infant during cardiopulmonary resuscitation use brachial artery near the axilla, CPR to infant use 2-3 fingers for compressions, depress sternum half-one inch, and perform at least 100 compressions per minute. Femoral, carotid, and apical pulses may be difficult to palpate.

Thumb sucking is normal and expected behaviour in the toddler 24 months period.

Genetic abnormally female having only one X chromosome condition is *Turners syndrome* (45 chromosomes).

Vitamin E is given to premature infants to prevent oxidation of red blood cells.

Asthma is chronic inflammation disorder of the airway, allergies is one of the predominant factor causing asthma, bedding often triggers childhood allergies which could precipitate the attack. Pillow of foam or dacron should washed weekly in hot water.

Adolescents have an increased need for nearly all nutrients because of their rapid growth and high activity.

DRUG

Lithium toxicity lethargy, ataxia, slurred speech, tinnitus, severe nausea and vomiting, seizures, arrhythmia, and hypotension–that may lead to coma and death if it is not properly recognized.

Methylphenidate/*Ritalin* is prescribed for children with attention deficit, hyperactive disorders because it is a CNS stimulant. Which improve concentration and adaptive behavior.

A patient that drinks *alcohol* while talking *disulfiram/Antabuse* will experience sweating, flushing of the neck and face, tachycardia, hypotension, a throbbing headache, nausea and vomiting, palpitations, dyspoea, tremor and flash or weakness.

The patient should report tinnitus because *Vancomycin* can affect the acoustic branch of the eight cranial nerve.

Ritodrine hydrochloride for premature labor keep available as *antidote,* Propranalol that is *Inderal.*

When analyzing laboratory values of patient receiving *Clofibrate* , the purpose is to decrease levels of very low-density *lipids.*

Phenytoin/Dilantin 100 mg tid to seizure control. A rash may occur 10-14 days after starting, notify and discontinue medicines. Perform good oral hygiene, including daily brushing and flossing, receive necessary periodic blood work, report to the physician if any problem with walking coordination, slurred speech or nausea.

Tensilion—test for diagnosis of myasthenia gravis with 30-60 seconds following injection, marked improvement in muscle tone that lasts about 4-5 minutes.

Side effect *of potassium supplement* is peptic *ulceration*, even with newer tablet coatings; still it can cause damage to the GI tract during absorption.

The blood should be drawn just before the administration of the next IV dose of *gentamycin sulfate*. The serum level of the drug would be *lowest* at that time.

Ondansetron HCL/zofran 6 mg q 6 h give 30 minutes prior to start chemotherapy, side effect include constipation, diarrhea, fever, lightheadedness and drowsiness.

Adriamycin will cause tissue damage, after applying ice, monitor site closely because extravasation may be progressive, it is an antibiotic antineoplastic. Side effect include red urine, nausea, vomiting, stomatitis, alopecia, cardiotoxicity and bone marrow depression, check EKG, avoid infiltration, monitor vital signs and give good mouth care.

Respiratory infections are very common and cardiac defect are the leading cause of death in children with *Down syndrome*.

PSYCHOLOGICAL

Observing the parents behavioral responses to their newborn, including holding and interacting with the infant, gives some indication of a healthy or pathological response to the child, early observations to identify infants at risk due to parental isolation, financial stress, or parental illness, referral to appropriate follow-up service may help to the establishment of a *healthy parent child relationship*.

Rape

The acute phase disorganization-includes reaction such as shock, denial, and disbelief. The survivor is also identified as embarrassed, degraded, fearful, angry, and vengeful.

Continued reality based orientation is necessary, so it is appropriate to use the patient's name in any interaction. Structured activities can help the patient refocus and resolve his delusions.

Nocturnal emissions (loss of seminal fluid during sleep) are found in the *adolescent male*.

Poison

Ingested toilet bowl cleaner, *Paint*–Initially the mother should be interested in taking care of the poisoning episode, the child needs a medical treatment, minimizing his guilt about the episode, and this is not a time for learning about poisoning but rather a time for helping the child get better. Why it occurred and how to prevent further. To learn ways to divert his interest in oral activity into other.

Impetigo infection can be caused by group B hemolytic streptococcus, the same organism responsible for glomerulonephritis.

Aspirin has a potent platelet inhibiting action that leads to an increased risk for bleeding, such as gastrointestinal hemorrhage, that would be the most life threatening.

Flank steak, green leafy vegetables and prune foods provide *iron Fatigue* is a complication of anemia, arrange for patient to have a bed on the first floor, encourage patient to balance rest and activity.

The patient has developed *osteomylitis*, a potential complication of bone marrow aspiration; fever and yellow purulent discharge from the site are signs of osteomylitis.

AIDS complaining of diarrhea decrease roughage in the diet. Avoid foods that stimulate intestinal motility, such as vegetables and fruits, fatty spicy and sweet foods, alcohol and caffeine.

Confusion due to AIDS, dementia, use short uncomplicated sentences, orient to daily activities by explaining the activities while they are happening, keep soiled laundry in a plastic bag hamper. Energy conservation technique, sitting and while washing is also helpful, place frequently used personal items within patient's reaches.

Serious health hazard for children with spina bifida due to repeated exposure, also at risk are health care workers and people who routinely use *latex* condoms, reaction can range from contact dermatitis, asthma to anaphylaxis.

Hemophilia

It is a sex linked recessive trait transmitted to mates by female carriers deficiency of factor VIII; abnormal bleeding in response to trauma, signs include easy bruising, joint pain with bleeding and prolonged internal or external bleeding, instruct pt to institute supportive measures when trauma occurs- rest, ice, compression and elevation, applying ice to his knee and evaluating his leg is the most appropriate action to take initially because it will help to stop the bleeding and decrease the swelling, will also help to alleviate the pain help to alleviate the pain. IM injections should be avoided, contact MD, avoid nasal packing.

Hematocrit measures red blood cells to fluid volume man- 42-50% woman 40-48% child 35-45%.

Pernicious Anemia

Vitamin B_{12} obtained from dietary sources is normally absorbed by means of intrinsic factor found in the stomach, from there it is carried out to the ileum, patient lacks the intrinsic factor so an oral preparation of the vitamin would not be absorbed. Pernicious anemia needs injection B_{12} rest of life.

Sickle Cell Disease

It is a severe hemolytic anemia resulting from defective hemoglobin, hemoglobin becomes sickle shaped in the presence of low oxygenation; symptoms caused by hemolysis and thrombosis and include pain and jaundice; infection and dehydration can precipitate a sickle cell crisis. Every person entering the room should wash hands thoroughly; person with URI should wear a mask when entering the room. Dehydration precipitates sickle cell crisis, patient should take in at least 200 cc/ bd by oral or parenteral route, do not offer caffeinated beverages.

Anemia

It is a condition of a decrease in the number of erythrocytes or reduction in hemoglobin; symptoms include dyspnea, chronic fatigue, paleness, severe palpitations, sensitivity to cold, profound weakness, iron deficiency anemia caused by blood loss. Major cause of iron deficiency anemia in adults is bleeding; assess the GI system, character of emesis, stools, diarrhea, anorexia, nausea and vomiting. Obtain a stool specimen to test for occult blood. Liver and onions, spinach, and rice pudding with raisins contains high amount of iron.

Schilling test- to be successful , the patient must comply carefully with collecting his urine over a 24 *hour urinalysis*, instruct pt to void and discard urine, test begins at this time, save all urine during specified time in one container that is refrigerated or kept on ice, label container with exact date and time that collection started and ended.

Administer *epinephrine* subcutaneously as soon as patient having *anaphylactic reaction*.

Polycythemia Vera observes for dark, flushed face, blood in tissues is incompletely oxygenated; intense itching due to vasodilatation occurs; blood moves slowly due to increased viscosity.

Oncology

A common site of metastasis from *breast cancer/ mastectomy* is the bone, indication of bone metastasis include pain and local swelling. Do not use affected arm to take blood pressure, draw blood or give injections, elevate affected arm to decrease swelling and discomfort. There is no relationship between begin disease and developing breast cancer. Mammography is X-ray of the soft tissue can detect cancer that is not palpable; size of the breast does not matter.

Gastric cancer abdominal discomfort relieved with antacids, other indications include indigestion, loss of appetite, bloated feeling, and weight loss.

Myelogenous *leukemia*—Patient is immunocompromised and at risk for infection; obtain temp q 4 h; inspect wounds, skin and mucous membranes for redness, swelling and drainage, notify physician. Hepatosplenomegaly an enlarged liver and spleen, causing abdominal pain. Do not dig in the garden or work with house plants in acute myelogenous leukemia. Weigh the patient's pads and tampons before and after use. Due to excessive bleeding better to determine the amount of blood loss, report the physician. Patient with WBC count below 10,000/mm placing him at high risk for developing a life threatening infection. When receiving *chemotherapy* if you are immunocompromised. Life threatening side effects of chemotherapy results in decreased leukocytes, erythrocytes, and platelets. Wash hands before touching any object in patient's room. Losing hair is temporary, new hair may be a different color, texture, and thickness. Should not take medications that contain aspirin due to danger of bleeding; Alka Setzer contains aspirin. Chemotherapy causes bone marrow depression. Include in meal and snack selection as much as possible, foods that are appealing, offer small, frequent feedings of nutrient dense food. Receiving chemotherapy for breast cancer develop myelosuppression avoid people who have recently received attenuated vaccines, avoid activities that may cause bleeding, wash hands frequently, avoid crowded places such as shopping malls. Patient's platelet count falls- normal 140,000 to 400,000/ul that are known as *thrombocytopenia*.

Cancer of the cervix place all linens in a special lead lined hamper, sheets are not radioactive, save all dressings and bed linens in the room until after the implant is removed, dispose in the usual manner. Restricting the patient's motion will decrease the chance of the radioactive implant becoming dislodged, since this includes minimizing use of bedpan, enemas may be given. *Radioactive implant-* visits must be limited and brief during treatment. Visitors and staff should decrease and time spent and keeps a safe distance form. *Pap smear* an important concept for the treatment, stage one indicates that cancer is confined to the cervix.

Laryngeal cancer—hoarseness, difficulty swallowing, color changes in the mouth or tongue, and oral lesions that do not heal are warning signs of laryngeal cancer. Risk factors developing chewing tobacco, pipe smoking, marijuana, voice abuse lifelong use of alcohol. *Laryngectomy* patient will not have an audible laugh after the surgery. Loss of verbal communication-alternative methods of communication postoperatively, patient will use speech board, then use artificial larynx, and then learn esophageal speech. Validates the patients concerns and encourage verbalization of surgery. After operation receiving radiation to the head and neck-often produces dry mouth/xerostomia, irritation of the oral mucus membranes/ stomatitis, and diminished sense of tast/dysgeusia.

Pancreatic cancer—whipped procedures is removal of head of pancreas, distal portion of common bile duct, the duodenum, and part of the stomach, performed for treatment of it. NG tube inserted to prevent stress on anastomosis sites, drainage should be serosanguineous, clear, colorless, bile tinged drainage or frank bleeding may indicate problem with anastomosis–sites–contact physician.

Skin cancer—over the age of 60, light skinned, and works outdoors are all risk factors for cancer. The sun is at peak strength during those hours–apply sunscreen.

Advancing age—single most significant risk factor 50% of all cancers occur in people older than 65 years of age.

Brain tumor—patient's violence is most likely due to increased intracranial pressure, the nurse should stay with her to help her regain control by talking in a calm, quiet manner, in addition, summon help quickly to facilitate medical treatment, the physician must be notified.

Diet high in fat is a risk factor for the development of *colon cancer*, does not matter weather fat is saturated or polyunsaturated, limit total fat intake to less than 30% daily intake. Animal fats, broiled meats and fish and concentrated sweets.

Right mastectomy measure and record the amount of drainage; change dressing around the drain as needed.

Stomatitis— assess, examine pts mouth thoroughly every 4 hrs; document size, character and drainage for blisters, sores.

Cancer of the lung—with severe headache, nauseated, vomiting, drooling, should perform neurological assessment and contact the physician. Undergoing radiation use a patting motion to dry the radiated area, dry with soft towel, wear soft clothing that does not rub. Use a soft bristled toothbrush, do not floss and avoid hard foods. Lobactomy for lung cancer chest tube connected to water seal chamber for drainage system.

Terminal stage cancer—*hospice care-* focus of care is on control of symptoms and relief of pain, a multidisciplinary team –possibly consist of nurses, physicians, chaplains, aides and volunteers provides care, bereavement care is provided to the family. It is based on need, not on the ability to pay.

Bladder cancer—surgical removal of bladder with construction of an ileal conduite mucus membranes are used to create conduit- dusky appearance of the stoma, stoma protrusion from the skin, sharp abdominal pain with rigidity.

Pressure ulcer—shearing force increase the risk of ulcer, they can occur as patient slide down in bed or are pulled up in bed, to reduce force, instruct patient to use overbed trapeze, keep head in bed no higher than 30 degrees.

Credes maneuver procedure is done to patient who has lower motor neuron damage who has difficulty with urination, gentle pressure over lower abdomen to empty the bladder.

Milk, custard and vanilla ice cream- *full liquid diet.*

Quadriceps sets are an *isometric* exercise to strengthen the muscles used for walking but no change in muscle length and no joint movement.

Psychological needs— assess and document the behavior and the enquiries continued–use of restraints, tie the restrains in quick release knots, ask the patient if he needs to go to the bathroom and provide range of motion exercise every 2 hours.

Let's talk about your mother's illness and how it will progress, you sound like you have some questions about your mother dying, lets talk about that, tell me how you are feeling about your mother dying.

Physical findings about *abuse* in medical record is essential, document the patient's statement and complete a body map indicating the size, color, shape, location and type of injuries, assist the patient in developing a safety plan for times of increased violence, provide patient with telephone numbers of local shelters and safe houses.

According to Kuble Ross, the five stages of *death and dying* are denial and isolation, anger, bargaining, depression and acceptance, loss, grief and intense sadness indicate depression.

Silence is a therapeutic communication technique, take a seat next to the patient and sit quietly, say to patient you are feeling upset about the news you got about the *transplant.*

Part of patients family are all the people whom the patient views as family, people who provide the physical and emotional needs of the patient.

Respect the patient's *cultural beliefs,* consider that nonverbal cues, such as eye contacts may have a different meaning in different cultures, ask the patient if he has cultural or religious requirements that should be considered in his care.

Hemicolectomy for Colon Cancer

Illness of one family members can affect all members, a family member may have more than one role at a time in a family, the effect of illness on a family depends on the stage of the family life cycle, changes in sleeping and eating patterns may be signs of stress in family.

Advance directive is a Legal document that provides instructions, living will and names, a durable power of attomey for health.

Alzheimer's disease spouse is too exhausted to continue providing care all alone- recommending community resources for adult day care and respite care, encouraging spouse to talk about difficulty, asking weather friends or church members can help with short period of relief.

Enalapril maleate/vasorec for treatment of hypertension avoid salt substitutions, advice the patient to report facial swelling or difficulty breathing immediately, advice the patient not to change position suddenly to minimize orthostatic hypotension.

Closed head injury—phenytoin/ Dilantin 100 mg IV every 8 hours for seizure prophylaxis-administer an IV bolus no faster than 50 mg/ minute, monitor ECG, blood pressure, and respiratory status continuously when administering this drug, know that early toxicity may cause drowsiness, nausea, vomiting, nystagmus, ataxia, dysarthria, remorse, and slurred speech.

Acute myocardial infarction patient with history of type 1 diabetes *metoprolol/lopressor IV-* monitor glucose levels closely, monitor for heart block and Bradycardia, monitor blood pressure.

Rash on chest and upper arms –when did the rash start, are you allergic to any medications, foods or pollen, what have you been using to treat the rash, have you recently traveled outside the country.

Cardiovascular Disorders

Raynauds disease—results from reduced blood flow to the extremities when exposed to cold or stress. It is commonly associated with connective tissue disorders such as SLE systemic lupus erythematosus, signs and symptoms include pallor, coldness, numbness, throbbing pain and cyanosis.

12 lead ECG—a patient experiencing an inferior wall myocardial infarction–following ECG changes, T-wave inversion, ST-segment elevation, and pathologic Q- wave–all are signs of tissue hypoxia–inadequate blood supply reflected by T wave inversion.

Patient with left ventricular myocardial infaraction/ left sided heart failure-signs are dyspnea, crackles, tachycardia.

Dizziness, headache, and hypotension are all common adverse effects of ACE inhibitors of *lisinopril/zestril.*

Patient with acute chest pain radiating down left arm indicated; *Laboratory studies;* Creatinine phosphokinase CPK, Troponin-T and troponin, elevated because of cellular damage, Myoglobin elevation is an early indication of myocardial damage.

Obesity, stress, high intake of sodium or saturated fat and family history are all risk factors for *primary hypertension.*

Gastrointestinal Disorders

Adverse reaction of *gentamicin* includes ototoxicity and nephrotoxicity. Monitor hearing, urine output, and serum calcium level.

For upper *GI endoscopy* tell the patient not to eat or drink for 6-12 hours before the procedure. Inform the patient that he will receive sedative before the procedure.

Neonates born with *esophageal atresia*- cyanosis, coughing, choking, occur when fluid from the blind pouch is aspirated into the trachea.

Inflammatory bowel syndrom/Crohn's disease—corticosteroid therapy, antidiarrheal medications part of care plan.

Integumentary Disorders

Scabies—Signs and symptoms include gray brown burrows, epidermal curved or linear ridges, and follicular papules, severe itching that occurs at night, areas of finger, webs, and flexor surface of the wrist and antecubital fossae.

Melanoma— The ABCDs of it is asymmetry of the lesion, borders that are irregular, colors that vary in shades and increased diameter. Fair skin with a history of sunburn and the location of the lesion on the leg are common site in women are risk factors for melanoma.

Stage 2 pressure ulcer—The ulcer is superficial like a blister; there is partial thickness skin loss of the epidermis.

Nursing care for pressure ulcer—Use pressure reducation devices, reposition every 1 to 2 hours, teach the family how to care for the wound, clean the area around the ulcer with mild soap.

Operation of partial thick skin graft—Elevates the left arm and provides complete rest of the grafted area.

Administer pain medication every 4 hours as ordered for pain in donor site, monitor the pulse arm every 4 hours.

Immune and Hematologic Disorder

In the classic pupus rash, lesions appear on the cheeks and the bridge of the nose, creating a characteristic *Butterfly* pattern.

Normal saline solution is used for administering blood transfusions.

HIV transmission—I&II–wear a mask gown, and gloves when splashing of body fluids is likely, I will wash my hands after client care.

Supportive, *nonpharmacologic measures* for the rheumatoid arthritis- applying splints to inflamed joints, selecting clothing that has Velcro fasteners, applying moist heat to joints.

Endocrine and Metabolic Disorders

After the removal of the *thyroid gland*, take thyroid replacement medication as ordered, watch for changes in body functioning such as lethargy, restlessness, sensitivity to cold and dry skin and report these changes to the physician.

Sings and symptoms of *diabetes insipidus* include extreme polyuria, excessive thirst, low urine specific gravity.

In hypothyroidism the thyroid replacement therapy has been inadequate when indicated prolonged QT interval on ECG, low body temperature, bradycardia.

Alcohol consumption, missed meals and strenuous activity may lead to hypoglycemia; symptoms of it include shakiness, confusion, and headache. Hypoglycemia can become a life-threatening disorder involving seizures and death to brain cells.

Graves disease/hyperthyroidism, is a hyper metabolism state that is associated with rapid, bounding pulses, heat intolerance, mild tremors, nervousness.

Addisons disease for an adrenal crisis- discuss with physician, steroid needs before dental work, weak or dizzy, obtain and wear a medic alert bracelet.

Goiter—can result from inadequate dietary intake of iodine associated with changes in foods or malnutrition. It is caused by, insufficient thyroid gland production and depletion of flandular iodine. Signs and symptoms enlargement of the thyroid gland, dizziness when raising the arms above the head, dysphasia and respiratory distress.

SIADH—syndrome of inappropriate antidiuretic hormone–decrease in body weight, increase in urine output, decrease in urine osmolality.

A patient with a *Parahormone deficiency* has abnormal calcium and phosphorous values because it regulates these two electrolytes.

Musculoskeletal Disorders

Osteoporosis is a degenerative metabolic bone disorder in which the rate of bone resorption accelerates and the rate of bone formation decelerates. It is common in females after menopause. It is a degenerative disease characterized by a decrease in bone density, it can cause pain and injury. Patient may report a gradual loss in height after menopause.

Patient with *gout* should avoid foods that are high in purines, such as liver, cold, and sardines, also avoid anchovies, kidneys, sweetbread, lentils and alcoholic beverages like beer and wine.

In a hip fracture, the affected leg is shorter adducted, and extermally rotated. Movement away from the body or midline is called abduction.

Neurosensory Disorder

The Glasgow coma scale assesses level of consciousness by testing and scoring three observations are spontaneous eye opening, obeying motor command, and orientation to time, place, and time.

Bacterial meningitis signs of meningeal irritation include nuchal rigidity, positive brudzinski's sign, positive kernig's sign, and photophobia.

Complete spinal cord injury notes flushed skin, diaphoresis above 15, and a blood pressure of 162/96, patient has severe, pounding headache, elevate the head of the bed 90 degrees, looses constrictive clothing, assess for bladder distention and bowel impaction, administer antihypertensive medication.

Cranial nerve XII, the hypoglossal nerve control tongue movements involved in swallowing and speech. The tongue should be midline, symmetrical and free of tremors.

Trigeminal neuraligia is a painful disorder of one or more branches of cranial nerve V that produces paroxysmal attacks of excruciating facial pain. Precipitated by stimulation of a trigger zone on the face. Triggering events may include light touch to a hypersensitive area, a draft of air, exposure to heat or cold, eating smiling, talking or drinking hot or cold beverages. It occurs most commonly in people older than age 40.

The occipital lobe is responsible for the interpreting visual stimuli.

Pneumothorax—air in the plural space is potential complication of all central venous access device. Sings and symptoms include chest pain, dyspoea, shoulder or neck pain, irritability, palpitations, lightheadedness, hypotension, cyanosis and unequal breath sounds. A chest X-ray reveals the collapse of the affected lung that results from pneumothorax.

Jaw thrust—If a neck or a spine injury is suspected, the jaw thrust maneuver should be used to open the patients airway. To perform this position yourself at the patients head and rest your thumbs on patients lower jaw near the corners of the mouth. Then grasp the angles of patients lower jaw with your fingers and lift it forward.

Bronchophony is an assessment on patient with pneumonia with stethoscope voice sound heard clearly over his lobe, e.g. ask patient to say ninety-nine several times.

Pulmonary embolus presents with low grade fever, tachycardia, blood tinged sputum.

Typical findings for patient with COPD include dyspnea on exertion, a barrel chest and clubbed fingers and toes.

Tension pneumothorax results when air in the plural space is under higher pressure than air in the adjacent lung. Decreased cardiac output, hypotension, and tracheal deviation to the opposite side.

Oxygen, diuretics and vasodilators are among the common therapies used to treat pulmonary hypertension. Others include fluid restriction, digoxin, calcium channel blockers, beta adrenergic blockers and bronchodilators.

Stress incontinence is a small loss of urine with activities that increase intra-abdominal pressure such as running laughing, sneezing, jumping, coughing or bending. These symptoms occur only in the daytime.

Hypocalcemia is a calcium deficit that causes nerve fiber irritability and repetitive muscle spasms. Signs and symptoms of hypocalcaemia include-trousseaus sign, cardiac arrhythmias, diarrhea, increased clotting times, anxiety and irritability. The calcium phosphors imbalance leads to brittle bones and pathologic fractures.

Urinary System

The *urinary system* is ultimately responsible for maintaining fluid and electrolyte balance by excretion or retention based on body's needs.

Osmosis is the diffusion of water—Prostate gland is a tubuloalveolar gland shaped like a ring with the urethra passing its centre. After indwelling catheter an interruption in normal voiding habits when catheter removed, the body must adapt to functioning once again. An enlarge prostrate constructing urethra, interfering with urine flow causing retention. The length of urethra is shorter in female than males.

Females develop cystitis because of proximity of urethra and anus, it is at risk of becoming contaminated, urethritis–obtain a urine specimen for culture and sensitivity to isolate before starting antibiotic therapy in urinary tract infection in patient with hematuria observe for gross blood in the urine–indicates progressive increase in kidney damage. Sharp, severe pain (Renal colic) radiating forwards the genitalia and thigh is caused by urethral distention. Urine is strained to determine weather any calculi has been passed.

Lithotripsy to break up renal calculi, cystomithectomy refers to the removal of bladder stones. If calcium exertion is still elevated on the test diet, dietary influences can be ruled out. Recurrent infection and inadequate fluids contribute most to formation of calculi- most stones are calcium oxalate in nature. Calcium oxalate renal stones can be prevented by low in calcium and oxalate, acid ash.

Dysuria, nocturia and urgency are all signs of an irritable bladder after radiation therapy. Disadvantage of ileal conduit is that the ureteries are implanted in a segment of the ileum, and urine drains continually because there is no sphincter.

In renal failure metabolic acidosis develops as a result of inability of renal tubules to secrete hydrogen ions and conserve bicarbonate receives low protein diet – the reduced amount of metabolic waste products will decrease stress on the kidney. Patient complains of tingling of finger and toes and muscle twitching caused by calcium depletion causes tetany. Patient will be confused and irritable because an elevated BUN indicating uremia is toxic and CNS causes mental cloudiness, confusion and loss of consciousness.

Chronic renal failure CAPD (continuous ambulatomy peritoneal dialysis) treatment uses the peritoneum as a semi-permeable membrane to clear toxins by osmosis and diffusion. Remove toxins and metabolic wastes from the blood into the dialysis solution. The failure of the kidney to maintain a balance of potassium is one of the main indications for dialysis. Due to hypokalemia hemodialysis done. Because an external shunt provides circulatory access to a major artery and vein, special safety precautions must be taken to prevent disconnection of the canula. Disconnection can cause unimpeded excessive blood loss and death. Clamps should be carried at all times by the patient in case this emergency should arise. So most serious problem of external shunt is Exsangulnation, insertion of AV shunt breaks the 1st line of defence against infection. It can be avoided by use of strict aseptic technique when gives shunt care.

Acute cholecystitis with biliary colic intolerance to foods high in lipids

Cholecystectomy assessed sign of bleeding – blood clotting may be hindered by lack of vitamin K absorption, 8 hrs. After colostomy the absence of drainage from the colostomy is normal.

The cessation of renal function is evidence by decreased in output less than 400 ml/24 hours.

Hypokalemia occurs in renal failure because kidney damaged, the body does not excrete potassium K+.

The waste product of protein metabolism is the main cause of uremia, protein restriction.

The presence of Fat in the duodenum stimulates painful contractions of the gallbladder to release bile, fat should be avoided.

Glaucoma – lost vision can't be restored, is permanent and progressive if the disease is not controlled.

Total hip arthroplasty – keep an abduction pillow between the leg at all times to maintain position of the prosthesis and avoid dislocation.

Bronchial asthma– raising mucus secretion for the chest – it interfere with gas exchange in the lungs.

Certain diagnostic test CBC, urine analysis, chest X-ray done preoperative to rule out health problem that could increase the risk involved with surgery.

Myasthenia gravis asses for Diplopia (double vision), drug for it will be periods when bed rest will be needed and times when fairly normal activity will be possible, swimming helps.

Potassium administers slowly to avoid cardiac arrest.

Deficiency of the glucocorticoids causes hypoglycemia in the patient with *Addison's disease.* Signs of hypoglycemia include nervousness weakness, dizziness, cool, moist skin, hunger and tremors. Because of diminished mineralocorticoid secretion patient with Addison's disease is prone to development of hyponatremia, the addition of salt to the diet is advised.

Burns—observe a loss of sodium and increase in blood potassium and, intake 6000 ml, output 1200 ml because of fluid loss via the burned area and sodium reabsorption by the kidneys which pull fluid, urinary output is diminished, output 30 ml/hr or less considered a sigh of shock.

Myocardial infarction salt limited, it produce a diuretic effect and reduce the circulating blood volume.

Oropharyngeal suction the presence of secretions in the upper airway produces gurgling sounds that interfere with the free flow of air with each breath.

Varicose veins—Leg fatigue they tend to develop increased hydrostatic pressure in the vein.

Hospice care attempts to break the cycle of anxiety, fear and pain. Pain medication given on regular basis free the patient from fear related to pain.

Neck surgery gives a high fowler to reduce edema at the operative site. After broncos copy with biopsy patient evaluate the presence of a gag reflex. To loosen secretion when patient has endotracheal tube – administering humidified oxygen. Pneumonectomy patient should be positioned on the operative side at the back, head slightly elevated.

Portable wound drainage system maintaining compression of the drainage system.

With a *suprapubic prostatectomy* an incision is made directly into the bladder via the abdomen so that bladder abnormalities can be corrected concurrently with prostate removal; other prostatic surgery uses the transurethral route. - use green vegetables to prevent constipation- no prolonged sitting–it increases the risk of bleeding.

The parathyroid gland regulates serum levels of calcium, calcium would be mobilized from bone in hyperparathyroidism and the serum calcium level increased demineralization of bone.

Cardiac arrest – administer sodium bicarbonate.

Ulcerative colitis + constipation chronic irritation and slower fecal transit are risk factor for cancer of the colon.

Standard precautions include gloves, gown, mask and gaggles should be worn when there is a risk for exposure to blood or body secretions. it is also used in communicable disease.

Primary symptoms of hypertension–occipital headache, particularly in the morning.
- The inability to withdraw from a painful stimulus indicates the greatest neurologic impairment (extending – use of Glasgow coma scale).
- Peritoneal dialysis complaining respiratory difficulty – drain fluid from the peritoneal cavity to reduce pressure of diaphragm.
- All patients who are confined to bed for any considerable period risk losing calcium from bones.
- Cancer of the prostate is rare before age 50 but increases with each decade, black men develop it twice as often as white men at an early age.

Jaundice – complains of pruritus itching associated with an accumulation of bile salts in the skin.

Varicose vein – increase hydrostatic pressure in vein

Herniation of lumber disc – pain radiating to the hip and leg

Phobia reactions occur when patient comes into contact with the object faced.

Antisocial personality disorder is generally unable to postpone gratification.

The gland that regulates the rate of oxygen is thyroid gland.

The medulla center for – Fat metabolism, temperature regulation, water balance

Risk of osteoporosis increased when a patient receives long term steroid therapy.

Isolation of patient with bacterial menisitis for 48 hrs after antibiotic therapy.

Communication ties people to their social surroundings.

Reyers syndrome – bleeding and ecchymosed from liver involvement

Tetracycline – tooth enamel defects in children under 8 yrs of age and in the maturing fetus.

Most spontaneous abortions are caused by germ plasma defects.

Prescribed sodium diet and diuretic reduce BP by reducing circulating blood volume.

Control uremia–limit protein *Crisis* outcome is unrelated – a high level of anxiety continuing for more than 3 months (a crisis would be resolved in 6 weeks). The specific circumstances surrounding the perceived crisis situation is an important assessment. Patient in crisis needs assistance with coping. I will be here for you to help you figure things out. Many parent's experience feelings of resentment towards their children. It is vital to help parents realize this. Too early too strict toilet training results in ambivalence because his needs and physical abilities are in conflict that need parental demand.

Developmental level is essential to understanding a child's response to a crisis situation. Child that genetic disorder parent's ability to talk about problems their infant may have in the future. Crisis short term – restore the patient's psychological equilibrium. Attempting to discover what is bothering the patient, various aspects of hospitalization and diagnosis could cause patient's anxiety. Assist the patient to acquire more effective behaviour. Employing an attitude of concern that is not intrusive.

Asses the patient's behavior in a non threatening manner; Acknowledgement of the patient's behavior will help lower anxiety reduce guilt and encourage discussion of feeling. (it must have been very difficult to care for him.) Each person is unique (not to dehumanize), accepting the patient's individuality. Have restricted questions to those relevant to the situation. Any other action would be an invasion of privacy. The nurse must know and understand personal feelings about terminal illness and death, feelings about the situation.

Calling for help during a suicide attempt demonstrates the patient's unconscious will to live or be stopped from dying the contrasting feelings of wanting to die and yet wanting to live demonstrate ambivalence.

Explaining procedures and routine decrease is patient's anxiety about the unknown, explaining what behaviour is expected. You are wondering how other will react to you now? Safeness provides security. Confused patient provide familiar environment.

The 1st step in the problem solving process would be exploration. Depressed patients are potentially suicidal. Ensure that all treatment options have been explored. Working with families encountering problems–nurse to have a sense of self and empathy for others. First interview with patient in clinic – most productive is exploratory.

Vitamin C strengthening capillary walls are structural tissue by depositing cementing material to build collagen from ground substance and thus prevent tissue hemorrhage.

A pathophysological change underlying the production of symptoms in leukemia is proliferation and release of immature WBC into blood.

Intracellular fluid is potassium:

Rare complication of pinworm infestation is appendicitis.

Nephritic syndrome – edema around the eyes and dark forthy unrine.

Angina pectoris – decreased O2 supply to heart cells associated with pain.

Patient with liver dysfunction have high serum ammonia levels.

Glycogenolysis is the production of glucose from glycogen stored in liver.

Function of B cell lymphocytes is to make antibodies.

Phogocytosis a process by which a particle is ingested and digested by a cell.

Specific immunity is the second line of defense against infection and is able to identify specific antigens.

Diabetic insipidus – insufficient production of anti-diuretic hormone

Patient with renal failure do not manufacture adequate amounts of erythropoietin

Aging process glomerular filtration rate decreases.

When potassium retention increase kidney excretes more sodium.

Normal serum amylase level is 25 – 151 unit/dl.

Normal serum ammonia level 35 – 65 mg/dl.

Insensible losses occur daily through the skin + lungs 800 ml daily.

Normal serum calcium level is 8.6 to 10 mg/dl, 12 is high.

Health and Internet

In today's fast forward ultra modern life, nurses too have to progress in her day today knowledge and get access to the internet to make a world of difference to her skill and personality, which is the need of the hour. She cannot just be satisfy herself with whatever she knows but get in touch with the advances made in science. If she wants to be component with the world of medicine, she will have to plunge into the updated knowledge. That not only will make her self-confident but much more efficient and capable in her field.

There are client-oriented sites as well as medico-specific ones. With increasing usage of the www by everyone all over the world, telemedicine, client support groups and health-focussed information has become freely available to everyone. Clients more than ever before, are better informed and have access to various databases. It therefore becomes important to keep abreast of the various health-info sources available on the net. It offers tremendous opportunities for the medical profession to serve humankind. We get latest information.

The internet has already changed the way we live. It has changed the way every important activity, weather commercial or academic, is translated. For the health professionals, it represents a big opportunity, not only to stay updated on the latest in the world of medicine, but also to get connected to the medical fraternity across the world as never before. A person with wide experience in both the field of health care and computer is important. It is a powerful tool. In the earlier days when a doctor could do nothing more for a critically ill person, the family would start praying. Now they turn to the internet, which provides a wealth of information for clients that can be very useful for the care of a critically ill client. People with medical conditions use the internet to communicate with each other in support groups and to compare experiences. Therefore, Internet is a resource that should not be ignored today.

Medical education on the internet- medicine is the only discipline, which requires a formal continuing education process. With advance of the internet, the newest modality of learning is the information technology you can participate in continuing medical education at websites. There you find visuals on the human body; research reports and lets you explore the amazing world of senses, nervous system, brain imaging and scanning techniques.

Learn about your topic as you search. It gives you subject categorization or you may be able to find a database on your subject. Multiple database searching lets you search in all of information categories at once. It is very convenient, searchable database, very worthwhile for many topics and for references. To see alphabetical list on everything available through search.com; which is comprehensive, informative and useful, easily found.

General sites of medical and pharma interest you have health and medical news, information on hypertension, dialysis and clinical nephrology, the alternative and complementary medicine center, hospital sites directory- international and national, anesthesiology, ayurveda, cardiology, clinical, dentistry, dermatology, emergency, to name them few Health care professionals providing for the exchange of ideas and opinions with experienced professionals.

Today nurse is not merely attendant in the ill room but also a educator and researcher. It is applied science to establish certain laws and principles. It requires sound knowledge. The better the scientific background the safer and more intelligent care provider she becomes. Thus, she utilizes the skills and techniques to meet the whole person in its totality that is considering all the aspects of physical, psychological, spiritual, social, economical, and intellectual.

Her profession promotes human and social welfare. She has to be up to date with the knowledge of physical and biological sciences, social science, and medical science, etc. to become a good nurse.

Today's nurses do various functions in the hospital as well as in the community. For this she needs to be adequately prepared and learn new ideas by lot of in-depth extensive reading, and attending latest conferences to fulfill her responsibility of the nurse who is responsible to conserve life and promote health, nature and nourishes her profession on continues research work. This will help her to maintain health, promote health and prevent diseases. That will help her to come up the level of accuracy and able to respond to the challenges. When she keeps her knowledge up to date, she can maintain a highest standard of care, current in the nursing practice. She will be able to plan her work in a purposeful way. Thus, she will do her work skillfully to provide relief and comfort to the client.

While caring the patient when she comes across a confuse terminology or a diagnosis or a diseases she can turn to the net and get the information to have better understanding of the condition as well as she will be better equipped to respond to the client. Knowledge is a power and an asset. It is the greatest weapon of our times. Good sound knowledge of a subject one can deals with situation in appropriate manner and it will take the person to the high test ladder of achievement.

Today we are served with so many good things only one has to have interest and access to right kind of information to know where and how to get it. Medical health is a vast giant subject and one can never dive into its depth, the more one knows the more thirst felt as there is so much to explore it is never enough. So together with your work and study go on and on getting in touch with the latest.

Keep informed yourself everyday. Because, even after few years of study, one knows something yet you are just like a drop in the ocean. Due to vast subject, you specialize in particular subject you are more interested in and go on exploring into that line to develop your specialty and your identity. Internet provides students and there teachers to easy to implement educational materials to spark an interest an interest in all manner of subject. You are a new age nurse with challenges and opportunities to gain skills.

Nurses with today's rapid and unprecedented changes, new urgency has been added to the critical need for a body of knowledge specific to nursing. Knowledgeable nursing services are indispensable to public safety. Humanitarian values add a further imperative to the search for understanding man and his world. True focus of the profession is on patient health care needs. Applying and teaching all we know for patient's highest potential for healthful living.

Nurse is a person who has completed a programme of nursing education, qualified, and authorized to provide responsible and competent professional service. Her responsibilities to promote health to prevent illness, to restore health and to alleviate suffering. Public health nurse most directly concerned with giving health education and care to individual and families in the community. To shoulder new tasks and responsibly and to much wider role she plays in society. She acts as a sheet anchor of total health care system. For the purpose of promoting, maintains, monitoring and restoring health. She is a key person and the back born of health care delivery system.

There is growing need for community-based health care. As more and more health care delivery shifts into the community, more nurses are working in a variety of community based settings, such as public health department, ambulatory health clinics, long-term care facilities, prenatal and well baby clinics, hospice agencies, and industrial settings as occupational nurses, homeless shelters and clinics and clients homes.

Here they must be self-directed, flexible, adaptable and tolerant of various lifestyles and living conditions. Here often it is an Independent decision-making, critical thinking, assessing, and health education. It focuses in maintaining the health of the population and of preventing and minimizing the progression of diseases. Here direct care is given to the entire community. So here she needs added knowledge to deal with multidimensional situations and problems that arise in health field.

In Critical thinking- using ones own reasoning or thought process while thinking refine-thinking skills, high level critical thinking within nursing process. Goal orientated activity, truth seeker with an open mindedness to the alternative solutions that might surface. Reflective, insightful, analyze information, questioning all findings, creative methods of proceeding. Knowing to interpret information and knowing what it tells her.

Today sophisticated *technology* can prolong life well beyond the time when death would have occurred in the past. Expensive experimental procedures and medication are available for use in attempting to preserve life, this has an influence on all stages of life, e.g. genetic screening in vitro fertilization, the harvesting and freezing of life, premature infants are given a chance for survival because of technical support. Children and adult who would have died a result of organ failure are living longer because organ transplantation. Technological advances have also contributed to increase life expectancy and better quality of life. The nurse as a teacher is challenged to focus on the educational needs of society. Nurses must seize opportunities both inside and outside of health care settings to facilitate wellness. Taking responsibilities for oneself is the key to successful health promotion. The possibilities are endless and the opportunities are countless. In addition, for people with drive and ambitions the world is truly not enough.

Nursing is a profession with much wider and greater than the world ever knows. Today they are sheet anchor. It has transformed the narrow confines of traditional nurses to professional nurses with wider responsibility. We have to equip them with better skill and higher education. Today Curriculum is reviewed, revised and restructured for improving the quality of human life. In this new dispensation they will become resource to people and the essence of community health. Nurses works like magic and give client considerable relief from mental anxiety. As hungry man needs food and water, so a sick client needs care and medicines. And the mediator and bridge, link, forming chain in this great nurse is a key force in providing.

Folded computer and television screens come closer to reality. Computers that can be folded up to be in the pocket and television sets that can be ended to view may soon be a reality, thanks to the efforts of researchers from Sony, beginning of a technological revolution for screen display. Such technology can also lead to the mass production of moving image posters for display systems that let readers to upload daily news to an easy to carry display contraption, the researches say. For example, no mean feet- researchers helped create *prosthesis for an athlete* who competed at the Paralympics; plans include similar devices for other disabled people. For example, follow the A, B, C, D, E -that is Avoid alcohol, smoking, Blood pressure control, Cholesterol, Diabetes, and Exercise. Before they seek you, you seek them with early detection. Due to globalization, all advance technology of west available in India but cost factor is more.

Remote diagnosis—on a computer monitor with hightech hub radiologist examines a scan of the skull of a six-year boy who fell off his bicycle. A few minutes later, thousands of miles away, doctors at a hospital in Philadelphia prepare the boy for surgery after receiving an urgent email diagnosing a subdural hemorrhage in the child's brain. India faces an acute shortage of radiologists even as teleradiology clinics sprout up. We can act as extended arm, teleradiology is just the beginning, telecardiology, telepathology, teledermatology, telepathology, and robotic telesurgery are possible in the very near future.

New artificial intelligence dupes people into thinking they are talking with fellow humans-bridging the divide between man and machine. All this only means computers are getting better in conversing with humans, reducing the gap between man and machine.

There was a time not so long ago when getting a second opinion almost always meant going to another qualified doctor that is spending more money, time and effort. Today internet available at home to look for health information at home on line. Up to 75% of online patients with chronic problems have search and taken decision to treat illness or conditions. Recent surge in high speed, always on broadband connectivity has enabled much more frequent and in depth information search which is particularly attractive if something important is at state. Patient go back to doctor with new questions regarding drug, diets or alternative procedures, they also post technical advice on line about managing a certain diseases beside offering advice on how to communicate with health care providers.

Such expanded level mean patient empowerment and more democratization of health care with information no longer following only one way from an erudite doctor to an untaught sufferers. It is certainly better than being very dependent on a physician, surgeon or specialist praising clinician. Largely because of time constrains makes patient full fledged and equal participation in the entire treatment procedure and the system as a whole. Causation, misinformation generated this way can harmful specially taking decisions without supervision or worse self-medication.

The mind is meant to absorb information, transform it into knowledge and lead it into action. Action and speech determine the quality of life. Wise men say that most peoples minds are as hard as rock. Just as rock is impervious to water, information that falls on a hard mind bounces off without trace. A hard mind offers immense resistance. It is full of previously absorbed information that prevents the flow of new knowledge and action. Our mind must be soft as sponge for maximum absorption; just as water, can easily absorb.

Moreover, Computer improves efficiency, decrease expenditure; convey a modern image to patients.

Modern health care delivery system has become very complex and there is need to obtain continuously up dated information that is efficient information transmission. Used in right time for the purpose of solving patients care problems. The development of electronic devices has given added impetus in problems that are difficult to tackle earlier; now detect accurately and rapidly. Today's nurse needs to communicate with people as well as with machines.

Computer technology has undergone significant changes from its inception. Health care institutions must also keep pace with the changes constantly with the invasions of internet essential latest technology. Because it improves efficacy at work, improves the services to the patient, provides better professional care to the patient, and improves profitability, efficient utilization of staff resources, time management.

In clinical too it helps in professional work, data handling, diagnosis and decision, prescriptions, statistics and reference and number of ways. It is useful in mental health and psychiatric nursing. Its technology is widely used. It has potential in continuous medical education and distance learning programme. With the help of internet, worldwide latest information with regard to diagnosis, treatment modalities and other therapeutic measures can be made available. In addition, for clinical conference, storage of information for long and the gigantic database that it can hold and allow to access in variety of formats, helps to undertake any future activity. It is time saving and money saving by reducing stationary costs, better planning of resources information of new drugs, materials and therapies with advancement of science, with the help of internet and multimedia detailed information obtained. It helps to improve the skills or levels of knowledge so that each employee is better equipped. It helps in desired medications in the skills, attitudes to perform job efficiently and effectively.

Every patient has right to know the nature of his illness, its prognosis, its treatment, its preventive, promotive and rehabilitative aspects. In addition, the health problems that he may have to face in the future for that the relatives also should be aware of these facts in order to help the patient. A long life is a gift –if it is a healthy one. Learn how to live better and how to manage the condition that creep up on your body interne, computer too can guide you how to go about. Dialogue with your doctor and ask him to explain the diagnosis and the course of treatment. If you do not get convincing answers, do some research in the internet about the illness, and be armed with information so that you can have a meaningful dialogue with your doctor.

Your health is too important to be left to the experts. Detection of illness is critically important in effective cures. Do research on internet on health issues. Getting older does not interfere with your ability to use a computer. You can enter the world of technology at an awkward age too. New technologies and economic opportunities are influencing the essence and quality of life. Fast changing lifestyle, western culture influence, and electronic media is urgently needed. Better late than never, where hope grows, miracles blossom, fear ends, faith begins. Awareness is power.

Computer influence every sphere of human activity and bringing many changes in education, health care, scientific research, social science, law, music and painting. Uses of computer save the time, economizes energy and help the nurses to provide quality nursing care. You just keep getting better every day. Your best is always the next one. Learning and assimilation what is learnt what remains and becomes basis for future growth and enters into personality. Reconstruct ideas and enlarge interest. Human being has the upper hand on technology.

Many of the places nurses are isolated and all alone aloof working in a place where she has no opportunity to update herself can approach internet and she will be united to the rest of the world nurses and she will come to know what is happening latest in nursing field and where she stands and she needs to pay attention and can improve. Rather than get stagnated and be satisfied with old ways of doing things and not open to see the world around wherein has reached. If she wants to widen her horizons she needs to make personal effort to inform herself with such knowledge.

So many machines and monitors are equipped in certain areas of her department but nurse who works know only the routine function and if she does not explore the possibility that this same machine can be operated differently and has many more information to provide .

If she does she will be enriched and will be assets to her working place. So nurses need to update and be in touch with internet and all that is happening in and around the medical field. Because it is everyday new challenges and new discoveries and researches are being done which are useful for her to know and save life entrusted to her. Because world is moving in fast space and there is so much to know that perhaps one life is not enough only for those who thirst for such knowledge. Knowledge is greatest weapon and the power in today's world and if nurses develop nursing profession will grow and will change radically. Nursing field is progressing yet it needs to progress still faster rate and that will happen if all the nurses develop in the areas of there work with skill and technology.

Surgery Nurse and Client

Nursing is a pillar on which the modern medicare is based, where nurse catch a vision of the challenges of nursing. The marvels of the human body so perfectly the creator has created. Therefore each nurse needs to seek the guidance of the creator, the source and original life giver in caring for his beloved creation who has been entrusted under her care. May it medical or surgical

Surgery, surgeons and nurses have changed considerably in a century, suffering continues the same. Surgical treatments are under taken away from patients own home. The nurse can do much to ally and alleviate the inevitable anxieties of the surgical patient all through, technical competence and anatomical knowledge, in surgeon and nurse alike, no operation could be a success surgery which results in altered body image requires much compassion and understanding.

Every day we see some new development in surgery, and the speed with which these developments occur makes it impossible to comprehend all the update. In addition, progress brings with its own problem. However sophisticated the equipment and no matter how advanced the surgical techniques, clients will continue to need understanding and skilled nursing care when they are ill. There are areas where equipments that are more modern are not available especially in remote areas; the sections on sterilization by boiling and open drop unaesthetic techniques have been retained.

Surgery is one of the most ancient arts in the world. It is almost as old as the world itself. Every person living and working in different surroundings and in different spheres of activity have unique chemistry. They are all different in outlook, in character, different in their reactions to the same diseases. Appreciation of this variation is fundamental principle of good nursing.

Surgical treatment is usually undertaken away from the clients own home. The client's mental outlook, his hopes, will play important part in treatment. The patient and families are free to accept or refuse the surgery. As all the surgical procedures, carry a risk to the patient's life.

Risks are affected by many factors such as age, nutritional state, fluid and electrolyte balance, general health, mental health, attitude, medication taken. Also younger babies because incomplete development of some of the body system. Elderly person too is more likely to have poor circulation, limited heart function, poor nutrition and limited energy. Risk of surgery of obese person is likely to have over worked heart and high blood pressure. Incisions of fatty tissues are more difficult to suture and are more prone to infection.

Malnourished person has a risk of deficient in protein, vitamin, calcium and iron which are necessary for blood clotting, wound and tissue healing. This affects his ability to tolerate surgery and recovery. Patients who have upper respiratory infection make anesthetic problem. A Cardio-vascular disease too increases risk. Good liver function is necessary in the healing process and for the detoxification. Diabetes mellitus has infection risk, smoking irritates the lung complication, and alcohol has many chemical effects in the body altering the action of the nervous system. Emotional health and attitude have definite relation to the out come of patient likely to have an uncomplicated, rapid recovery.

A nurse's comfort and being a sympathetic, reassuring, and listening, her attitude, her explanation, and her attention increases patient's confidence.

In *emergency* when there is an immediate threat of life from hemorrhage, respiratory or intestinal obstruction, or a spreading infection not likely to be controlled by conservative measures alone surgery done.

Planned/elective can be undertaken when clients general and local conditions are controlled to the maximal degree. Timing is an important in surgery. Accurate diagnosis is the corner stone of treatment.

What are the psychological aspects of surgery? What is the duty of a nurse in the operation theater? What are the hazards in the operation theater? What types of anesthesia and what are its complications? What are the surgical instruments commonly and specifically used? Why do we need a theater dress, headwear? How the surgical hand-washing procedure is done and what is its importance? How is the theater cleaning done? How is the theater prepared to receive infected cases? What are the methods of sterilization and disinfections of equipment used? All and more question a surgical nurse need to ask herself and learn all the theatre techniques?

The psychological aspect of surgery is also very important, the importance that of compassion is rooted in the fact that illness creates anxiety, which is heightened if a client is forced to put his life in the hands of people who seem unsympathetic and indifferent. It is too easy to treat a client as just another case that must fit into the pattern of the day's activity, rather than a human being who is perhaps facing the most frightening experience of his life and simply terrified of the impeding surgery.

Nurse should be always alert to the needs of the client. Understanding another person depends on feeling the emotion he feels in a particular situation. Illness deprives him of normal life and work and makes him dependent on others for help. People differ from one another in many ways and not all react to their new environment in the same way. You need to be extra sensitive to children because for them it is a traumatic time.

In preparation of client—consent *signed* by the client before any operative procedure can be undertaken. A careful *history* is important single part of diagnosis. His family history, previous medical history, the exact complaint, the nature of pain, site, should be obtained.

Clinical evaluation—facts discovered by examination, *inspection* reveals at a glance–clients anxiety or distress, fright, depression, indifference, stupor, a flush, pallor, cyanosis, a swelling, a rash can be observed just by looking at client may be informative. Previous scars, dilated veins or any abnormality to be reported.

Palpation done gently with hands can reveal tenderness, stiffness, spasm may be discovered. The presence of the increased peristaltic sounds of intestinal obstruction may be heard with the stethoscope. The nurse's special contribution to diagnosis in careful observation, accurately recorded, is of great value.

Particular attention should be paid to hemorrhage, increase pulse rate, falling blood pressure and subnormal temperature together with cold and clammy are essential to record. There is greater liability to mistakes, for this confirm again is this same client? Is this the correct injection, tablet, blood? Make sure identification of the client.

Surgery, whether elective or emergency is a stressful, complex event. Even today, with advances in surgical techniques and instrumentation as well as in anesthesia, emotional feelings continue. Recent technologic advances have led to more complex procedure, more complicated microsurgical and laser technology, more sophisticated bypass equipment, increased use of laparoscopic surgery and more sensitive monitoring devices, surgery might now involve the transplantation of multiple human organs, the implantation and mechanical devices or the reattachment of body parts.

Advances in aesthesia have kept pace with the newer surgical technologies. More sophisticated monitoring and new pharmacologic agents, such as short acting anesthesia and more effective anti-emetics have combined with improved postoperative pain management techniques to reduce procedures and recovery times.

Concurrent with technologic advances have been changed in the delivery, it is now common for a client to be admitted to the hospital, receive general anesthesia and be discharged home to the care of the family on the same day.

Surgery may be performed for a Varity of reasons. It may be *diagnostic* such as when a biopsy is obtained or an exploratory laparoscopy is performed.

It may be *curative* such as when a tumor mass is excised or an inflamed appendix is removed.

It may be *reparative* such as when multiple wounds must be repaired.

It may be *reconstructive or cosmetic* such as when a mammoplasty or a face-lift is performed.

On the other hand, it may be *palliative* such as when pain must be relieved or a problem compensates, e.g. when a gastronomy tube is inserted to compensate for the inability to swallow food.

Surgery depends on the degree such as emergency, urgent required elective or optional type.

Surgeries are major which are extensive, involves significant, serious risk, may involve significant loss of blood, serious complication may result.

Minor surgeries minimal, few serious complications, involves minimal loss of blood

Optional surgeries performed simply for patients preferences and is not needed

Elective performed for the patients well being but not absolutely necessary.

Surgical procedures are performed to enhance the lives of those receiving them. The patient undergoing surgery hope to have whatever problems they are experiencing corrected so they can live normal life. There are times; however, problems cannot surgically corrected such surgical procedures results in a poor outcome or possibly death. No surgery is without risk even for the healthiest patient. Nurse's responsibility is patient's safety, confidentiality and dignity must be maintained.

Nursing intervention during surgery is to assist anesthetist, if arrest occurs, respond immediately to assist in establishing airway, provide cardiac arrest tray, emergency drug , syringes, long needles, assist surgeon with cardiac massage. Monitor vital signs and effects of CNS depressants for 24 hours after administration. Keep patient warm during recovery, watch for shivering, temperature, blood pressure, respiration, monitor liver function after surgery and observe urine output closely.

Observe allergic reactions, COPD, hepatic/renal dysfunction, record vitals, heart rate, strength, respiratory rate and depth, oxygen saturation, skin color.

She should be aware of what operative procedure was performed. What pathological disorders encountered during surgery. Did the patient suffer any complication during surgery and what interventions were insinuated. Was cancer or other unexpected problem discovered.

Nurse must always be focused that Surgery and anesthesia places client at risk for multiple complications or adverse events. Team works collectively to implement professional standard and care, to foster high quality of client outcome.

Client may feel relaxed and prepared or fearful and highly stressed. They may develop the fears about loss of control, fear of the unknown, fear of pain during and after, alteration in body structure or functions and death. He is subject to multiple risks as all major body systems are disturbed by anesthesia and surgery.

Although most clients can effectively compensate for surgical trauma risk including drug toxicity, faulty equipment and human error, over sedation, infection, nerve damage, and cardiac problem can take place.

The intra operative nurse maintains surgical standards of care, identifying existing risk factor and assist in modifying complicating factors to help reduce operative risks.

The circulating nurse monitors and documents specific activities throughout the operative procedures to ensure safety and well-being. Health hazards associated with the surgical environment includes safety in operation theater exposure to blood and body fluids. Hazards associated with laser beams and exposure to latex, radiation and toxic agents.

During the postoperative period, nursing care is directed at re-establishing the client's physical equilibrium, elevating pain, preventing complication and teaching client self-care. Collection of specimen, and bowel, pain and sleep, diet, oxygen therapy, breathing exercise, drainage, care of wound, removal of stitches, early mobilization are some of the points to bear in the postoperative period. Prevent thrombophebitis and improve circulation flex the knee, raise the foot, coughing and deep breathing exercise aids in preventing lung infection. Watch for airway obstruction, change position, assist with ambulation, promote comfort, rest and sleep, watch for chilling, attention to hygiene and care of surgical wound is important. Ongoing care in the community through home care, clinic visits, follow-up facilities an uncomplicated recovery.

Bacterial contamination continues to be the greatest hazard of surgery. Infection is the state or a condition in which the body, or a part of it, is invaded by pathogenic microorganisms. Surgical sepsis results from many factors, one of which is bacterial contamination. Strict aseptic discipline must be applied at all times and no amount of drugs, devices or architectural innovations can compensate for this.

All infections are caused by microorganism. These are divided into bacteria, viruses, fungi and protozoa. Organisms, which cause disease, are known as pathogens. Infection is the successful invasion and growth of micro-organism in a body tissue. The severity or mildness of the resulting diseases depends upon the dosage and virulence of the organisms and the resistance of the client. Inflammation is the response of the body to an irritant, the irritant may be burn, a chemical, a wound or a micro-organism. Restoration of full function and health should be the aim of the nurse. The client is more likely to continue treatment until cure is effected and to cooperate if nurse doctor treat him with human understanding tact and compassion.

Admission to hospital has always exposed the client to the risk of infection. Infection prolongs convalescence, increases morbidity and, if sufficiently severe, will start a chain of events which ultimately may result in death. Prevention of infection which is the most demanding of his requirements is the most difficult to satisfy. Sterilization is the destruction of all microorganisms and spores. It demands constant vigilance. Microorganisms are found everywhere. Asepsis is the underlying principle of surgery by which organisms are denied accesses to the client.

Poor technique in the handling of sterilized instruments and materials may infect the client. Faulty packaging of disposable articles and faulty storage may result in infection. The nurse should be clean in her person, her hands kept free from cracks fingernails kept short. The duties of a theater nurse, duties of the circulating nurse responsible for specific assigned jobs. The nurse must always be conscious of the client's feelings, a friendly word and a sympathetic ear will do much to help the client and allay fears.

The nurse must practice good surgical asepsis, thoroughly document care, and emphasize client safety in all phase of care. To ensure quality outcome and prevent the complications effective discharge planning needs to be done. The continuing care that is convalescence to home based which requires education and follow up of filmily for positive surgical outcomes. The discovery of anesthesia 1840s revolutionized surgery. Surgery classified according to seriousness, urgency and purpose.

Nurse must learn technical terms used for different surgeries and procedures such as- Hysterectomy that is used for denoting removal or excision of a structure.

Endoscope inspection of the interior of an organ or passage by means of special instrument, usually carrying light.

Gastrostomy constructing an artificial opening into an organ.

Laparotomy incising and opening the abdomen.

Arthroplasty an operation designed to increase the amount of movement at a joint.

Arthrotomy making an opening into a joint for drainage or exploration.

Curettage removing tissues by scraping.

Episiotomy incision of the perineum in the second stage of labour, to prevent extensive laceration.

Lithotripsy/litholopaxy crushing a vesicle urinary bladder calculus by means of an instrument.

Nurses will have to learn elements of theater; control of infections, sterilization and disinfections of equipment, types of anesthesia and its complications. Handle surgical instruments and know the different types of surgeries such as operation of nose, ear, throat, ophthalmic surgery, traumatic surgery, radium insertion, orthopedic surgery, neurological, vascular, gynecological, genitor urinary tract, etc. That will increase her efficiency and give her a job satisfaction of the theater nurse and can make a significant contribution to improve client care.

Types of anesthesia–IV anesthesia are most common method. Drugs are used in sufficient dose to produce light sleep or in drip to provide prolonged sleep. E.g. short acting Thiopentone 2.5% given and long acting Pentobarbitone 2.5% is given.

Spinal and epidural anesthesia is given by injecting a solution into the cerebrospinal fluid through a lumber puncture needle so that, it bathes a portion of the spinal cord and associated nerve roots. Common drug use is cinchocain one in two hundred often dissolved in C.S.F.

Epidural entails injection in large volume solution into the space outside the durra, thus affecting the nerves as they transverse the extradural space to escape from vertebral column. Xylocaine 1-2% common in use. Both techniques cause fall in blood pressure if the drugs reach thoracic levels.

Inhalation agent used which includes Nitrous oxide Cyclopropane gases, Ethyl chloride which is all volatile liquids.

Rectal instillation method of induction is used for children. A warmed solution is introduced with either a catheter and syringe or a suppository. In this way child within 15-20 minutes goes to sleep.

Local anesthesia injection Novocain, Xylocaine 0.25% to 2.0% injections is used. Client is awake throughout procedures.

End tracheal anesthesia- intubations assure a patent airway and can provide a gas and watertight connection between client and machine. Proper size tube passed via vocal cords in to trachea with aid of laryngoscope.

Indications for end tracheal intubations are:

- Client with risk of regurgitation of stomach contents, or blood in the airway–this procedure is done.
- Client to be artificially ventilated that is those on muscle relaxants for thoracic and abdominal surgery.
- Operation on the head and neck, to remove the anesthetist from the immediate field of operation.
- Client with pre-existing respiratory obstruction.
- Client with whom it is difficult to maintain an airway using a mask, client lying in prone position and those with anatomical abnormalities of the face or neck.

Variety of tubes sizes with number available, different needles and cannula available.

During anesthesia client once put to sleep must be kept asleep for the duration of the operation and yet wake as soon as possible afterwards and recover all his protective reflexes.

There is apparatus for inhalation anesthesia. Oxygen is often blown under the mask through tube:

– Black and white shoulder contains oxygen cylinder.
– Blue contains nitrous oxide.
– Orange cone contains cyclopropane.
– Grey green contains carbon dioxide.

Each gas has a different pin-index fitment, which will connect only to its own reducing valve. Thus, only cylinders of the correct gas can be fitted into the appropriate yokes each gas pass its own flow meter.

Management of Cardiac Arrest

Sudden cessation of cardiac action in a client not expected to die need not be lethal. If oxygenated blood is artificially pumped to the brain within three minutes, then life can be maintained until heart resumes normal action.

Cardiac arrest is of two kinds that is total absence of cardiac contraction where there is uncoordinated twitching of the heart muscles which pumps no blood into the arteries. In addition, I in 10,000 adrenaline, 10% calcium gluconate and 8.4% sodium bicarbonate injection required.

Ventricular fibrillation requires external electrical defibrillation. Repeated shocks at increasing voltages with message continued until normal rhythm is re-established. Same above injection is given.

Diagnosis by sudden cessation of respiration with cyanosis.

Absent pulse in major arteries and pallor.

Widely dilated pupils.

Treatment

Ventilate with pure oxygen, intubations mouth to mouth ventilation, set up IV drip, ECG re-recording, organize timekeeper to call out half-minute intervals. External cardiac massage, defibrillator and resuscitation trolley

Some surgeries involve major extensive significant serious risk. Check wounds drain sites, open wounds, central venous pressure low bleeding usually in peritoneal or pleural cavities or retroperitoneal areas, sepsis, cardiac arrest, drug sensitivity, pulmonary embolism, adrenal failure. The nurse plays a critical role in the postoperative care of the patient. Today surgery rang is from OPD procedures to complex IPD procedures. No matter what type of surgery is performed, however, the patient needs a great deal of expert nursing care. The quality of that nursing care can determine whether the patient has a successful preoperative experience.

Categories of surgical procedure as mentioned above is diagnostic -is to confirm a diagnosis; to estimate the extent of disease and to confirm a diagnosis, to remove or repair damaged or diseased tissues or organs. Emergency-performed to maintain life, maintain organ or limb function, stop hemorrhage. Imperative requires surgical intervention within 24-48 hours. Exploratory, Curative, Reconstructive-partial or complete restoration of a damaged organ or tissue to its original appearance and function.

Constructive—repairing of a congenitally defective organ by improving its function or appearance. Palliative-relieves symptoms but does not cure underlying disease.

What operative procedure was performed? What were the patient's vital signs in the operation room? What were the patient's blood loss, fluids or blood infused and urine output? What was the patient's general condition? What are the patient's medical diagnosis, patients medical history and daily medications? What anesthetic agents, narcotics, muscle relaxants, antibiotics and steroids has the patient received? Did the patient suffer any complications during surgery? What interventions were instituted? What was the outcome? What pathologic disorders were encountered during surgery? Was cancer or some other unexpected problem discovered? When will the patient be told that the cancer is present? Are there any specific symptoms or complications to observe? What symptoms should be reported immediately? Are there physician's orders to be carried out immediately?

Anesthetics are drugs that are used to bring about a state in which painful surgical procedures can be performed painlessly and safely. Some gases and vapors of volatile liquids are administered by inhalation, IV rout. Depending on type of surgical procedures that is to be performed. Sensory blocks, the looses of pain perception. Mental block a state in which the patient is unaware of what is going on and is later totally unable to recall what took place. Lock of reflexes, peripherally, in order to reduce various involuntary responses that might adversely affect the patients respiratory, cardiovascular, gastrointestinal functions. Motor block of the spinal reflexes that maintain muscle tone is often desirable during abnormal surgery.

Local anesthetic drugs that are used to cause a loss of feeling especially pain, without making the patient unconscious. They temporarily interrupt the production and conduction of nerve impulses. Certain local anesthetic are employed mainly to relieve itching and pain caused by skin disorder.

These are some of the responsibilities and basic knowledge that an nurse must know towards patient who undergoes surgery.

Nurse's Responsibility in Keeping Surgical Asepsis Principles

Always face the sterile field, do not turn your back or side on a sterile field. Keep sterile equipment above your waist level or above table level. It is considered as margins of safety and promote maximum sterile field. Do not speak or cough over a sterile field to prevent droplet infection. Never search or cross a sterile field gravity causes micro-organism to fall into sterile field. Prevent excessive air circulation as micro-organism travel in air. Keep unsterile object away form sterile field and keep it dry surface. Never assume that an object is sterile. Always check the expiry date, wrapper. Avoid sweeping and dusting when sterile objects are open. Remove the cover of the container when necessary and only for a short period.

CHAPTER 7

Research-Nurse's Role with an Eye on the Future

The purpose of this chapter is to strengthen the knowledge of nurses regarding the concept of research, research process is to enable her to utilize her research findings to provide quality care. As nurses are available when and wherever wanted by the needy and who closely follow the scientific nursing practice.

Scientific research in nursing- knowledge acquisition is essential in contributing to scientific research in nursing. The expansion of technology, change in health care delivery system. A person continuously takes in information and through the process of critical thinking evaluates numerous process of information to understand experiences. Nurses interested in acquiring knowledge about a wide range of human needs and responses to health problems. Identification of clinical problems in nursing practice, by assisting with organizational data collection, approximately using research finding in clinical practice.

Nursing research improves the practice of nursing and raises the standard of the professional involvement in nursing research takes place in many ways. Designing, studying, being part of research team, collecting data, using researching finding to change clinical practice, improving physical outcomes.

A scientific investigation is an orderly, planned and controlled way and study reality that can be applied to general situation and contribution to the testing and theory about people, places or life events. Nursing research is conducted to study the physical and psychological responses of people of all ages in health and illness.

Research finding have rapidly expanded last few years, advancement of nursing science, the multidisciplinary nature and the nursing profession changes nurses to be knowledgeable concerning current research in the discipline of nursing, it is means for improving the health and welfare of people. It is a way to identify new knowledge, improve professional education and practice and use resources effectively. Research based intervention. Research as a basis for practice.

Research is scientific approach which is a logical, orderly and objective, e.g. to help a patient to sleep nurse uses methods to help him sleep like back rub, making clean and comfortable bed, dim light, talking to worried and anxious patient frequently, which measures are considered in greater depth with scientific approach, a patient uses relaxation exercise to reduce postoperative pain. Pain severity rate of wound healing and body temperature, body change can be measured.

Read the nursing literature, especially when there are different views on the same subject. Ask for help if you are uncertain about an aspect of patient care. Report any problem immediately. If your knowledge cause's you a question a physicians order be thorough in whatever you do. Look for different approaches if interventions are not working. Always ask why, a clinical signs and symptoms can indicate a verity of problems, explore and learn more about so as to make right clinical judgment. Recognize when your opinions may conflict with those of a patient, review your position and decide how best to proceed to reach mutually beneficial outcomes. Recognize when you need more information to make a decision. When you are newly assigned to a clinical division and you are unfamiliar with the patient ask to be oriented to the area. Keep updated on new approaches of care, practice hygienic skills before giving hygienic care. Modify nursing care plan.

Are there any areas that need to be improved or changed? What will influence your ability to adopt any need changes? Are the risk factors present that could be modified? What resources are available to you? What level of quality health care, or how will you plan discharge care better. Develop a vision for nursing, making communication a priority advanced educational and management practice. Goal setting, time analysis, set periods, education, quality management.

Continuous quality improvement, team work, group interaction skill, belief in people, clarify current knowledge of process redesign the process, **re-evaluate.** Scope and key aspect of clinical areas monitor outcome, establish criteria for measuring quality of nursing care, education and research.

Goal of nursing is to facilitate the body's reparative process by manipulating patient's environment. To develop interaction between nurse and assisting patient gains independence quickly as possible assist patient in overcoming obstacles to reduce stress and help in recovering process, to maintain maximum levels of total wellness by purposeful interventions, to respond to human needs carrying as a central focus on human being as living unity.

Nursing is rooted in helping individuals to regain, maintain or improve their health, prevent illness, find comfort and retain their individuality and dignity. In the face of rapid change, nursing must lead the way and retain its values for client care while meeting the challenges of new roles and new responsibilities in the health care environment. The future of health care needs to find ways of redesign their services, and reduce unnecessary costs, improves high quality client care.

Low socioeconomic status people who live in poverty are more likely to live in hazardous environment, work at high-risk jobs, eat less nutritious diets and have multiple stressors in their life. They lack finances, unavailable transportations, have chronic health needs. Nurses need to help them to promote and increase their ability to improve their health statues.

Research provides a solid foundation on which nurses base their practice. **Research means to search again or examine carefully.** Through the use of systematic process provides a scientific basis for nursing practice and effective nursing intervention. Identify new knowledge and use resources effectively. **Research based practice is essential if the nursing profession** is to meet the needs of society for safe, effective and efficient care.

The scientific method is the foundation of research. It is the most reliable and objective of all methods of gaining knowledge. Scientific method is a systematic step-by-step process. Conducting an investigation are undertaken in a systematic, orderly fashion. Problems are studied in depth. Nurses are interested in acquiring knowledge about a wide range of human needs and responses to health problems. Nursing research uses many methods to study clinical problems.

Nurses often need to find research articles on subjects that interest them, research activities. Knowledge is acquired through tradition, from authorities, in a field through experience, through problem solving and critical thinking and through application of the scientific method. Nursing research is conducted to study the physical and psychological response of people of all ages in health and illness. To determine whether research findings can be used as a basis for nursing practice, the nurses should consider the scientific worth of to study the substantiating evidence provided in other studies, the similarity of the research setting to the nurses own clinical practice setting, the status of current nursing.

We are living in an era of fast scientific changes affecting our lives and working conditions. New technologies and economic opportunities are influencing the essence and quality of life. This is the space and nuclear age and is full of changes. These changes have greatly influenced the society and the life style of our people. Such technological changes have brought about tremendous development of biomedical science resulting in newer diagnostic equipment, newer drugs and new monitoring system in all field of health all over the world.

We need to increase our knowledge in all areas of nursing care. So that, the profession will grow in stature and lay down a base of perfect knowledge for future generations of nurses to come

Rapid scientific progress is an important reason for continuous educational program. **Everyday some new knowledge, new discoveries are added**. Interventions in many branch of science makes changes in medical practice. These changes are so rapid that it is difficult to keep pace with them. You will need to increase knowledge and improve performance as changes that taking place in medical science.

Research in nursing plays an important role in development and progress of nursing profession. It is a **systematic study of problem using scientific technique, which can provide with facts and solution to the problem.**

Its purpose is to find out a valid answer to problems. It is a quest for new knowledge. It is a systematic technique to the solution. It requires brode knowledge based on promoting human health, aided by specialist areas of health care practice. It gives new direction to the nursing care practice.

Steps- identify the problem, determine the purposes of study problem, review the literature for reference on similar problem, develop a theoretical frame work, identify the study assumption, acknowledge the limitations for the study, formulate the hypothesis/research question, define study variable, select the resources design, identify the population, select the sample, conduct a pilot study, collect the data, organize the data for analysis, analyze the data, interpret the findings, communicate the finding.

In modern era, research has been part of development process in every field.

Clinical research education has unique advantages due to the collaboration- opportunity to gain a global perspective and have an edge over others. Research in clinical and biomedical sciences, Educational opportunities enables you to be competent, consistent and confident at the highest level; Enhances knowledge and your personality to create.

Show the way- invest in *education for* a better tomorrow. One good teacher can teach millions of children through technology. The teacher should just inspire, and use interactive electronic media to teach science, geography and other subjects. The corporate sector should come forward to provide teaching soft ware. Investigating in education is not survival but business. Human resources will be the biggest problem tomorrow, so cooperators must invest in education today. We must focus on the 70% population in rural India where educational infrastructure is abysmal. No English education to rural masses. In India is to be world player. It is crucial that the masses learn English. English gives us an edge.

Every business house wants to grow by leaps and bounds and this would ensure that they have their own trained, focused, loyal labor force. It is not charity; it is a long-term investment. We talk in terms of millions of graduates, but by international standards, many are not employed. We are a mixed bag. We have capability to cross the economic threshold we are at, but only with the right kind of focus and inspiration. Our quality education is extremely poor to reach full potentials. We need vibrant economic activity that translates into jobs for education. Nearly 3.5 millions children in this country do not go to school. Education is the only way can make a difference. The youth will lead us into the future. Youth are our future.

Research—tiny microscope to revolutionize diagnosis. A pocket sized microscope diagnosing diseases like malaria. Built on to a single image-sensing chip and does not need any lenses. The whole thing is truly compact, it could new put in a chip phone and it can just sunlight for illumination. Health workers in rural areas could carry cheap, compact molds to test individuals for malaria. An implantable microscope analysis system can autonomously screen for an isolate cancer cells in blood circulation, thus providing important diagnostic information and helping arrest the spread of cancer.

In many health care settings, nurses are responsible to provide meaningful information with the development of sophisticated technology that allows measurement of functions in the body. Broader research to validate nursing diagnoses and nursing interventions for clients with spinal problems is needed. Certain diseases nursing research has been limited. Further nursing research is needed to answer the possible questions for further nursing research.

Assignments and Findings

What are the best preventive measures to avoid in back injury?

How can the nurse best meet the psychological needs of the client with spinal cord injury?

What are the best pain relief medications that the nurse can use for the client with a vertebral or spinal injury?

How can the nurse collaborate most efficiently and effectively with physical and occupational therapists in providing holistic care for the client with a spinal injury or disease?

What are the best interventions to prevent restlessness and agitation in the client with Alzheimer's disease?

How can a nurse maintain positive self-esteem and body image with Parkinson's diseases?

Do client with sudden vision loss and those with chronic vision loss use similar and difficult coping mechanism?

Are clients with learning problems at an increased risk for isolation during hospitalization?

Are clients aware of medication actions that affect the ear and hearing?

What are the consequences of hearing impairment for the client and his family?

What is the effect of hearing loss to the physically and psychologically needs of the elderly?

What nursing measures best decrease the recurrence of otitis media in young adult?

How can the nurse effectively help a client with an amputation improve body image and self-esteem?

What is the best method of immobilization a fractures hit in a disoriented elderly client?

What factors motivate client to adhere to a regimen of dental and oral hygiene?

What barrier exists to seeking early health care for client with gastric symptoms? What are the nursing strategies are effective in reducing these barriers?

How can the nurse best help the client with a body image disturbances related to having an ilestomy/colosomy?

How can quality of life be measured after transplantation?

How can the nurse asses the degree of jaundice in dark skinned client?

How can the nurse help the client with pancreatic cancer prepare for the poor prognosis associated with the diseases?

What are the behavior and feelings about food and weight in elderly clients who refuse food or who have a very low weight?

How can the nurse best provide emotional support for the obese client during a weight loss program what strategies can nurses use to help diabetic client develop and maintain life long healthy behavior?

What is the relation between perceived emotional stress and the course of skin disease?

What type of community programmes is best for teaching burn prevention?

What pain relief measure work best for the client with urinary calculi?

How do client with a known family history of renal diseases cope with the uncertainty of renal failure?

What should include on tools to identity the woman at high risk for psychologic difficulties after breast surgery?

What nursing interventions promote self-esteem in positive client with a reproductive dysfunction?

What is the most effective method of teaching clients about risk assessment?

What are the long-term psychologic effects of chronic STD infections?

SCIENTIFIC RESEARCHES AND NEW TECHNOLOGICAL DISCOVERIES

Here there are some of the scientific researches and new technological discoveries which will help you understand better the concept of researches undertaken; and many months and years gone by to come to this stage of research as you see in front of you.

- *Scar free*—A new procedure allows doctors to extract a donors kidney through the navel, thus preventing scarring, technique may also be employed in other operations, with single incision in belly button, will reduce recover time less and no scars. The operation involves making a three quarter inch incision in the interior of the belly button and inserting a tube like port with several round entry points, which allows for the further insertion of a camera and other tools into the belly. The belly is inflated with carbon dioxide to provide maneuvering room. The kidney is then freed from connecting tissue, wrapped in a plastic bag and removed through the naval when the blood supply is cut. A donor is one of the most altruistic people you will ever meet, he is giving kidney, so they decrease anything you can do to make it better for that patient.

- **Passing it on** *Genetic* **clues** to what run in the family according to new science, known as epigenetic, your ancestors diet, smoking habits, obesity could be affecting you today. In turn, your lifestyle could affect your children and grandchildren. For millions of people choosing to delay parenthood this raises new moral questioners. If we drink heavily, take drugs, get fat or wait too long to reproduce, then epigenetic might start tying up some of the wrong genes and loosening the bonds on others. Sometimes those changes will affect sperm and egg cells.

- *Research*—development effective **new computer** *controlled inhaler* that is far more effective than the traditional one. Inhaling a drug in aerosol form is an increasingly common way of treating cancers, Aids, diabetes and asthma. However, inhalers are notoriously ineffective because at best, they deliver 20% of their load into the lungs and at worst; they deliver less then 5%. The rest is left in the mouth and throat or are blown back out into the air- particularly if the user's intake a breath is not well synchronized with the aerosol jet. The inhaler measures airflow around its nozzle to determine the best moment to release a powered drug such that it achieves maximum penetration into the lungs. The new type of inhaler can target specific areas of the lungs with a drug. This is done by injecting power into different parts of the airflow, aiming the drug towards the right or left lung or even areas within each lung.

- Two innovations may make *dentists drill and toothbrush obsolete:* a method to make teeth heal themselves, and a new mouthwash that cleans teeth when exposed to light. Get ready to bid adieu to the dreaded dentists drill and floss-creating toothbrush, a radical *new inventions* by British dental researchers that could change the way we take care of teeth. Scientists have come up with a solution that can mimic the bone forms new teeth, which would do away with drilling and filling by making it possible for the teeth to repair themselves. Along with this discovery, the researchers have also formulated a mouthwash that kills plaque-causing bacteria when a light is shone into the mouth.

- *Self-repairing-teeth:* We looked at a way to treat early decay and avoid drilling, a new protein that would make it possible to repair holes naturally in the enamel on the surface of the tooth. This works by creating a scaffold, which attracts the minerals that form enamel, just like the body creates new teeth. The substance can be painted on teeth in the early stages of tooth decay, to fill up tiny holes before they become large holes full of decay. In fact, this treatment could also be used for filling tiny holes in the teeth's dentine, which causes intense sensitivity to hot, and cold food or drinks. Safety checks are already under way for the protein used in the treatment, as it is absolutely new. In addition, they hope that it can enter trials early next year aiming to gain a license within five years. We feel confident that this is a major step for the future.

- The other **invention is** *mouthwash* using a molecule that is absorbed by bacteria in the mouth. This molecule destroys the bug from within after being activated by a bright light- a method called photodynamic therapy. There is no risk for client in case mouthwash is swallowed, as the molecule is completely safe. It is safe alternative way of improving oral hygiene for those clients for whom brushing is not feasible. The methods also could be used for gum diseases, which is the major cause of tooth loss. It could be inserted below the gum line by a hygienist during a routine checking up, with a tiny fiber-optic light source to destroy the bacteria. More research is still on.

- Now, a **painless** *"micro needle"* that mimics a mosquito's bite will be soon in the market, which too will enhance to control *malaria* researchers say.

- *New mesh* could help eradicate *malaria*. Now Germany based chemical company has developed the interceptor- a net coated with the insecticide fen Dona that remains effective against malaria causing mosquitoes for several years. Brief contact with the net is sufficient to seal a mosquito's fate. Within as little as 5 minutes after contacts the insect drops paralyzed to the floor, the effect known as knock down. Moreover, almost all mosquitoes die.

- *Malaria*—way to keep RBC alive found in malaria parasites secretes a 'glue' which causes red blood cells to stick to the blood vessel walls, so that they cannot be cleaned by the spleen. Now, researchers have found that removing just one protein can prevent the infected cells from sticking.

- *Mosquitoes*—prefer men, says study two Mumbai based doctors two years study concludes that mosquitoes are attracted to male sex hormones, men of 15-40 years are more susceptible fundamental research has established that and its explanation found in their sex hormones. Doctor Shobbona Sharma, an expert in malaria and professor of biology at TIFR Tata institute.

  Virus can wipe out malaria mosquitoes can 'instruct' the insect to die before it transmits the disease. Medical break through discovered that a virus which they claim is infectious to the **Anopheles** Gambia mosquito that is responsible for transmitting malaria. According to them, the virus could someday be used to pass on new genetic information's to anopheles mosquitoes to control malaria. As part of stages to control malaria. Which kills over one million people worldwide. In theory, we could use this virus to produce a lethal toxin in the mosquitoes or instruct the mosquito to die after 10 days, which is before it can transmit the malaria parasite to humans. However, these concepts are many years away.

  Did you know the first effective treatment for malaria was the bark of the cinchona tree-growing on the slopes of the Andes in Peru, which contains quinine. The inhabitants of Peru to control malaria used this natural product. In the 1640s, the Jesuits introduced this practice to Europe, where it was rapidly accepted.

- *Tuberculosis*—**rapid** *diagnostic test* relief for tuberculosis patients MDR-TB. The new technology is a revolutionary breakthrough fighting killer cough. TB is contagious and spreads through the air. If untreated, each person with active TB infects 10-15 people every year. One third-2 billion of the world's population is infected with TB. One person is infected with TB every second. TB kills 4400 people everyday. 1.7 million People died from TB in 2006. There were 9.2 million new cases of TB in 2006. Multi drug resistant / MDR-TB is difficult and expensive to treat and fails to respond to standard first line drugs. Every year, an estimated 4.9 lakh new MDR TB cases occur causing 1.3 lakh deaths. Five percent of all new cases are MDR TB in India. India has 3.8 million TB at any time. India records 18 lakh new cases of it annually and over six lakh Indians are unaware that they suffer from TB.

- *New drug trial* may be in India. Scientists have identified Moxifloxacin as a drug with potential to cut the length of treatment for TB from present 6 months to 4 moths. There is increased TB globally, urgent need for treatment combination of shorter duration. Reduction of treatment time to 4 months would mean less exposure to drugs for the patient and interaction with health services therefore reducing their workload.

  For mere living is not a good, but living well. Accordingly the wise man will live as long as he ought, not as long as he can. He always reflects concerning the quality not the quantity of his life. it is not a question of dying earlier or later, but of dying well or ill. And dying well means escape from the danger of living ill.

- *Breakthrough may lead to new drug against TB-* scientist have figured out how TB tricks the immune system, a discovery that could lead to new anti-TB drugs. Drugs that cure tuberculosis have been available for decades, but the poorer counties TB continues to ravage.

- For a *model, pregnancy* researchers have used video game technology to create precise 3-D models of pregnant women; study can help in safer, more accurate and more effective therapy without harming the fetus.

- *Research-**Cardio mobile device**-* to keep a tab on heart attack rehabilitation scientists have developed a cardio mobile monitoring system that acts as a mini ECG helping heart attack rehab patients to keep a check on their heart signal at any time and place. The program allows people who have been in hospital for a heart attack or heart surgery to undergo a week walking exercise rehabilitation program whenever it is convenient, while having there heart signal, location and speed monitored in real time. If there is any problem with the heart signal we can immediately contact the patient, and consult with the cardiologist if needed. In addition, if there is an emergency we can direct the paramedics to the exact location immediately.

- If the *heart* is compared to a house, a heart attack can be put down to a plumbing problem. Sudden cardiac death, in which the heart stops working abruptly and without warning, is like a short circuit.

Sudden cardiac death (SCD), is also called cardiac arrest, is used to describe a situation in which the heart abruptly and without warning stops working, so no blood can be pumped to the rest of the body.

It is responsible for half of all heart disease deaths. It is a catastrophic presentation in a variety of cardiac diseases and on some occasions, happens without an obvious structural heart disease.

Heart attack is the result of a sudden blockage of an artery supplying blood to the heart muscle leading to muscle damage, pump failure and its consequences. Sudden cardiac death occurs due to electrical system malfunctioning of the heart leading to complete cessation of heartbeat or a chaotic beating, which is not compatible with life.

If the heart is compared with house, a heart attack can be put down to a plumbing problem. Sudden cardiac death can be due to an electrical problem. The heart has a built-in electrical system.

Who is at risk? Seventy-five percent of people who die of SCD show sign of previous heart attack. Eighty percent people have CHD. The signs of SC arrest have an abnormal heart rate arrhythmia, tachycardia, episodes of fainting.

Prevention of SCD, living a heart healthy life, which includes exercising regularly, eating healthful foods, maintaining reasonable weight and avoiding smoking. Treating and monitoring diseases and conditions that can contribute to heart problems, including high blood pressure, high cholesterol and diabetes is also important. Taking regular medications and doing tests.

High blood pressure or arterial hypertension is generally a persistent elevation of systolic blood pressure of 140 mm of Hg or above and of diastolic pressure of 90 mm of Hg or above. Increased BP level is related to increased severity of arteriosclerosis, stroke, nephropathy.

- *Research—**Indian doctors use robot for the chest surgery**-* all the patients were suffering from myasthenia gravis, a disease characterized by nervous and muscular weakness, walking and chewing problems, and double vision. To cure the disease, the thymus gland needs to be removed. The thymus gland is deep inside the chest. Earlier, we used to tear apart the ribs for the operation. Now with the robotic assistance, the same operations can be effectively performed.

- New chips to allow home tests for illness' lab-on-a-chip' tool may soon make a new generation of instant home tests possible for food contamination and toxic gases. 'Lego like kit that brings micro fluidic devices to the masses. The kits that operate with tiny drops of liquid allow researchers to conduct quick, efficient experiments. They can be engineered to mimic the human body closely, and are useful in growing and testing cells, among other applications.

- *Meditation slows AIDS progression* in just a few weeks, perhaps by affecting the immune system, US researchers reported. Findings could offer a cheap and pleasant way to help people battle the incurable and fetal condition. Tested a stress-lowering program called mindfulness meditation. Avoid thinking of the past and worry about the future. CD4 counts measured after and before. The meditation classes included eight week two hours sessions a daylong retreat and daily practice.

- *Cigarette smoke* worsens family, other viral infection, often mild in non-smokers, can seriously hit smokers, scientist explain smokers die with COPD, chronic obstructed pulmonary disease.

- *Eye examination* is not required only when you need glasses. By viewing the health of the blood vessels inside the eye, one can spot serious conditions while they are still in the early stages. E.g. a high blood glucose level can weaken and damage the tiny blood vessels next to the retina a tiny leak from damaged blood vessels that is one of the indications of diabetes. High blood pressure, glaucoma, macular degeneration, brain tumor, eye cancer can be detected early by this will save your sight and life.

- *IVF test tube infertile couples-* the treatment involves surgically removing eggs from a woman's ovaries and combining them with sperm in the lab, doctors then pick the best embryos one or two and implant them in the women's uterus.

- *Excessive cell* usage may lead to cancer, experts have warned.

  *Investigations—***red alert on** *cell tower radiation-* radiation levels emitted from phone towers dangerously high across city. People are exposed to the gravest possible health risk. What radiation can to your health- constant headache, sleep disorders and heart problems? They have been known to intensify in many a case into leukemia, brain tumor and other cancers. Known effects to the brain include in ODC activity and decreases in the brain metabolism. Special risks lie to pregnant women and children. Children due to thinner skulls and increased mitotic activity in their cells, and pregnant woman because the EMR continuously reacts within the developing embryo. Also at great risk are, clients carrying pacemaker, which the radiation may interfere with to a point of fatality.

- New research could lead to drugs that help *erase traumatic memories-* researchers have identified the brain mechanism that switches off traumatic feelings associated with bad memories- a finding that could lead to the development of drugs to treat panic disorder. They found that a small brain protein called neuropeptide S is involved in erasing traumatic responses to adverse memories by working on a tiny group of neurons inside the amygdale where those memories are stored. These findings can help the development of new drugs to treat conditions in which people are haunted by persistent fears, or other panic disorders.

- *Researchers* ***put Exercise in a pill****—*US researchers have developed a new drug that that emulates the effects of exercising; could help in treating obesity and diabetic in future. For all who have wondered if they could enjoy the benefits of exercise without the pain of exertion, the answer one day may be, yes, just take a pill that tricks the muscles into thinking they have been working out furiously.

- Here is couch potato's dream; what if *drug* could help you gain some of the benefits of exercise without working up a sweat? The drug in the new study appears to act especially on a process in muscles that boosts endurance. The experiment on mice is done and been successful; and the result likely to apply to people, who control muscle tone with the same underlying genes as do mice. If the drugs work and prove to be safe, they could be useful in a wide range of settings. They should help people who are too frail to exercise and those who with health problem. Researcher Ron Evans holds a vial of a drug that boosts the effect of exercise in mice, which he touts as exercise in a pill. The drug held promise for treating disease and help in treating diabetic and obesity. For majority of people she said it would be better to do exercise than to take a pill.

- *Discovery-which under further research- and further studies on biological science still on- New pill may let dieters* eat normally-scientist in the UK may have discovered a new anti-obesity pill that could free dieters from eating restrictions and also slow down the aging process. The pill may lock in the benefits of dieting, allowing dieters to return to normal eating without putting on weight. The pill- dietary supplement called alpha-lipoic acid also slows aging, which is a known effect of low-caloric diets. It indicates that by following a calorie restriction diet for six months and then taking this while eating, normally people will experience life extension effects.

- *Nerve cells grown from new-style stem cells*- ordinary skin cells taken from clients with a fatal and incurable nerve disease have been transformed into nerve cells in a first step toward treating them, the US researchers reported. They transformed the cells from two clients with amyotrophic lateral sclerosis into motor neurons. Now we can make limitless supplies of the cells that die in this awful disease. This will allow us to study these neurons. We can generate hundreds of millions of motor neurons that are genetically identical to clients own neurons. This will be an immense help as we try to uncover the mechanisms behind this disease and screen for drugs that can prolong life.
- Device scans for moles that can trigger **skin** *cancer*. Mole mate is a non-invasive, rapid and painless mole-screening device that can enable a medical practitioner to quickly scan ones moles. It may make it possible to detect the early stages of skin cancer by allowing doctors to screen and evaluate mole within a seconds. Doctor can say weather moles are harmless or refer them to specialist thus providing early diagnosis. The device uses light waves to break in two months beneath the skin. The researchers can then use the differences light waves that return to detect potentially harmful changes in colour, blood flow, the skin pigment melanin and collagen that may signal progression to cancer unless treated. Scared if that mole on your face could turn out to be a skin cancer?
- Did you know the average human head has about 1, 00,000 *hair follicles.* The average hair loss is about 100 strands a day, while each follicle will grow an average of about 20 individual hairs in a person's lifetime. Approximately 25% of men begin balding by age of 30, while two thirds begin balding by the time they are 60.
- With advances in medical technology, ***congenital heart disease*** is easily treated. Parents need not panic, as there is treatment available for the complication. People with pacemakers enjoy a normal life.
- Research moot daily pill to keep HIV at bay. Can a pill daily help prevent HIV infections that virus that can cause AIDS? Findings of the safety of efficient drug research are on.
- *A cure in sight*- scientists are looking at implantable lenses to treat lazy eye-an optical disorder affecting millions worldwide which is difficult to detect, and may lead to virtual blindness. This could be written off as a blind eye. up to 5% of worlds population have Amblyopia commonly called lazy eye. Where one eye is so much strong than the other eyes that the brain learns to ignore the weaker eye. Untreated at early stage the proper neural connections for vision do not form, eventually rendering that eye useless.

Problems with early treatment is tricky, kids do not realize they are seeing clearly out of only one eye, and often won't squint or other wise signal there is a problem. They red perfectly, they are normal active children. if they have vision test can this be decide early or else will remain unnoticed.

Experimental therapy implantable lenses are put on top of a natural eye lens that cannot focus properly, thus helping sharpen vision.

They have certain risk as surgical infections, inflammation and are very expensive for an eye. However, the upside is that lenses can be removed if there are problem. Repkas own research shows that it can be possible to treat lazy eye after age 9.

- *Findings—**Bionic eyes*** may soon be a reality, thanks to a new eye-shaped camera; research could also obtain clear pictures from current cameras. Borrowing from one of natures best designs, US scientists have built an eye shaped camera using standard sensor materials. They say that technology could improve the performance of digital cameras and foreshadows artificial retinas for bionic eyes, similar to those in the movie, it is cured surface to make it look like a human eye. The device could be used to make better imaging equipment, such as curved sensors to monitor brain, activity that follows the contors of the brain. It could even be used in the development of an artificial retina or a bionic eye. If you want to develop an eye to replace a human eye, certainly you want the shape to look like a human eye.

- *Smoking* can accelerate wrinkling of skin. Smokers have dull and shallow looking skin and often require intensive skin care. Over time, facial skin of people who smoke starts to get contaminated resulting in poor blood circulation, thinning of skin and blocked pores. Since nutrients are blocked from penetrating the skin surface, smokers tend to have dull, shallow and wrinkled looking skin compared to non-smokers. A typical smokers face can be distinguished, added vitamin C is essential, laser photo facial can reduce wrinkles. Peeling for rejuvenation of facial skin, peeling sensations can be opted for. Peeling can be done with the use salt and enzymes. The procedures can be undergone only under care of a qualified medical cosmetologist.

- *Cosmetic, plastic and laser surgery*- body researching; permanent fat and weight loss, obesity treatment, boggy eyelids, nose reshaping, lip rejuvenation and reshaping, threat life, breast implants and reshaping, baldness, hair transplantation, laser face rejuvenation, fractional laser-botox-fillers, laser hair removal, lesser removal of black and red, pigmented birth marks, spots, acne scars and tattoos.

- Running **slows** *aging scientist* discovered the people over 50 who ran regularly over several years suffered fewer disabilities, had a longer span of active life and reduced the risk of dying early by 50% compared to those who were inactive. To study has a very pro exercise message. The health benefits of exercise are greater than we thought. He attributed this to the fact the runners have leaner body mass and generally healthier habits.

- Scientist has long grappled for ways to cure the ***common cold***. According to researchers, the cold busting pill, known as BTA 798, could be used to clear up stifles in healthy people and prevent any kind of life threatening infections in asthma, cystic fibrosis sufferers. In fact, the drug works by latching on to cold- causing HRV preventing them from breaking into the body's cells and causing infection in a double attack, it stops any infection from spreading. It is a significant milestone in treatment of HRV (human rhinovirus) in high-risk client. In laboratory tests, the drug killed large quantities of cold virus within a couple of hours. Moreover, trials on volunteers have started to determine whether it could prevent people from catching a cold. If successful, the drug could hit the markets in few years time, the researchers said.

- Edible sensors-researchers designed ***biofriendly optical sensor*** that promise myriad applications in food, medicines and health. It could be placed in production bags to detect harmful levels of *bacteria* and consumed right along with the veggies or an implantable glucose in your blood for a year, then dissolved.

- *Heart- what is entopic cordis?* It is a birth defect in which the heart is normally located in the most common form; the heart protrudes outside the chest through a split sternum. This condition is usually fatal in first days of life. In some cases surgical treatment is possible. The entopic heart is not protected by the skin or sternum; other organs may also have formed outside the skin.

- Australian scientist had mapped a blood cell structure which could hold the key to improved drug treatment for diseases such as leukemia, asthma and rheumatoid arthritis. They have created the first 3-D image of a protein receptor in WBC which, when malfunctioning, can cause Leukemia. It is called a receptor because it interacts with a hormone when something goes wrong with receptor, is what happens in cancer with discovery of new receptor what it looks like and works, they can design new drugs to target the deadly abnormal blood cells. At the moment, many leukemia are treated with chemotherapy that destroy the diseased blood cells and bone marrow as well as normal cells. The particular protein receptor had been involved in some of the most aggressive and deadly forms of *leukemia*. It will help to target disease that is just difficult and untreatable.

- Indian scientist work towards *creating vital part of human eye-* half a dozen eye hospitals in India are collaborating with the research center in Chennai to create the inner layer of the cornea, the vital window of the human eye. The findings that the endothelium of the cornea contains stem cells have triggered worldwide reaches creating corneal cells for therapeutic use. The eyes have three parts. The first is the cornea, which is the transparent light into the eyes. The other two are the lens and retina. During eye transplantation, only the cornea is taken from the donor, not the whole eye. The back corneal portion of the eye has an outer layer, a middle portion and an inner layer known as the endothelial layer. Eye fluid keeps the cornea alive for up to six hours, allowing time for harvesting it and transplanting it. With the new technique, when comes the specimen from eye donor is recovered, it could be used for 5-10 needy clients. The research center is hoping to begin phase one clinical trials on humans in six months.

- Your *skin cream* can lead to *cancer*, scientists urge more research as creams used by millions of people cause tumors in mice. Researchers found several creams caused skin cancer in the specially bred mice, which had been pre-treated with ultra violet radiation. The cancers are not melanoma, the deadliest kind of skin cancer. Such tumors are slow growing highly treatable and only fatal if client fail to have them removed.

- *Electronic devices* get smaller and more complex every year. A new report has predicted that the *human brain* may be the battlefield of future wars, including pharmacological land mines and develops directed by mind control. US leading scientist were asked to examine how a greater understanding of the brain over the next 20 years is likely to drive the development of new medicines and techniques. They found several areas in which progress could have a profound impact, including behavior-altering drugs, scanners that can interpret a person's state of mind and devices capable of boosting senses such as hearing and vision. Products in this market could also alter the concept of torture. It is possible that some day there could be a technique developed to extract information from prisoners that does not have any lasting side effect. The report highlights one electronic technique, called

Transcranial direct current stimulation, which involves using electrical pulses to interfere with the firing of neurons in the brain, and has been shown to delay a person's ability to tell a lie.

- *Achalasia* is a condition characterized by worsening dysphasia. Elderly is different than in the younger population. The research compared two groups of people. Nurses need to be aware that health problems do not always present in the same way in older adults. Therefore, she should remember the differences and do accurate assessment.
- *A stroll on the beach may damage your lungs*- if you think that a short stroll on the beach is good for your health. A new study suggests that sea air could actually leave you breathing in noxious chemicals which damage lungs.
- An international team has carried out the study and found that smoke from vessels at sea or in the port affects the air quality of many costal cities across the world, which in turn is airing the health of many beach walkers.
- According to the researchers, primary sulfate in ship emissions consisting of tiny sulfur particles less than 1.5 microns across can harm the lungs when beached in and pose a serious health hazard.

In this study, the researchers analyzed the contribution of ships to the air pollution and it should be ignored the risk of beach walkers.

Did you know *aerobic exercise* might be one of the best ways to improve memory, as it increases the supply of oxygen to the brain study found that walking for three hours each week suffices, as does swimming or bicycle riding? This increases the number of neurons in brain and the number of connections between neurons.

- *Using humans skin to test drugs* – discarded human skin can be used to test new drugs and cosmetics, a researcher has found, most people would go to rats and mice for lab testing, butt when it comes testing new wound or products and cosmetics that go on human skin, pig skin is our closed alternative and is most often useful. This is expensive test there are ethical problems to consider. Skin science exhibition- skin collected donated by consenting clients who have had surgery resulting in a surgical off-cut and the skin is then processed in lab to isolate the cells, once they are growing healthily again, they are brought back together and create the multi-component skin equivalent in the lab. So deconstruct the skin off cuts themselves, as those cells are dying and we need to get the cells back to a state where are growing healthy again.
- Cesarean babies more prone to diabetes- but now, scientists have also found that another agent, besides insulin, can be used for a cure.

Babies born by caesarean section have a significantly higher risk of developing diabetes in childhood. Although the reason for the link is not clear. Scientist believe exposure to hospital bacteria may be involved. Childhood infections, along with genetics, are known to play an important role in the development of type 1 diabetes.

The diseases are an auto immune disorder in which immune system attacks insulin-producing cells in the pancreas.

Type 1 diabetes occurs in childhood and has to managed with life-long insulin injections. Type 2 diabetes on the other hand is different disease, and is linked to lifestyle. Researchers found children delivered by caesarean were 23 per cent more likely to develop the disease than those who had natural births.

However, there is a hope- the leptin a hormone produced by the body's fat cells also lowers blood glucose levels, and maintains in a normal range for extended periods. Clinical trials are within next years will give accurate information.

- *Re-walk*- Israeli boffins develop human exoskeleton suit to help *paralyzed* people walk again with a dim mechanical hum. The device, called re-walk is the brain child of engineer Amit goffer, founder of Argo medical technologies people paralyzed below the waist to stand, walk and climb stairs. The system which requires crèches to help with balance consists of motorized leg supports, body sensors and a backpack containing a computerized control box and rechargeable batteries.

The user picks a setting with a remote control wristband stand, sit, and walk descend or climb and then leans forward, activating the body sensors and setting the robotic legs in motion. It raises people out of their wheelchair and lets them stand up straight. Goffer said, it is not just about health, it is also about dignity.

- *Research—Cosmetics* lead to breathing problems, cancer, manufactures big and small go to town with heir wider range of cosmetics and hair dyes promising the moon- right from making you fairer overnight to wiping away your scars and making you look younger. However, can you really rely on these publicity campaigns? Experts warned against use of cosmetics in general saying they may cause major health problems in the long run. Excessive use could lead health problems. The market is flooded with products claiming to be made with a herbal base. People from pharmaceutical and cosmetics industry, dermatologist, plastic surgeons and regulatory authority must sit together to assess the safety norms and lay down strict guidelines. The ill effect of cheap cosmetics.

- *Research—Water birth*- a trend at present popularly practiced, was first introduced in 1970 in UK. Specially designed birth pools were introduced to use for prolonged immersion in water throughout labour. The depth of the birth pool is enormous different from normal bathtub where more space to mother to move freely in the tub and it help to adopt different position. Warm water naturally helps pregnant woman to reduce the pain, relax the pelvic ligaments that stretch during labour, softens and relaxes perineum, reduces the strains on joints, muscles. Pleasant dim lights and aromatherapy oils accompany water birth, which aids in mind relaxation. Water birth is natural aid to relaxation, release tension and anxiety, help to cope up with expulsive painful contractions. With less anxiety, body produces fewer hormones such as adrenaline and noradrenalin. This allows the natural painkillers the endorphins to be released it promotes the sense of well being. The atmosphere in the water birth is less rushed, in the second stage of labour takes longer duration and strain imposed on the mother to push is less imposed. It is a low tec way of conducting the labour and has only fewer obstetric interventions. Heart rate of the baby monitored using held Doppler with waterproof. Temperature of water should be comfortable for mother and it should not rise above 370°C, it will be carefully measured and recorded regularly.

Researches conducted for both mother and newborn, almost all the results portrays that mother experienced less pain enjoyed the water birth and so far no neonatal problems reported.

Potential disadvantages can be tackled by proper obstetric intervention. Neonatal water aspiration, maternal hyperthermia may contribute to fetal hypoxemia, blood loss estimation and assessment is difficult in the water.

Maternal water embolus. Medicals problems like diabetes mellitus, kidney disease or chronic mental illness. Mother with very high blood pressure, less weight of fetus during pregnancy, last week of pregnancy vaginal bleeding, mother with previous cesarean section. Multiple pregnancy or twins, breech position, premature baby. Mothers will be asked to leave the pool if baby's heart beat is slow. Need for strong pain relief, labour progressing very slowly, start bleeding during labor, mother feel faint.

Water birth is peaceful. In future mother may feel her pain and enjoy the birth water.

- Soon, breathe tests to **detect cancer-** a new tool that would help in detecting cancer in early stages by analyzing the client's breath. Scientists are working to create a sensor with mild-infrared lasers to detect biomarker gases exhaled in the breath of a person with cancer. It has already been shown that dogs identified breast and lung cancer clients with accuracies of 88-97%. It is possible to develop easy to use detection devices for cancer, particularly for hard-to detect cancer like lung. Research continues and may take 5-10 years for these devices easily available.

- **Babies can read emotions in faces.** You may be well aware that your baby recognizes your face, but a new study has revealed that the toddler can also recognize the way you smile or frown. Researcher at London found that babies as young as four months are able to recognize emotions in faces of people, in face; they are able to notice non-verbal signals adults use to communicate before they start talking. According to them, infants use the same brain regions that adults do when they look at the gaze of another, a base for social interactions that often appears critical for social development.

- **Incense sticks linked to cancer-** burning incense may create a sweet scent, but regularly inhaling the smoke could put people at risk of cancer of the respiratory tract. Link between heavy incense use and various respiratory cancers. Incense are used in many cultures religious and special ceremonies. It is derived from fragrant plants, materials, like tree bark, resins, roots, flowers and essentials.

- **Tiny ultrasound probe to provide clear tissue images.** A new ultrasound probe small enough to sit on a catheter tip can provide physicians with clearer images of soft tissues minus risks associated with X-ray catheter guidance. Biomedical engineers have designed and fabricated the ultra sound probe, which is powerful enough to provide detailed 3-D images. It works like an insect's compound eye, blending images from 108 miniature transducers working together. The 3-D ultrasound machine is on wheels and can be moved easily to a client's room.

- **Woman whose legs weight 95 kg,** only amputation will save her life. The size of her legs makes walking difficult and client needed crutches just to go around in house. Her whole weight is about 127 kg of which are her legs. She uses an electric wheel chair when she gets out. Her mobility getting worse day by day which she has no control. It could be called *sellers syndrome* the medical book named after her. She will go down the history while amputation is inevitable. *Proteus syndrome* is a congenital disorder that causes skin overgrowth and atypical bone development. often accompanied by tumors. 200 cases so far confirmed of such diseases worldwide.

- Doctors claim cure for high blood pressure during pregnancy- nearly 15-20% of women usually have normal blood pressure develop high blood pressure during *pregnancy*, generally after the 20 weeks. The cause is unknown. Symptoms- the woman may suffer swelling of her hands, legs or face and blood pressure reading spike up. This syndrome is called pre-eclampsia. Danger-if it worsens, the pregnant woman could have swelling of the brain and suffer fits and slip into unconsciousness. It is the cause of 20-25% of maternal mortality causes. It affects the fetus too. New therapy- doctor injected bone marrow stem cells into the woman's uterus and claimed that 14 out of 15 showed significant improvement.

- *Mobile phone*-like device could diagnose *cancer* in 15 minutes. As scientists have developed, a new biosensor technology that they claim provides results within 15 minutes. The technology uses antibodies to detect biomarkers-molecule in the human body, which are often a marker for disease- much faster, then current testing methods. They are trying to develop small device similar to mobile phone into which different sensor chips could be inserted, depending on the disease being tested for. The technology could be used in surgeries for more accurate referral to consultants and in hospital for rapid diagnosis.

- *Cell phone* use ups brain cancer risk in kids. Kids and teenagers today are an increased risk of developing brain cancer. If they use mobile phones according to an alarming new research. Kids are five times more likely to get brain cancer due to mobile use. The research raises fears that today young people may suffer an epidemic of the diseases in later life. People who started mobile phone use before the age of 20 had more than five fold increase in glioma, a cancer of the glial cells that support the CNS. The extra risk to young people of contracting the diseases from using the cordless phone found in many homes was almost as great at more than four times higher. Five times more likely to get acoustic neuromas begin but often disabling tumors. This is a warning sign and it is very worrying. We should be talking precautions.

- *Brain cancer* in children is becoming a problem worldwide. The incidence rate of brain tumors in children across the world is increasing by about 2.7%/per year. The survival rate is approximately 60% but this varies with the age of onset and cancer type with young and children having higher mortality.

- ***Put on your thinking cap***- they say the spark of genius lurks within all of us. Now, a group of researchers is developing a thinking cap that can make the reality unlock the potential of the brain. The revolutionary device works by switching on and off certain sections of the brain, there by unlocking its hidden potential. Wearing the hairnet like cap for a few minutes improved artistic ability and proof reading skills, trials found.

Scientist have developed new stimulating **headgear** that could unlock the hidden genius in you. How it work- a cap containing a magnet that is connected to an electric current is placed on the head. The magnet in the shape of an eight is made up of a bundle of interviewed wires, and is located near the left ear. The headgear generates tiny magnetic pulses that disturb the electric circuits on the left side of the brain, which is known to see the bigger picture. The stronger left side usually suppressed the detail hoarding right side. Since the right side remains undisturbed, details filed there come to the force to create a burst of creative, mathematical, or other relent.

- New nipple shield helps protect breast-fed babies from contracting *HIV*. It could be a breakthrough in AIDS prevention if successful, a simple shield to block mothers transmitting the HIV virus to their babies while breastfeeding. HIV mothers who have no option but breastfeed the scientist have long fretted over how to stop it. More then 91,000 children n India have HIV, with nearly 21,000 new infections occurring every year.

  The new study pushes back origin of HIV by several decades, virus began spreading at the turn of 20th century.

- Are bad times good for your health? People drink more, eats fat-laden meals, and skip exercise and doctors appointments in boom time. Most people are worried about the health of the economy. However, does the economy also affect your health? People work more hard does less of the things that are good for them, like cooking at home and exercising.

- Now, a shortcut to making *stem cells* from skin. Researchers trying to find ways to transform ordinary skin cells into powerful stem cells. Harvard stem cell institute team used two genes to transform ordinary human skin cells into stem cells. Stem cells are the body's master cells, giving rise to all he tissues, organs and blood. Embryonic stem cells are considered the most powerful kinds of stem cells, as they have the potential to give rise to any type of tissues.

- *No more evolution-* from monkeys to men, but what's next? One geneticist believes that man will not evolve any further because he no longer has to struggle to survive. Man in developed world has stoped *evolving*, because he no longer has to struggle to survive and natural selection does not come into play any more. We now know so much about the process of evolution that we can make some predictions about what might happen in future. Natural selection and mutation drive evolution. *Genetic mutations* create trails, which if helpful, give individuals a competitive edge over rivals.

- No race for survival- takes natural selection. Before modernity, life was so tough that most children died before they reached adolescence. It was race for survival and only the strongest made it, making out a case for natural selection. This means babies with genetic mutations that made them more resilient had better chances of survival as well as passing on their genes to their offspring.

- In modern world central heating and plenty of food, the same mutation is far less likely to give a child any advantage. A baby born today can expect to live long and healthy life, which in turn works against the evolutionary tool of natural selection. Older means sperm detoriates and contains more genetic mistakes which in turn can lead to mutations in their children. Cell division in males increases with age. Every time there is a cell division, there is a chance of a mistake, a mutation, an error. Small populations that are isolated can change at random, as genes are accidentally lost. Worldwide all populations are becoming connected and the opportunity for random change is dwelling. We are mixing into global mass. Breeding between the races is becoming more common as the globe becomes smaller.

  Future evolution scientist believes humankind will struggle to evolve from its present states. Only by interbreeding and bioengineering can a new species emerge.

Genes do not stay in one place for very long in evolutionary terms.

- *Greek philosopher* **Anaximander** of the 6th century BC is considered, as evolution is most ancient proponent. He claimed that life sprang out of the sea as fish like animals, and conjectured that humans earlier had to live inside the mouths of big fish to protect themselves from Earths humid climate. Once dry land emerged on earth, humans came out in open air and lost their scales.
- *Genetic health*—study of hereditary diseases Genes are the units of heredity. They contain the hereditary information, they affect development and function both normal and abnormal. It is said that we inherit about 50,000 genes father and 50,000 from mother. Since genes are contained in the chromosomes, genes also occur in pain. Genes are usually stable, but sometimes normal genes may be converted into abnormal ones. This change is called mutation.
- *Chromosomal abnormalities*—alteration occur from time to time in human beings.

Non disjunction—by an error in nuclear division a pair of it may fail to separate and both are carried to one pole. Wrong attachment and wrong detachment and lost. Duplication, some genes may appear twice in same chromosome.

Genetics and its relation to community health—the study of the traits are passed on from parents to children are known as genetics. The study of heredity innate capacity of an individual to develop traits, e.g. body size, skin, and hair color, intellectual capacity, susceptibility to certain disease possessed by ancestors determines in the chromosomes of the fertilized ovum from which an individual develops. Children resemble their parents and to there brothers and sisters.

Genes contain the hereditary information encoded in their chemical structure for transmission from generation to generation. Brown eyes from one and blue eyes from other parent one will dominate. Genes occur in pairs. Each ovum and sperm has 23 plus 23 total 46.

Inheritance of diseases- sickle cell anemia, high blood pressure, anterio-sclerosis, mental illness as schizophrenias, mania, psychosis, epilepsy, hemophilia, glaucoma, diabetes, have an inherited tendency. Thalassemias, asthma, cancer, coronary heart diseases, Alzheimer disease.

More than 300 numerical and structural types of chromosome aberration have been described. A significant portion of embryonic and fetal wastage.

Klinefelters syndrome affects male with non functional tests. Spermatozoa are absent in their ejaculation. The growth of hair on face, axilla and pubes is scanty.

Xyx syndrome- the male with extra 'y' chromosome have tendency to anti- social, aggressive and often criminal behaviour, exceptional height serious personality disorder leading to behavioral disturbances. One in thousand male found.

Turner's syndrome—They have increased risk of dying in the neonatal period. Have 45 chromosomes instead of 46; missing chromosome clinically patients are short stature, infertile and have primary amenorrhea, show congenital defects such as coactions of the aorta, pulmonary stenosis, renal malformations and mental retardation.

Supper females—3-5x chromosome extra have greater risk of mental retardation and congenital abnormalities, e.g. under developed external genitalia, uterus or vagina.

Relating to Autosomal—Recognized by short stature and small round head, narrow tilted eye-slits, malformed ears, short broad hand, lax limbs mental retardation internal congenital defects, cardiac defects, atresia of alimentary tract.

Mendelian diseases sex linked-50; 50 affected-hemophilia, Thalassemias, blood grouping and diseases, Sickle cell anemia, blood grouping determined by genes, cystic fibrosis.

Multifactor disorders-such as high pressure, mental retardation, schizophrenia, duodenal ulcer, ischemic heart disease, diabetes, congenital malformation, family cancer.

DNA technology- mutation implies a change in the genetic material results in new inherited variation. The cause of spontaneous mutation not known certain external influences such as ionizing radiation.

Natural selection process harmful genes are eliminated from the gene pool and genes favorable to an individual tend to be preserved and passed on to the offspring.

Genetic counselling, early diagnosis and treatment ad rehabilitation is important.

Stem cells are the body's master cells with the power to transform into any cells. Sterm cells obtained from the patients themselves instead of embryonic or cord blood cells. Embryonic cells have ethical issues as well as the threat of cancer. Cord blood cells are expensive to process. Stem cell from the patient's bone marrow is simple to process and without side effect. The procedure is long, they are extracted from the patients marrow, analyzed and processed before being injected back into the site of the injury, the surrounding as wells as C.S.F. All this takes five hours. Patients are in waiting list.

- A simple screening of proteins in human saliva was able to accurately detect a common type of **oral** *cancer;* a finding may led to a painless new diagnostic test.

- Researcher's study effects of healing touch therapy- often mothers touch lulls her bawling baby into quietude and restfulness. By restoring balance within the energy system, you create an optima environment for healing.

- Making headway, scientists are using a ***brain pacemaker*** to treat OCD, headaches and other neurological disorders. DBS deep brain stimulation. Drilled two coin sized holes in skull and insert the electrodes about four inches into the brain. A connecting wire from the electrode run under the skin to a battery implanted near the collar born. Today DBS devices also known as pacemakers for the brain used in treatment of Parkinson's, it improves tremors. Still this novel treatment is not without adverse effects. Jotting sensation, numbness or tingling the face or hand, dizziness, muscle spasms, slurred speech, double vision and depression noted. However, the benefit outweighs the risks. When there is side effect, we can turn the device and reverse them.

- Deep brain stimulation for ***Parkinson's*** **disease** is a surgical procedure in which a thin wire is implanted deep within the brain to deliver an electrical current. The current helps to block abnormal brain activity that causes the tremors and other symptoms that are the hallmark of Parkinson's disease. While it is not a cure, it is effective in improving the quality of life for people with this disease. Other than the dangers of the surgical procedures itself, it seems to carry fewer side effects than the medications that have traditionally been used for the disease. Journal of medicine confirms these findings. Deep brain stimulation has generally only been available to those with the most severe symptoms of advanced Parkinson's.

- *Hormone therapy and hearing loss*- a new study finds that older women are taking hormone therapy that included progestin may suffer hearing damage. No studies of hearing in the younger age group using those medications, has been done. Talk with your doctor and have your hearing evaluated by a professional.

- *COPD patients need physical activity*- researchers have founded that even a small amount of physical activity can improve the health of patients suffering from chronic obstructive pulmonary disease/COPD. Those who engage in exercise and activity have a fewer hospitalization and have lower risk of dying. COPD is a group of diseases, very often caused by years of smoking that restricts the airway and makes the breathing more difficult. Many patients are depended on oxygen most of the day. This study found that even light activity like walking three days a week could help.

- *Facing death brings positive thoughts*- when thoughts of death intrude; the human mind isn't paralyzed with negativity or fear. Instead, the brain instinctively moves toward happier notions and images, a new study suggests.

  The findings supported the notion that people are stronger, emotionally, when faced with their own or a loved ones death than they may have ever thought possible. It again speaks to how resilient humans are and how this tendency to cope with threats is some sort of indicator of mental health. Humans are the only animal known to have a clear understanding that their life will end. On the surface, this knowledge could prove psychologically paralyzing-why complete, learn and grow if these achievements will end? Scientist believe that as humans developed an awareness of death, they also evolved what is been called the "psychological immune system" during crisis, this mechanism tilts thoughts and attitudes toward positive-even when the grimmest of events intervene.

- Magnetic beam to drive away the blues- brain stimulator a device that beams pulses through skull to combat depression. It does not cause the risk of surgically implanted electrodes or the treatment of last resort, shock therapy. A non invasive procedure to help fight depression called Tran cranial magnetic stimulation of TMS uses a magnetic pulse to stimulate brain cells that control moods.

- **Computer** *heart model* recalls da Vinci's sketches- intricate drawings transformed understanding of the human heart promises to do the same for modern-day cardiac care. The model so realistic its four chambers beat in the same asymmetrical rhythm on screen, as does a real heart in the human body-is the work of the British doctors who say the creation will improve both training and care during surgery. The three-dimensional models intricate details coupled with life like animation make the cyber heart unique. We can slice it, spin it around and look at it from any angle. We have reproduced the timing of the human heartbeats to within 20 milliseconds. The new model will lead to better care; it opens up to new approach to the understanding of cardiac structure. Recreating was not easy, I took four years of tapping the expertise of dozens of doctors who each specialized on the different parts of the heart. Said the researcher doctors of UK have created a visual heart model of the organ.

- Dr. Paul Gnanayutham developed this new mind reading system- *Screening thoughts-* brain injury patients, who are unable to speak or move, are finally able to communicate using a new computerized system that translates their thoughts to a computer screen. People who have suffered brain injuries and unable to move or speak, are given a chance to communicate just the power of thought and a laptop loaded with sophisticated algorithms, a new software developed by this doctor computerized research in UK uses patients brain waves, eye or muscular movements to move a cursor on a computer. Using a prototype device, paralyzed patients can point a cursor on a screen that could include options such as yes, no, thank you, a switch to turn on a TV set, are even a link to an internet page of the patients choice. The system is noninvasive and works by attaching probes to a band than can be worn around several places on head EEG pick up brainwaves on muscles MG or sound on forehead to pick up eye movement signals that is EOG/electrooculography.

  These signals are then fed into an amplifier; signals of a person wearing electrodes are transmitted to the serial port. So the computer just sees the brain body inter face as the cursors control. Hospital staffs look after these people feeding them, washing them but these patients do not have the voice. They have no way of saying please do not turn off the lights because I want to stay awake for another hour, or no, I do not want visitors today added the researcher. It is first time patient have such option with this technique with simple words yes, no is the first conversation they have had with their loved ones in years. Researchers want to give back patient there voice. Only when will it be a real success.

- Japanese research- brain tissue created from stem cells. A world first that has raised new hopes for the treatment of disease for mental illness like *Alzheimer*. Stem cells taken from human embryos have been used to form tissues of the cerebral cortex, the supreme control tower of brain. This research have potential to save lives by helping to find cures for disease such as cancer, diabetes or to replace damage cells, tissues and organs. Embryonic stem cells are harvested by destroying a visible embryo a process that some find it unacceptable.

- **In a first, cancer genes decoded mutations found**- using cells donated by a woman in her 50s who died of leukemia, the scientists sequenced the entire DNA from her cancer cells and compared it to the healthy skin cells. Then they zeroed in on 10 mutations that occurred only in the cancer cells, apparently spurring abnormal growth and enabling them to fight off chemotherapy. This would help doctor to make better choices among existing treatments, based on a detailed genetic picture of each patient's cancer. The same technique can be used to study other cancers.

- **New ice slurry technology can save *heart attack victims*.** Brain cells start to die in a span of few minutes without the ability to obtain fresh oxygen from blood pumped through the body. US researchers have developed a new: *cooling; technology* that can reduce the brain and other organs demand for oxygen, giving doctors extra time to treat critically ill.

  Current medical guidance says that if you want to save the brain, you have to lower the temperature to 4-5 degree celsius with 5-10 minutes of cardiac arrest. Team has created an ice slurry that can easily pumped directly into patients blood stream through a small iv catheter using the slurry doctors can chill the targeted organ, e.g. in the heart attack the slurry would be delivered to the lungs through an endotracheal tube. Paramedical would then administer chest compression which would force blood through the cold lungs from there; the chilled blood would flow into the brain, cooling it rapidly. They say that by understanding the interactions between the slurry and the vulnerable organs, we can optimally induce protective cooling and save lives.

- Scientists are developing a new *'field hospital on a chip'* that will monitor *soldier's* well-being, and administer drugs and treatment on the fly. A field hospital on a chip. The sense and treat system uses a minimally invasive biomedical sensor to continuously monitor a soldiers sweat, tears or blood for biomarkers that signal common battle. Field injury such as trauma, shock, brain injury or fatigue. Once a problem is detected, the system will administer the right medicine to the soldier using the drug delivery device. Professor Joseph Wang holds up a flexible electrode, one of the components of his hospital on a chip project. We hope that our system will revolutionize the treatment of injured soldiers and lead to dramatic improvements in the survival rate.

- Scientist's have developed a small new smart; i pill' that is, when swallowed enables doctors to target precise areas in the body and administer accurate doses of medicine. Enabling new therapies for debilitating and life threatening digestive tract disorders such as Crohn's disease, colitis and colon cancer.

    By delivering the required drugs directly to the site of disease, side effects could be reduced; I pill or the new intelligent pill electronically controls drug delivery specific areas in the body microprocessor contains a wireless radio pump and a drug reservoir to release medication that combine electronics with diagnostic and therapeutic properties will open up the possibility of targeting almost any kind of drug to a specific location in the intestinal tract.

    The I pill is a capsule 11 × 26 mm in size that can be swallowed with water normally and is then carried along by the normal movement of food through the gut. It can also be electronically programmed to control the delivery of medicine. The ipill locates in the intestinal tract by measuring the local acidity of its environment. Armed with information and data location in the gut determined with good accuracy.

- *Bone marrow* **transplant, cures *AIDS*** in patient- from a donor with a natural genetic resistance to the Aids virus has suppressed the IV infection in a patient for two years. Bone marrow transplant, normally applied in curing leukemia, to cure a 42-year-old AIDS patient. 20 months after the treatment the patient was still free of HIV virus. They are still skeptical of the therapy. The virus is tricky. It can always return, it could inspire researchers to pursue gene therapy as a means to block or suppress HIV.

WHAT IS UMBILICAL CORD BLOOD BANKING

It is the collection and storage of blood from the umbilical cord and the placenta. In 1970s, researchers discovered that umbilical cord blood was rich in blood forming stem cells. Diseases that can be treated with cord blood, currently, a multitude of malignant and non malignant disease including sickle cell disease, bone marrow failure syndromes and congenital immuno-defiency syndromes are treated with stem cells. Used to treat disease like leukemia, lymphoma, Thalassemias and blood disorders in the infant.

Artificial pacemakers powered by ones own *heartbeats and implants* to monitor. Your blood pressures that produce their own electricity may soon be a reality. Imagine a small sensor embedded in your body which keeps altering you through a mobile phone about your blood pressure levels or consider a futuristic pacemaker that uses surplus energy from heartbeats to power itself. Self-powered-small-scale generators are now enabling the development of a new class of hi-tech self powered, wireless sensing systems. The devices could gather information, store and transmit the data all without an external power source.

The generator is capable of producing electricity by rhythmic contraction and relaxation of very thin wires of zinc oxide. The wires around a hundred times thinner than human hair are encapsulated in flexible plastic base with two ends of the wire bonded together. When the device is mechanically stretched and released, it produces up to 45 milli volts of electricity by converting neatly 7% the energy.

- **Safe cure for** *sickle cell disease* found a research team said led by an India origin scientist. A new form of bone marrow transplantation; that can prove safe and effective in curing, sickle cell disease. It is the only one known care for such a disease.

- *Overnight hemodialysis* **cuts** death risk- undergoing dialysis 8 hours overnight 3 times a weekly reduces the risk of death by nearly 80% they increased in appetite, gained weight and their serum potential albumin levels increased. Many patients are able to return to work.

- *Hormone free contraceptive* pill a side effect of today's contraceptives pill is that they disrupt hormone production in women, but zp3, scientist have found a protein target, which could prove the way for contraceptives that does not tinker with a women's hormones. The protein called zp3 is present in the coating of mammalian eggs. It plays a crucial role in contraception, as the sperm must bind to zp3 if they are to burrow through the coating and fertilize the egg. Scientist found that female mice engineered to lack zp3 do not have this coating.

- *Cell phone chip* promises to counter radiation. The Ewave phone chip is a small circular gadget that sticks on the back of a phone to neutralize harmful rays.

Infecting the Infector

Research have successfully lab-tested a new way to fight *dengue fever.* By cutting the short lifespan of mosquitoes that, transmit the deadly diseases. A mosquito borne virus that each year harms up to 100 million people and kills more than 20,000.

The effectiveness of a new way of limiting the lifespan of mosquito that spread this fever.

They have done with infecting the dengue mosquito, Aedes aegypti, with a bacterium that is harmless to human and other animals, but halves Aedes lifespan. This has the potential to greatly reduce dengue because only old mosquito is effective transmitting the virus to humans.

There is no vaccine or cure for dengue fever, which is a painful and debilitating diseases also known as 'break bone fever' dengue hemorrhagic fever can be lethal. The virus is of great concern in tropical parts of the developing world, globally outbreaks are being more common and climate change will place people at risk.

Reduce the lifespan of mosquito which must be approximately 12-15 days of old before they can transmit the virus. Be passed by females to their offspring's and spread into mosquito population.

It would be several years before the technique would be tested.

Lack of Good Nights Sleep Can Lead to Paranoia

A new study has found that almost 70 percent of people who admitted to suffering from paranoia had difficulty in sleeping. The study also showed that over 50 percent of psychiatric patients who experience feelings of persecution, suffered from moderate to severe insomnia. Tracking the problem of insomnia could help cut the risk of paranoia.

Researchers synthesize human bone marrow for improved drug testing.

Lab on a phone- new cell phone-based technology allows for portable monitoring of HIV and malaria patients, and also for testing water contamination in disaster areas.

Forget clinic, consult physician online–To be introduced soon, E-service will reduce waiting time and may prove crucial in emergency.

America well, a web service that puts patients face to face with doctors online. The services are for people who seek easier access to physicians because they are uninsured or do not wait for an appointment or go to clinic.

Patient use the service by logging on to participating health plans websites. Doctors hold 10 minutes appointment, which can be extended for a free and can fie prescriptions and view patients medical history through the system.

It is well suited for Remote Island, and places where it takes time to travel and is difficult for the state to recruit doctors in rural areas.

Drawback is that doctors will miss important symptoms if they do not see a person. Certain diagnosis, e.g. sore throat is a virtue or a strep infection, are difficult using a web cam.

Sci-tech

An insider's view- entering from a tiny 1.5 cm incision, a new wireless camera will provide surgeons with a better view of the insides of the body during minimally invasive surgeries.

During an MIS procedure, such as laparoscopy, multiple small incisions are made in the abdominal wall for various devices-the most important of which is the camera the 'the eyes' of the surgeon. The tiny device ill ultimately enables high resolution emerging, auto focus, optical zoom, sophisticated image processing and wireless transmissions of code images. The new camera, a light source and surgical instruments to enter the body, without incisions, through a single point of access-thus further minimizing trauma to the body wall.

Disadvantages is the movement of any instrument in the tube also move the camera resulting is an unstable image which can even change optical room of auto-focus capability and requires a heavy cable of connect it to the video screen.

With these above many example of medical research done can give you an idea how the research is conducted and new discoveries are done. After having, understanding let us once again turn to the continuation of topic. What is research?

Research is a systematic process of finding answer to question. Here a data is collected systematically and analyzed to find answer to the scientific question, which trouble us. It is a logical reasoning and scientific method to explain activities and solve the problems. The conclusions reached as a result of research must always be logical.

Because nursing is profession requires skills and practice. As it, one or the other way influence clinical practice. Research is a search for new facts and adding to the existing body of knowledge to provide effective care.

As health care is changing at a faster pace, keeping the eye on the future and changing with the changing times, nursing too must keep up with changing pace for the future health care. To make the difference to the health care and improve quality care there is absolute need for research. Nurses who are involved in care and encounter a problem can start reasoning, organizing, formulating and verifying ideas adding new knowledge by systematic planed investigation is ultimately lead to great discovery that is research.

A nurse observes a particular behavior of a patient study in detail. Traditions that are passed from one generation to another can also lead to action. Develop and intuition, reflect your unique experience as experience not reflected is a lost experience and something new findings may be born. In addition, that data or information can lead to research. In your practice if you notice a particular observation of more than few people you can take up as a challenge and see if it can be used in other similar setting on many more people. This can help to find certain answers, which are not touched, or partially solved. It can help to improve existing techniques and develop new discoveries.

As you read in above chapter, so many researches are done and published in journals but how many of them are particularly materialized into concert action. To use in ordinary setting for a common person to understand and follow, therefore research done should be scientific and useable in practical life of people.

In nursing field, one draw back, I experience is how many are open to accept new ideas suggested where they have fixed protocol; if you try to do a bit different in new way, you are questioned. Sometimes it could bring revolution. In that way many growing talents and creativity are suppressed and have no outlet is given. Trial and error should be allowed when it is not harmful and cause no danger to life. Otherwise always ask why you want to conduct a study like that? It discourages blooming enthusiastic budding nurses to withdraw into cocooning discourage her from proceeding. Therefore, a climate of shared interest is needed. The stagnated and just satisfied doing a bit of routine will drag this field of research.

As research is important to improve the practice to give better service. It helps to improve her care with most current principles of practice. Redefining the existing theories and discovering new theories can broaden the knowledge and give new measures for nursing practice and improve the standards of nursing education. Your search should be new and not already existed or else it will be loss of time and energy.

As it will need farsightedness and vision for the goal, you have in mind, which needs careful designed framework. Accurate reliable observing. Which needs to be recordable, reportable and scientifically measurable? It takes handwork and at time many years to complete a particular finding to become acceptable. It is as if gold is tested in fire or a diamond is polished to get the shine.

It needs intellectual thinking, reasoning, e.g. a particular drug studied in pharmaceutical company and after testing and going through all the process is put into market. Now a nurse who administers a drug after physician has ordered finds a particular indication or side effect. She notes and whenever she has given this drug, she finds a particular effects, which she after referring the books, etc. is not found anywhere. She needs to look into this new fact observed and follow the steps. She also can put this finding into a net where world over nurses give there opinions and feed back is shared could be a beginning of new discovery. It will help you to give better care keeping in mind do's and don'ts.

Knowledge will give you power and it will help to change your attitude, e.g. new challenges and areas we can research is heart diseases increasing in youth, effect of menstrual pain and coping methods. For research nurse needs a support, needs time release, financial support, materials, tools, validity, format preparation, etc. therefore a support and encouragement is a powerful motivating force. Nurse can research in particular areas of work and interest of specific group, e.g. a school children-growing obesity or recent diagnosis of diabetes, etc. follow the data collection, different types of questioning like open ended question, closed ended questions, structural or unstructured interviews, discussions, evaluation.

CHAPTER 8

Remarkable Structure of Human Body and its Importance to Nursing Care

The human body is made up of trillions of cells. Different parts of our body are made of different kinds of cells. Your brain is like a computer, and controls your entire body. Your heart beats about 70 times a minute, and each time it beats it pumps about a cupful of blood, an adult human heart weighs about 10 ounces and beats over 100,000 times a day. There are 206 bones in your skeleton; about half of the bones in the human body are located in the hands and feet. Every one has 32 teeth. Your muscles make up about one half of your body weight. If you were to remove your skin, it would weigh as much as 5 pounds; about 70% of your body weight is water.

Nursing links body and mind. It is a human relations field, all ages, of all socio-cultural economic backgrounds. Nursing is an integral part of our education system. There is limitless scope for development where nurse has vital part to play in evaluating health care system. Having nurses at the center means improved access to care, help patient manage chronic condition to live longer and healthier lives. She knows the needs of children, families, homes, work and at play. She is serving as the connecting link between individuals, families, communities and health care provider. Those qualities are why she is backbone of health care the world over.

The human body has many enemies, large and small. The most dangerous are far too small for human eye to see. These are the germs and viruses.

The human **heart** is a marvelous organ. Its function is to move the living stream of blood through all parts of the body, never stopping even for a moment in its endless activity. Although the heart is one single organ, it actually consists of two pumps, right and left. The right side of the heart, with its two chambers, receives blood from all parts of the body and propels it to the lungs. Each side of the heart operates independently of the other, but act together in keeping the blood circulating normally. The walls of the heart consist of powerful muscle fibers that have the power to contact or beat rhythmically. This constant rhythmic beating keeps the circulation going.

Heart does an enormous amount of work. It beats over one hundred thousand times a day, continually pumping the blood through more than 60,000 miles of tiny blood vessels.

The **tiny capillaries** are only a tenth of an inch long, but if they could be placed end to end, they would stretch two and a half times around the earth at the equator. To maintain the right pressure, all these vessels must be filled with the right amount of blood; otherwise the tissues of the body would waste away and die.

Breathing is the first law of life. No one can live more than a few minutes without an adequate supply of oxygen. We need fresh air to stay alive. To make this possible, nature has provided with a remarkable living pipeline-the trachea. If that lifeline were blocked or cut off, we could not survive more than few minutes. Air must be kept flowing in an out of the body. This is done by the expansion and contraction of the chest and abdomen.

Our **lungs** are most remarkable structures in the whole human body. They are light and spongy and capable of expanding and contracting into a narrow space. They are extremely elastic. Trachea brings air to the lung which is just below the voice box and extends down to the middle of the chest where it divides into two main branches called bronchi. They break up into numerous smaller branches called bronchioles. If they were spread out flat they would cover an area more than 1,000 square feet. This is more than 20 times as much surface as the skin on our body. Yet all these little air sacs are folded up and compressed into less than one cubic foot of space within our chest.

Every highly **complex machine** must have a control center-some place where all important decisions are made and where the activities are co-coordinated. For instance, a large jet plane has powerful engines to carry it through the air, and luxurious space for the comfort of all the passengers. The plain is so well equipped with food compartments, so that delicious meals can be served by charming hostesses who are constantly watching over the welfare of all on board. All the vitals decisions are taken by captain who works hard during a long flight, while passengers relax and rest, but they are on duty day and night, as long as the plan is in the air.

So it is with the **human body.** We have many important organs such as the heart, lungs, kidneys and liver, all hard at work. Over all this remarkable machine known as the human body we have almost efficient nervous system, consisting of brain, the spinal cord and the autonomic nervous system. This great nervous system is always on the job, ever alert to protect us from danger, and to guide us in all we do. Our most important decisions are made by brain. Here are the centers of memory, reason, intelligence and understanding. Here we decide what is right and what is wrong. Intelligent and understanding are the chief attributes that set man above the rest of the animal kingdom.

The **'nervous system'** (NS) are the basis for all human function. It is the center of thinking, memory, judgment, sensation, movement, cognition, communication, behaviour and personality. Disorders of the NS can range from acute life-threatening emergencies to chronic, long-term conditions resulting in significant impairments, disability or handicap. The brain and spinal cord are the major components of the CNS.

Role of Cardinal Nerves in the Body as Follows —

1. Olfactory for smell,
2. Optic for vision and are sensory nerves.

3. **Oculomotor** is extraocular eye movement, elevation of eyelid, pupil constriction and is parasympathetic motor nerve.
4. **Trochlear extraocular** eye movement is motor nerve.
5. **Trigeminal ophthalmic** division somatic sensations of cornea, nasal mucus membrane and face are a sensory nerve. Maxillary division somatic sensations of face, oral cavity, tongue and teeth are sensory. Mandibular division of lower face is motor.
6. **Abducens** for lateral eye movement-motor nerve.
7. **Facial-facial** expression, taste, salivation-parasympathetic nerve.
8. **Vestibulocochlear** for equilibrium sensory nerve.
9. **Glossopharyngeal** for taste, swallowing is motor.
10. **Vagus** for sensation in pharynx, larynx, and external ear is parasympathetic nerve.
11. **Spinal** accessory for neck and shoulder movement is motor.
12. **Hypoglossal** for tongue movement is motor.

Did you ever wonder how in the world all the various organs of the body know what to do and when to do it? With so many different parts working at the same time it would be easy to produce too much of one thing, too little of another. This is what happens when we are ill. Two major control systems regulate all the functions of the body one is CNS and the other Endocrine system which has highly important organs such as pituitary, thyroid etc.

The skeleton or bony framework of the body is truly a master piece of design and engineering. It consists of over 200 bones; the number varies according to person's age. All of the bones are important, for they not only provide strength and stability, but they also protect our organs. At the same time, they provide a vast storehouse of minerals, which are constantly being drawn upon to meet the needs of the body. Each bone, tailored by nature for the particular job it has to do. Our bones are built in a remarkable way similar to a modern steel and concrete building. The basic construction of the bone consists of a soft spiral type of reinforcing protein material which is filled in and surrounded by a complex mixture of minerals. These consist mainly of calcium and phosphorus, a veritable storehouse of mineral material. Calcium not only gives strength to the bones but also keeps the heart beating and the nervous system functioning properly.

To prevent *low back pain* use proper body mechanics with specific attention to bending lifting, and sitting. Use good posture when sitting, standing or walking. Avoid prolonged periods of sitting and standing. Keep weight 10% of ideal body weight. Ensure adequate calcium intake, stop smoking.

To prevent *Back injury* – when lifting an object, keep your back straight, do not bend at the waist, and lift with the large thigh muscles. Push objects rather than pull them. Sit in chairs with good support, sleep on a firm or semi firm mattresses. Avoid shoulder stooping – do not walk with high-heeled shoes for prolonged periods. Size up the load to determine the number of persons needed to perform task.

Some **neurological problems,** such as CVA/ cerebrovascular accident, head injury, brain tumor and brain abscess can cause increased intracranial pressure ICP a life-threatening complication. Through prompt recognition and aggressive management of this complication, permanent neurological dysfunction or death may be prevented, CVA commonly referred to as a stroke that is a, disruption in the normal blood supply to the brain. It often occurs suddenly and produces focal neurological deficits. The brain must receive a constant flow of blood for normal function because if deprived of its blood flow, the brain can be damaged irreparably within a few minutes.

Brain **Absences** is a purulent infection of the brain in which pus forms in the extradural subdural or intracerebral area of the brain. The causative organisms are most often bacteria, which invade the brain directly or indirectly.

Organisms from the ear, the sinus, or the mastoid are generally enter the brain by traveling along the wall of the cerebral veins and therefore may spread to any area of the brain. The organism from ear erodes the bone from a tract and directly enters brain. Septic emboli from the heart, the lungs, dental or peritonsillar abscess may break off and enter the systemic circulation. These organisms may become lodged in a cerebral vessel and produce a localized infection.

The **human** *eye* is not only beautiful; it is a masterpiece of design and expression, far more wonderful than the finest optical instrument made by human. Marvelous instrument, a living camera that can focus itself automatically according to the amount of light and the distance of the object we are looking at. We have two of these little cameras, each independent of the other, yet working together. Long before anyone dreamed of photography, motion pictures or television, the human body contained these magnificent twin cameras that not only give beauty and expression to the face but inform us constantly of what is going on around us. Before we are born our eyes were already formed.

The *eye is the sensory* organ responsible for gathering visual stimuli to assist people communicating with the world around them. Nurses need an understanding of the structure and function of the eye, and of the relationship of the eye to the body, when caring for patient with ophthalmic disorders in addition assessment of visual function is an important component. The eyeball, a spherical organ is located in the anterior portion of the orbit. The orbit, the bony structure of the skull that surrounds the eye, protects the eye, visual changes affect each patient in a unique manner, and the uses a holistic approach to guide the patient care. The need to investigate the impact of visual alterations is important.

The **human** *ear* is one of the most important and also one of the most beautifully designed organs of the whole body. We live in the world of sound. All through our waking hours and even during sleep our ears are alert. They play their part in protecting us from injury and they help us on guard and well informed of what is happening around us. The **ear** is the sensory organ of hearing and balance. Hearing impairment is common and onset may be insidious. Many medications affect hearing. Impaired hearing is a common health problem. Wax, physical disruption in the transmission of the sound waves, infection of the middle ear, formation of spongy bone around structures of middle ear leading to low-tone hearing impairment, damage of the structures important for hearing, age related degenerative changes in the ear, leading to decreased hearing acuity, hearing loss resulting from neural defects, such many disorders affect the ear.

Early hearing loss can be noticed when a person frequently asking people to repeat sentences, straining to hear, turning the head to favor one ear or leaning forward.

Also shouting in conversation, experiencing ringing in the ears, failing to respond when not looking in the direction of the sound.

We can also notice in person demonstrating irritability answering questions incorrectly. Raising the volume of TV or radio, avoiding large group are some of the symptoms.

Prevention of ear infection or trauma – do not use small objects such as cotton-tipped applicators, matches, toothpicks, hairpins to clean your external ear canal. Blow your nose gently, sneeze with your mouth open. Wear sound protection around loud continuous noises. Avoid activities with high risk for head or ear trauma such as wrestling, boxing, motorcycle riding and skateboarding, frequently clean headphones, telephone receiver that come into contact with ear. Avoid environmental conditions with rapid changes in air pressure.

Skeletal disorders include metabolic bone diseases, bone tumors and a variety of deformities and syndromes. The elderly patient is at the greatest risk for the development of many of disorders particularly metabolic bone disease, osteoporosis, osteomalacia, bone cancer.

Trauma to the *musculoskeletal* system ranges from simple muscle strain to multiple bone fractures with severe soft tissue damage. Fracture is a break or disruption in the continuity of a bone. Fracture can occur anywhere in the body at any age.

Every healthy person enjoys eating. This is one of the pleasures of life. Digestion begins the moment food is introduced into the mouth. Ptyalin is added to the food from the saliva which begins to break down the starches and it is a valuable enzymes.

GI Assessment–have you noticed changes in your bowel habits?

If, so, what are they

Have you experience a sudden weight gain or loss?

Do you smoke?

Do you have pain?

Have you noticed any skin change?

Has your appetite changed?

Do you have any problem with swallowing?

Have you have any indigestion or feeling of bloating of fullness?

Have often did the feelings occur?

Problems of the **oral cavity** pose numerous actual and potential difficulties for many patients. The basic functions of eating, breathing, and speaking can be severely impaired by diseases or trauma to the oval cavity, appearance of body image and self concept linked to it. Eat balanced diet, brush and floss your teeth everyday, maintain emotional health see dentist regularly, fit dentures properly.

Intervention for patients with **esophageal problems,** the esophagus severs as a food conduit, transporting the bolus of food from the mouth to the stomach. Esophagus is vulnerable to a variety of inflammatory structural, motor and neoplastic health problems.

GI disease heartburn regurgitation coughing, hoarseness or wheezing at night, dysphasia painful swallowing chest pain, belching, flatulence, nausea with vomiting unplanned weight loss; eat small 4 to 6 meals a day. Limit fatty foods, coffee, tea, cola and chocolate. Eliminate spice, alcohol and tobacco, eat slowly and chew food thoroughly to reduce belching, remain upright 1 to 2 hours after meal, never sleep flat in bed, do not wear constrictive clothing, avoid heavy lifting, straining and working in a bent over position. Nurses play a vital role to prevent complications, and promote comfort and provide health teaching.

Because of common symptoms among people with various types of intestinal diseases, inflammatory and infectious intestinal disorders are often difficult to differentiate. Some disorders are acute and easily treated; others are chronic and may be life-threatening. Appendicitis, peritonitis and gastroenteritis are the most common acute inflammatory bowel problems. If these disorders are not treated early major symptomatic complications can result.

The *liver* is the largest single glandular structure; and one of the body's most vital internal organs. It is located high up on the right side of the abdomen under the lower ribs and just under the diaphragm which divides the chest from the abdomen. Liver has many important functions to perform, for it is the great chemical laboratory of our body. When one is healthy the liver works so smoothly that you never give it a second thought. It performs more than 400 functions, which affects every system in the body. Most of the foods we eat are stored in the liver, after having been digested and absorbed from the gastrointestinal tract. Certain vitamins also are stored in the liver. When the liver can not perform its complex activities, hepatic failure result; Liver diseases range from mild hepatic inflammation to chronic end-stage cirrhosis resulting in death. Cirrhosis is a chronic progressive liver disease.

Prevention of *viral hepatitis:* Maintain adequate sanitation and personal hygiene wash your hands before eating and after using toilet. Drink purified water. Wash vegetables and fruits well. Do not share bed linens, towels, eating utensils or drinking glasses. Do not share needles for injection. Avoid all medications, including over the counter unless prescribed by your physician. Avoid all alcohol. Rest; eat small frequent meals that have high carbohydrate and low fat content.

Disorders of the *gallbladder* and the pancreas initially occur as single organ processes. If the primary disorder is untreated the inflammatory response may extend to other organs. The anatomic proximity of the liver, the gallbladder and the pancreas as well as the possibility of impeded flow of bile from the liver through the gallbladder ductile system, contributes to potential complications and multigrain involvement in diseases processes, obstruction of bile flow by gallstones, edema, structure and tumors can cause inflammation of gallbladder, the liver and the pancreas, depending on location of the obstruction in the biliary system.

Acute *Pancreatitis* is a serious and at times, life threatening inflammatory process of the pancreas, resulting in auto digestion of the organ by its own enzymes. The pathologic changes occur in variable degrees. The severity of pancreatitis depends on the extent of inflammation and tissue destruction, ranging form mild involvement evidenced by edema and inflammation to necrotizing hemorrhagic pancreatitis. This sever form of Pancreatitis is characterized by diffusely bleeding pancreatic tissue with fibrosis and tissue death. Many factors can produce injury to the pancreas. For example, alcoholism and biliary tract disease with gallstone, trauma from surgery pancreatic tumors, cysts and abscesses viral inflammation, toxicities of drugs, steroids and oral contraceptives.

In chronic pancreatic, clinical manifestation is intense abdominal pain, abdominal tenderness, ascities weight loss, jaundice, dark urine, diabetes mellitus are noticed. Avoid alcohol, eat bland, low fat meats, and avoid gastric stimulants such as spices. Eat small meals and snacks high in calories. Rest frequently restricts your activity. Nurse provides emotional support to client and family to deal with issues related to this life-threatening illness.

Eating disorders—Teach your children to eat in moderation from all food groups and to avoid an excess concentration of fats and sweets. Be a role model for your children by showing them healthy eating and dieting behaviors, foster self-esteem. Help select an appropriate diet that is within the calories limits allowed, take fluids to prevent constipation take foods in high fiber. Malnutrition and obesity are common nutrition problems.

Most invading germs enter the body through the nose and throat. Germs are often carried into the body on tiny droplets of water when air is drawn into the lungs. Food particles may also be infected with various types of germs.

The human body has been given a most beautiful covering the **skin**. Nothing is more lovely and attractive than a glowing, health skin. It is first line of Defence against the germs that might enter the body. *Skin* as the largest organ of the body, it regulates many physiologic functions, such as body temperature, fluid and electrolyte balance. It also acts as a physical barrier to invasion by harmful microorganisms. Throughout a person's life span the appearance and functioning of the skin may be altered by aging process, emotional stress, injury and disease.

Nurse to see appearance and texture of the skin, pain, itching heat, cold and pressure can provide patients well-being, skin problem medical-surgical history – family history.

Is there any family tendency toward chronic skin problems?

Is patient allergic to any systemic or tropical medications?

What drug reactions he has?

What is over the counter drug taken recently?

What is his occupation, has traveled recently?

Where body it begun, is it associated with itching, burning, stinging, numbness, pain, fever, nausea, vomiting diarrhea, sore throat, cold, stiff neck, new foods, new soups, or cosmetics, new clothing or bed linens, or stressful situation?

Does Anything Make the Problem Worse?

For example, Sun exposure medication heat or cold or a dry environment, improper skin lubrication, inadequate fluid intake, breaks in the integrity of the skin, skin changes linked to poor hygiene, low socioeconomic backgrounds. Excessive soiling, matted hair body odor, self-care deficits, dry skin is common problem in elderly patients, poor skin hydration, increased skin temperature, perspiration.

The **human body is a living engine**. Like any other engine, it burns fuel/food and requires a constant supply of oxygen, as well as water and various important chemical substances. Once the various food materials have reached the organs of the body they are quickly utilized for energy and for the repairing damaged tissues.

All of this means that there is a constant building up and breaking down of tissue, a process known as metabolism. In this process a considerable amount of waste material must be removed of the body is to stay healthy. Part of this waste material is given off through the lungs in the forms of carbon dioxide, other waste products being eliminated through the urine.

The *kidneys* filter metabolic waste products from the blood and excrete these wastes in excessive body water, structural or functional alterations in any part of the urinary tract may be life-threatening. Diagnostic test provides information, changes occur as a result of the aging process.

The **socioeconomic status** of the patient may influence health care practices. People with limited income or no health insurance often ignore physical ailments or delay seeking health care because they lack funds to pay for diagnostic test or treatment. They may have difficulty following medical advice. A patient's education level may affect his health-seeking practices. Recurring UTI often results from inadequate or incomplete treatment, including lack of follow-up, lack of money to pay for antibiotics or nutritious foods. Patient's health belief affects his approach to health and illness, cultural background and religious affiliation may influence the belief system.

The family history **of renal problem is significant** because some disease are genetically transmittal or have a familial inheritance pattern, history of diet and any recent changes in diet pattern, current health problem – nursing interventions are directed toward prevention, detection and management of urologic disorders.

To prevent UTI/urinary tract infection drink 2-3 liters of fluid daily clean your perineum, avoid irritating substances such as bubble bath, nylon underwear, wear cotton, burning or frequently, difficulty in urination notify health care provider. Empty your bladder regularly. Monitor bowel movement to prevent constipation. If urine is foul-smelling; if blood in the urine notify physician.

When UTI obstruction is present, pressure builds up directly on tissue, which can cause structural damage. The nurse assesses the patient for his emotional reaction to the alteration in renal function. Acute renal failure affects much body system. Chronic renal failure affects every body system. The abnormalities related to fluid volume excess, electrolyte and acid-base abnormalities accumulated nitrogenous wastes, hormonal inadequacies. CRF / chronic renal failure is a permanent, irreversible condition in which the kidney ceases to remove metabolic wastes and excessive water from the blood. When kidney function is inadequate for sustaining life chronic renal failure is referred to as end stage renal diseases.

CRF – Diminished renal reserve stage – I. Renal function is reduced, but no accumulation of metabolic wastes occurs. Ability to concentrate urine is decreased, resulting in nocturia and polyuria. Stage – II, Renal insufficiency metabolic wastes begin to accumulate in the blood because the unaffected nephrons can no longer compensate responsiveness of diuretics is decreased, resulting in oliguria and edema. Treatment is by dialysis or other renal replacement therapy, CRF results in serious abnormalities in many laboratory values. Values routinely monitored are serum Creatinine, blood urea nitrogen levels serum sodium, serum potassium, serum calcium, serum phosphate, serum bicarbonate, hemoglobin, hematocrit, frequent hospitalization for evaluation and modification of treatment plan.

AV FISTULA, AV GRAFT OR AV SHUNT—CARE

Do not take blood spressure readings using the extremity in which the vascular access is placed.

Do not perform vein punctures or start IVS in the extremity in which the vascular access is placed.

Palpate for thrills and auscultation for bruits every 4 hours while the patient is awake.

Assess the patient's distal pulses and circulation.

Elevate the affected extremity postoperatively.

Encourage routine range-of-motion exercises.

Check for bleeding at needle insertion sites or shunt tubing insertion site.

Keep small clamps handy on the dressing of the AV Shunt.

Assess for sign symptoms of inflammation at needle sites and shunt tubing insertion sites.

Do not allow patient to carry heavy objects or anything that compresses the extremity in which the vascular access is placed.

Do not allow patient to sleep with his body weight on top of the extremity in which the vascular access in placed.

The patient undergoing hemodialysis; weight the patient before and after dialysis. Know patient's dry weight. Discuss with the physician whether any of the patents medications should be withheld until after dialysis. Be aware of events that occurred during the dialysis treatment. Measure BP, pulse rate, respiration, temperature, observe for bleeding, headache, nausea, vomiting. Wash your hands, put on sterile gloves, remove the old dressing, and remove the contaminated gloves. Assess for inflammation, such as swelling redness or discharge around the catheter site.

What is Renal Transplantation?

Dialysis and transplantation are life-sustaining treatments for end stage of renal diseases [ESRD] transplantation is not considered a 'cure'. It is up to each client.

Candidates for transplantation must be free from medical problems that might increase the risks associated with the procedure. The usual age range for patients undergoing transplantation is 4 to 70 years. In patient older than 70 years, the risk of complications increases but patient older than 70 are considered on an individual basis.

A thorough body systems assessment of the patient is performed before he is considered for transplantation. The process of transplantation can place a life-threatening stress on the cardiac system in patient with advanced, uncorrectable cardiac disease. Other contraindication includes active infection, IV Drugs abuse, malignant neoplasm, severe obesity, active vacuities severe psychological problems.

Donor are living related donors and cadaver donors. Some use living unrelated donor who meet stringent eligibility requirements. The available kidneys are matched on the basis of immunologic similarity between the donor and the recipient clients and donors do not need to be matched for age, race or sex.

The size of the kidney is seldom a problem except in the youngest pediatric patients. Pediatric cadaver kidneys hypertrophy to accommodate adult needs within a few months, an adult kidney shrinks after placement in a child's abdominal cavity, increasing in size as the child grows.

Organs from *living related donors* (LRDs) provide the highest rates of renal graft survival. Donors are usually at least 18 years old because of legal requirements and are seldom older than 65 years. The physical criteria for donors include – the absence of systemic disease and infection, no history of cancer the absence of HBP/high blood pressure and renal disease. Adequate renal function as evidenced by diagnostic studies – living related donors must express a clear understanding of the associated surgery and a willingness to give up a kidney.

In *cadaver donor,* the brain-dead persons body is kept functioning by technical means until immediately before the kidneys are removed. The kidneys are specially preserved and transported immediately to recipient waiting in another operation room or in other hospital.

The transplant recipient usually requires dialysis within 24 hours of the surgery in addition the recipient often receives a blood transfusion before surgery. Current research favors donor – specific transfusion, in which blood from kidney donor is transfused into the recipient. This procedure has resulted in increase graft survival, especially of organs from living related donors.

Operative procedure the donor deprecatory varies between cadaver donor and LRDs. The cadaver donor deprecatory is conducted as a sterile autopsy in OT. All arterial and venous vessels and as long a piece of urethra is possible are carefully preserved. After removal the kidneys are preserved until time for implantation into the recipient. The technique for kidney removal from LRDs requires greater surgical care and is a delicate procedure lasting 3–4 hours.

A flank incision is used, and care is taken to avoid scarring. They need special nursing care and support for the psychological adjustment to loss of a body part. The transplanted kidney is usually placed in the usual anatomic position. This placement allows easier anastomosis of the urethra and the renal artery and vein and also minimizes postoperative pain. The recipients own nonfunctioning kidneys are not usually removed, unless chronic infection in one or both kidneys would compromise overall recovery in critical care unit.

Complication unfortunately, numerous potential complications are associated with transplant surgery.

Rejection is the most common and the most threatening complication of renal transplantation is a reaction occurs between the antigens in the transplanted kidney and the antibodies and cytotoxic T cells in the recipient's blood. These immunologic substances treat the new kidney as a foreign invader and cause tissue destruction thrombosis and types rejection: hyper acute, acute, and chronic.

What is the Importance of Breast Care?

The most common disorder of the breast is a lump or mass. The discovery of a lump in a woman's breast is often perceived as a sentence of death. 90% all breast lumps are benign;

she may think that the lump is cancerous. This fearful reaction accompanies the woman throughout the period of diagnosis decision making and treatment, what final outcome. Whether the disease proves to be benign or malignant and whether the care end after diagnosis, treatment or death the nurse is aware of both the physiologic and emotional factors involved to be effective in nursing care.

Identify the location of the mass by the face of the clock method.

Describe the shape, size and consistency of the mass.

Assess whether the mass in fixed or movable

Note any skin changes around the mass such as dimple, increased vascularity, nipple retraction or ulceration.

Assess the adjacent lymph nodes both auxiliary and supraclavicular nodes.

Ask the patient if she experience pain or soreness in the area around the mass.

Nurses collect health data, analyze, consider factors related to safety, effectiveness and cost in planning and delivering patient care.

What are the specific psychological and physiologic impacts of PMS/premenstrual syndrome on patient?

What nursing interventions promote self-esteem in patient with a reproductive dysfunction?

Technique of Moving a Lifting Patient

Once the nurse knows the diseases condition it will help her for moving and lifting a patient safely. A cardiac patient in ICU should be moved on the advice of a doctor. A very ill patient with low pulse and pressure should be moved without the patients help. Very ill patients should be moved as little as possible. While moving or lifting a patient you should avoid bending your back. Draw the patient to the side of the bed and bend your knees slightly. Lifting patient's hips have patient flex knees with feet flat on bed, place your hand under sacrum to raise hips and ask him to bear weight slightly upon his feet. Invalid or obese patient two or more staffs are needed. Care taken while moving or lifting a hip

While lifting patients, head and shoulder raise head with one hand bend your arm slightly, pass it behind the patient, place hand under his far shoulder fingers in axilla. The neck of patient should rest in bend of our elbow. When moving patient to one side of the bed one nurse pass one arm under patients neck and shoulder, the other under upper part of thigh and draw him towards you. Two nurses- one nurse support had and shoulder with one arm and slips other arm under back beside that of the other and the other arm under the thighs. Nurse may sand on the same side of the bed.

When turning the patient on his side cross patients legs slip left arm over his far shoulder to turn patient towards you. Slip other arm over his far hip, raise him slightly and turn him towards you. Keep pillow under his head.

When lifting patient upon pillow ask patient to flex his knees, pass left arm under upper part of thigh and knees. Have the patient put hands on bed, palms down and slightly bear his Weight on hands and push up with his feet. Make sure that your lifting corresponds with his pushing. If patient is unable to do this two nurses are required.

When carrying patient from bed to a stretcher place stretcher parallel to bed. Four persons are required. One starts on the opposite side of the bed. Three will have to reach across the stretcher. The person at the head and the foot end of the starchier may find it easier to step around the end of the stretcher. Grasp sheet beneath patient and support shoulder and legs separately. Coordinate lifting and swing patient by pulling the sheet and patient towards stretcher, quickly and gently. The sheet can be removed at this time by turning patient from side to side or wait until the patient has been transfer from the stretcher to the bed or table again. The opposite method is used when moving a patient from the stretcher to the bed.

CHAPTER 9

Nurse and Management of Cancer

The word 'cancer' frightens most people. Too many people this word means death. The term cancer is a collective term describing a large group of diseases characterized by uncontrolled growth and spread of abnormal cells.

20 years ago, cancer was incurable, today because of advance in early diagnosis and treatment more and more people are living longer. Nursing personnel's are involved in all phases of cancer experience that is prevention, detection, diagnosis, treatment, rehabilitation, survivorship, palliative and terminal care. Cancer clients are seen in the home, office, clinic, hospice settings.

Cancer to be world's top killer 2010 says WHO cancer will overtake heart diseases. Rising tobacco use in developing countries is believed to be a huge reason for the shift particularly in China and India. Where 40% of the world's smokers now live; Global cancer deaths are expected to reach 7 million according to WHO an annual rise of 1% cases.

Cancer strikes all ages, socioeconomic and cultural background and both sexes. The incidence rate for cancer reflects the number of new cases occurring in a given population at risk during a specified time. It gives current magnitude of the problem and helps to establish future priorities in control program.

Today all diagnostic methods are more precise than in the past and now they are correctly diagnosed. Cancer of the oral cavity, pharynx, liver, pancreas, colon have decreased, at the same time, the survival rate for Hodgkin's disease and prostate, testicular, bladder cancer has increased.

Despite significance advances in detection, diagnosis and treatment, cancer continues to be a significant health problem. Prevention and early detection of cancer is high priority to further decrease caner morbidity and mortality rate. The exact causes of cancer still unknown and it remains obscure. Researchers are actively pursuing the role of immunity in preventing, controlling and treating cancer investigators are trying to determine weather the immune system controls the spontaneous regression of tumors a mysterious phenomenon is provocative and unanswered question. Researchers suspect that cancer results from multiple agents working together.

The study of virus as carcinogens is one of the most rapidly advancing areas in cancer research today. They have proof that virus may be one of the multiple agents acting to initiate carcinogenesis virus have been associated with hepatic cellular carcinoma, T-cell lymphoma, T-cell leukemia and cervical cancer.

Some chemicals like tar, soot, dyes, and fuel oil are found to be carcinogens and usually workers in industries where these chemicals used cancer is found. Radiation and asbestos are physical carcinogens. Scientists have found relationship exists between hormonal secretion, action, tumor development and growth.

The incidence of different types of cancer varies on a geographic basis. People in certain jobs are more susceptible to certain cancer because of their greater contact with specific carcinogens. There are number of cancers that provide evidence of a heritable predisposition of cancer. The role of diet in the causation of cancer is unclear. Recent research suggests a strong link between stress and cancer. Physical changes can occur in the patient throughout the cancer experience. The malignant tumor itself may cause oblivious disfigurement or internal organ changes even prior to diagnosis.

Surgery as in the amputation of a breast or arms. Radiation therapy may cause change in body functions and skin integrity. Chemotherapy may lead to hair loss, weight gain or weight lost, and skin pigmentation changes. Although some of the physical, changes influence a patient's self-concept, self-esteem and general feeling of worth and acceptance remains intact. The fact that client brings with him his own set of values, beliefs, attitudes, resources and coping mechanisms to the cancer experience. Anxiety along with depression, each client diagnosed with cancer reacts to the diagnosis differently and has unique concerns and problems regarding diagnosis and treatment each on cops with cancer in his own unique way.

The diagnosis and treatment of cancer are expensive, medical intervention is technical and lengthy. The financial consequences of the illness are a major concern to the client.

Despite research advances, investigations still have unanswered questions about cancer. What is a cancer cell/ how does it differ from a normal cell? What are the factors that cause cancer cells to develop? Researchers are learning more about normal cells and their regulation at the genetic level. The walls of tumor cells are different from those of their normal counterparts. Distant lymph nodes may be affected later in the diseases. The blood vessels carry cancer ceils from the primary tumor to the capillary beds of the lungs, liver and bones. Metastasis spread to distant organs and tissues is usually the result of cells moving through the bloodstream.

Benign grows slowly, usually continues to grow throughout life unless surgically removed. It always remains localized, it never infiltrates surrounding tissues. Recurrence extremely unusual when surgically removed. Metastases never occur, it is not harmful.

Malignant usually grows rapidly, infiltrating surrounding tissues, recurrence and metastasis is common. It is harmful to the host. It depends on cell type and speed of diagnosis, poor prognosis indicated.

Prevention—Risk analysis and modification. Screening is ideal method of cancer control. Early detection is major tool in the fight against cancer to eradicate it early. Early detection could raise the survival rate to 50%.

Emphasizing the need for an annual physical examination by stressing the importance of yearly pap test, BSE/breast self examination, testicular self-examination, increasing public awareness of cancers warning signals. The seven warning signals such as-change in bowel or bladder habits; a sore that does not heal; unusual bleeding or discharge, thickening or lump in breast or elsewhere, indigestion or difficulty in swallowing, obvious change in wart or mole. Nagging cough or hoarseness, if you have a warning signal, see your doctor.

Physical examination for all people over 40 includes examination of skin, lymph nodes, mouth, thyroid, breast, testes, and rectum and prostrate. Avoid those factors that might lead to primary prevention such as cigarette smoking, sunlight, ionizing radiation, faulty nutrition. Risk factor for lung cancer is all types of smoking, air pollution, and family history of lung cancer. Similarly, breast cancer has family history, especially on maternal side and occurring before menopause, history of early menarche, late menopause, and birth of a first child after 30s. Cancer risk increases in obese person, high fiber food diet might help reduce risk of colon cancer. A varied diet containing plenty of vegetables and fruits rich in vit A and C may reduce risk for a wide range if cancers. Salt cured, smoked, and nitrite cured foods have been linked to stomach cancer.

Diagnosis is done to obtain family environmental history, through physical examination, evaluating laboratory test of blood, tissue, sputum, urine and other specimens, a digital rectal examination, procto-sigmoidoscopy. Health care professionals must face the difficulty of telling client in time about the diagnosis. Health teaching on proper diet, exercise, health habits, high risk women , that is abnormal uterine bleeding, estrogen therapy, history of infertility, diabetes, high pressure to advice to do test of endometrial tissues sample and fecal occult blood test. Effective test should be specific anatomic site, reliable, acceptance to client, and cost benefit.

Radiation safety precaution for internal implants: Place the client in a private room. Plan care well so minimal time is spent in direct contact with client with implant avoiding any close contact with unshielded areas. Use lead apron or lead shield. Health care personnel should wear appropriate monitoring devices, room marked with appropriate signs. Prevent undue exposure, prepare meals trays outside room and work quickly as possible to avoid unnecessary high amount of radiation.

The search to understand and manipulate the human immune system has fascinated scientists for decades. Evidence exists that under the proper circumstances, malignant tumors are susceptible to immune surveillance and subsequent destruction. This, the quest to isolate and identified effective biologic agents continues.

Cancer is a feared and dreaded disease for several reasons. It may present in an advanced stage with no symptoms. Cancer may recur after many years of remission; great variability exists in the effects of cancer on the lives of client and the families. Respond to cancer depends on client's psychological make up, family, social community, disability it may cause. Cancer affects intellectual functions, client's self-concept is affected by the physical changes such as laryngectomy, glossectomy; produce changes that may be humiliating and overwhelming to the client.

Cancer has impact on family and their daily life in changed with extensive, rigorous treatment without a guarantee of cure. Each cancer experience is unique and most clients experience fear of death first few months of treatment. Fear such as when will be symptoms relived, what will be the side effect of treatment, will I able to return to work? Some client withdraw into isolation, some laugh it off making situation light. Some distract themselves by doing some other things, are some of the coping strategies clients use.

Some avoid, feel helpless, powerless, guilt and hostility, blaming others, depression and denial are some of there responses. Some try to get social support, become hopeful, positive, self-esteemed, seek information's, and turn to God and religion. Nurses have to help them to deal with their emotions by listening actively and allow expressing negative feelings, doing counselling, putting up music and give antiretroviral therapy (ART), stressing relaxation technique and identifying the misconception and correcting it. Provide compassion, caring, sensitivity and understanding in time of uncertainty and threat.

After chemotherapy or radiation, support and bridge home health care. Function as a vital link, touch and say kind words which will provide comfort and solace. Advice him to eat small frequent meals, eat food at room temperature, avoid fatty and fried foods, spicy foods, take regular nausea medications so eating is possible. Drink lot of water to support blood pressure, flush the bladder and replace fluid that is lost in vomiting and diarrhea. Pay attention to mouth care, use soft tooth brush, keep lips moist and rise mouth after every meals, use prescribed medications, good hand washing and maintain body temperature to promote comfort.

In chronic cancer, the hope for cure becomes the struggle for existence. Be sensitive and alleviate complications assist them when disease enters the terminal phase of illness. Terminally ill 50% die with diseases. Provide support care until death occurs providing comfort and dignity during the dying process. The nurse is the witness to the essence of human life and the courage of the human spirit. Beyond what machines, medicines, and procedures can do for the client, the act of caring remains a powerful weapon in the fight against disease. It is one thing that medical technology can never replace. When everything is done, that can be done, compassion is the only thing that brings beauty and meaning to our lives. It is the irreplaceable gift. The nurse must be sensitive to the emotional aspect of their illness, be skilled with technical aspect of care, and anticipate client's needs. Caring can be just as successful as curing especially when such care is exercised during the final stage of life the last journey on earth.

Malignant cells—Mitosis leads to multiple daughter cells that may or may not resemble the parent. Multiple mitotic spindles, cells larger and grow more rapidly than normal. Heterogenous in size and shape; cells not as cohesive, irregular patterns of expansion Larger, more prominent nucleus, lack characteristic pattern of organization of host cells. Anaplastic, lack of differentiated cell characteristics, specific functions invade adjacent tissues. Proliferation in response to abnormal stimuli, growth in adverse conditions such as lack of nutrients.

Do not exhibit contact inhibition. Cell birth exceeds cell death. Loss of cell control a result of cell membrane changes, growth rate erratic. Able to break off cells that migrate through blood stream or lymphatic or seed to distant sites and grow in other sites.

Do not contribute to the well being of the host, parasitic, actually feed off host without contributing anything. If cells function at all they do not function normally, or they may actually cause damage. Develop antigens completely different from a normal cell. Chromosomal aberrantions occur as cell matures invades, erode and speed grow in presence of narcosis and inflammatory cells such as lymphocyte and macrophages. Exhibit periods of latency that vary from tumor to tumor.

Have own blood supply and supporting stoma.

Seven warning–change in bowel or bladder habits.

A sore that does not heal

Unusual bleeding or discharge

Thickening or lump in breast or elsewhere.

Indigestion or difficulty in swallowing

Obvious change in wart or mole

Nagging cough or hoarseness

An understanding of the basic principles concerning its development, prevention and early detection is essential.

Patient to be helped in coping by giving social support, positive appraisal, hopefulness, self esteem and problem solving ability.

Help him to avoid denial, powerlessness, gilt, despair and depression. It affects all levels of functioning. It has an impact on the entire family. Nurses have important role in the caring process of a patient's illness, especially during the final stages of patient's life.

Help patient and the family to elevate fear and misconception. Provide a quiet, calm environment. Provide an opportunity for patient to discuss concerns. Talking with skilled professional may further assist the patient with constructive problem solving.

Nursing care requires sharpened critical thinking skill. Nurse must be able to think through the complexities of using highly technical intervention and pharmacotherapeutics. To provide the best possible care through understanding, she needs to be assertive person. Nurses who work in such setting which they have large responsibility in helping the patient understand the possible results of radical procedures. You can help patient work through their feelings and offering supportive services and counseling.

Nurses see their patient in all stages of health and illness. Nurses are more aware of the whole episode of care, including post discharge issues. She is in unique position to reinforce teaching strategies. Patient well motivated will follow the instructions and medications. Nurses must be skilled in physical and psychosocial aspect when providing care.

Research—Vaccine without side effect- tobacco plant used in fight against cancer. Tobacco normally associated with causing cancer rather then helping cure it- could aid people with lymphoma in fighting the disease. US researcher said, the treatment, which would vaccinate cancer clients against their own tumor cells, made using a new approach that turns genetically engineered tobacco plants into vaccine. First time plant has been used for making a protein to inject into a person. The idea is no marshal the body's own immune system to fight *cancer*.

Now, a vaccine for lung cancer—Cuban scientists, first registered vaccine in the world designed to battle lung cancer, the vaccine based on two proteins triggers an immune response from the victim's body and has no side effects. The vaccine is available in Cuba.

Cancer catheter—Scientists create new biochip that can detect cancer before symptoms develop; that can save lives by diagnosing before patient become symptomatic. A tumor even in its earliest asymptomatic phases can affect proteins that find their way into a patient's circulatory system. These proteins trigger the immune system to kick into gear, producing antibodies that regulates which protein belong and which do not. This technique doctors could use to understand and fight cancer better.

The term cancer was coined by Greek physical Galen from coercions meaning crab, because of the similarity to crabs to some tumors with swollen veins. The oldest description and surgical treatment of cancer was discovered in Egypt and dates back to approximately 1600 BC. The papyrus describes either case of ulcers of the breast that were treated by cauterization, with a tool called the fire drill.

New video game puts cancer patients inside a virtual body to blast tumors; players show Improved adherence to treatment and increased knowledge of condition.

Brain cancer in children is becoming a problem worldwide. The incidence rate of brain tumors in children across the world is increasing by about 2.7% per year. The survival rate is approximately 60%, but this varies with the age of onset and cancer type, with young and children having higher mortality.

Cell phone—Radiation-exposure beyond a certain level of frequencies can be a health hazard. The invisible threat of gadgets like mobile and laptops are we paying huge price on such electronic items? Mobile radiation damage DNA- and low sperm count, TV, computer, vacuum cleaner, microwave etc. cordless phone, fax machines, hair dryers. High frequency EMFS - electromagnetic fields to digestive disorders, fatigue, high blood pressure, insomnia, irritability, low blood pressure, infertility in males, cancer, neurological and cardiovascular problems. Risk of leukemia, risk of brain cancer unshielded headsets, potentially self-harming antenna, holding the phone close to the brain regularly increases changes of brain tumor. What is further warring is the cell phone and their growing tissues are much more vulnerable to harmful radiation.

Cell phone use ups brain cancer risk in kids. Kids and teenagers today are an increased risk of developing brain cancer. If they use mobile phone according to an alarming new research, kids are five times more likely to get brain cancer due to mobile use. The research raises fears that today's young people may suffer an; epidemic' of the disease in later life. People who started mobile phone use before the age of 20 had more then five fold increase glioma, a cancer of the glial cells that support the central nervous system. The extra risk to young people of contracting the disease from using the cordless phone found in many homes was almost as great at more then four times higher. Five times more likely to get acoustic neuromas benign but often-disabling tumors of the auditory nerve, usually causing disease. This is the warning sign and it is very worring. We should be talking precautions.

TOP TEN FUN WAYS TO PREVENT CANCER THROUGH EXERCISE

The American Cancer Society recommends exercising 30 minutes a day, 5 days a week for cancer prevention. If you cringe at the word, "exercise" check out these fun ways for fitness. You will have so much fun; you will not even consider it to be working out!

Walking

Walking has many health benefits, such as cancer and other disease prevention. Instead of using the treadmill, walk outdoors. If you can find a safe sidewalk, or park, you can walk! Bring headphones and listen to music, or even an audio book.

Make it a family event! Exercise is important for children, too! Moreover, if kids are involved, they will not ever let you forget when it times to take a walk!

Yoga

If you have never done Yoga before, why not start a beginners' class? Yoga is a great physical activity and is a great stress reliever. Do not worry if you are not flexible; you will work your way up each class. Bringing a friend to class with you makes it easier and less intimidating. Once you learn the basic, you can do the exercises at home in your free time.

Dancing

Dancing can be the most fun way to meet fitness goals. You can dance in the privacy of your living room, or go to a club. If you have two left feet, try a dance class! Learn salsa, ballroom dancing or even the meringue! There are so many types of dance to learn, you can't go wrong.

Rollerblading

Rollerblading just is not for the kids! Make sure you have the proper protective gear like a helmet, knee and elbow pads, and have a go at rollerblading! It is very cardiovascular and works out all muscle of the body. Do not worry if you do not get it at first, practice makes perfect!

Tai Chi

Tai Chi is a Chinese martial art that promotes health through slow moving exercises and breathing techniques. It is also meditative. Classes can be taught in a group setting or in private classes. Many seniors practice tai chi for its health benefits.

Join a Team Sport

Joining a team sport like softball, volleyball, and soccer can be tons of fun! Organized sports are sometimes offered through the workplace and recreation centers. If your workplace does not have one, why not organize a sport? You'll meet new people and engage in healthy competition.

Swimming

Swimming is an excellent form of exercise! You workout out all muscles of the body, and it can be very cardiovascular. Many gyms or YMCA's offer poem swim sessions. If you don't know how to swim, lessons are available for adults. You can also try water aerobics.

Hiking

If you love the outdoors, hiking is for you! The scenery alone makes hiking worthwhile. Set a goal for yourself like distance or the amount of time you hike during each session. Not only are you challenging yourself, you are getting one of the best ways to get in shape!

Cycling

You can cycle at home while watching TV on a stationary bike or hit the outdoors with a traditional bicycle. Most adults prefer stationary bikes because it is convenient. You can also control the resistance and simulate biking uphill or downhill. Whether you bike in the home or outdoors, you are easily meeting the 30 minutes/5 days a week goal.

Dodge Ball

Do you remember playing dodge ball in high school gym class? Dodge ball is back! Gyms and race centers across the country are catching onto the new trend by offering classes and organized teams. It is also the ultimate stress reliever! Think back to when playing in school, how good it felt to get someone "out". Yes, its definitely a stress reliever!

Follow the above mentioned tips to lead a healthy and a happy life.

ALWAYS LISTEN TO YOUR FAMILY DOCTOR

I have learned that it's taking me a long time to become the person I want to be.

I have learned that you should always leave loved ones with loving words.

It may be the last time you see them.

I have learned that you can keep going long after you think you can't.

I have learned that we are responsible for what we do, no matter how we feel.

I have learned that either you control your attitude or it controls you.

I have learned that learning to forgive takes practice.

I have learned that there are people who love you dearly, but just don't know how to show it.

I have learned that just because some do not love you the way you want them to, does not mean they do not love you with all they have.

CHAPTER 10

Emergency Life-Line Care

HOW DO YOU HANDLE COMMON PROBLEMS IN NURSING?

How will you Manage Emergency in Casualty?

The casualty department provides the first impression on the patient, relative and friends who come along with the patient. The first impression must be positive one. Quick and competent care can save lives and reduce severity and duration of illness. Importance to pay attention to this area of service in causality; Sudden attack requires immediate attention, therefore avoid delay, be prompt and competent in giving treatment.

When a patient's condition is such that death appears imminent, family members need the support and the health care team. It is at this most uncomfortable time that nurses have the opportunity to speak to patients and their families. How does a nurse approach an upset or grieving family? It is an not easy task to discuss this matter with their families, but nurses should assess there patient. How can nurses serve as advocates for confused patients? Patient who are confused or comatose are vulnerable to injury.

Nurses provide a lifeline for this patient provide counseling when the patient and family face many difficult decisions. Nurses play an essential role in the prevention of further damage. For example, sudden paralysis of your one side of your body, experience sudden changes in speech, vision or hearing.

The nurses need to focus care on the management of clinical manifestations and prevention of complications, family support throughout the process of care is essential. Communication is key to successful care. Maintain constant contact with the patient, family members and other members of health care team to maximize patient outcomes also to entire needs being met. Nursing care should be same to all patient, strive for justice in nursing practice.

There is acute medical and surgical emergencies, e.g. acute myocardial infarction, shock, acute abdominal pain, snake bite, accidents, attending all medicolegal formalities will require maximum attention. Causality is most important area of care and priority. To be effective in such department you need to analyze how many patients are with injuries from accident, fracture, surgical acute attract of bronchial asthma, high fever, shock, coronary thrombosis will help you to organize better care. Qualified experience trained staff handle causality patients round the clock services and specialist available and well maintained and equipped emergency medicines and attention given without delay will save man lives . Time is of essence. Poor services, incompetents' staff, unable to cope with multiple emergency, communication delay, and inadequate amenities, improper documenting of medicolegal cases and incorrect action taken will affect the emergency services.

Emergencies are very challenging and rewarding. Know the principles of emergency care; nurse can function effectively regardless of the environment in which the care is delivered. Because of the variety of the emergency possibly encountered, nurses need to be responsible, and accountable for updating there knowledge and skills besides mastering psychosocial care to the patient and significant others. As a specialist emergency nursing provides stimulating professional opportunity. Emergency nurses are active in health promotion, prevention, education, research and emergency care. They are on the forefront of providing competent and professional care to a variety of patient and significant others.

How will you Manage Various Traumatic Injuries?

Trauma means injury. People may be injured single or many at a time, e.g. train crashes terrorist activities. Nurses should make sure the familiarity of such a major disaster plans as the efficient treatment of a large number of causalities presented in or very short time depends on a large extent upon the efficient organization of the medical staff. Life threatens conditions that threats to the airway must receive absolute priority. Patient with severe head injury require urgent resuscitation and attention to the air way. The nurse should always have the time to answer patient's questions and to keep the patient informed as much as possible as to why various procedures are necessary.

A skilled staff, equipment required to obtain highest level of medical and nursing care by day and by night. In severe injuries the initial treatment is directed towards saving the patients life. Particularly by attention to the air way and the replacement of any blood loss, accurate repair of damaged tissues, fractures, prevention of infection and restoration of the function.

Expert critical nurses embrace a holistic philosophy and caring that enables them to offer a level of comfort and support that is often intuitive, it is an on going process. Nurses play a key role in prevention and early interventions areas they can meet health promotion needs in all setting.

Chest trauma- maintains airway, breathing and circulation. Obtain a quick history. What happened? What was the mechanism of injury? How long ago did it happen? Where is the pain? Does it radiate? is thee anything that makes the pain better or worse/what does the pain feel like? How severe is the pain on a sale of 1 to 10? Is there any medical history?

Check for shortness of breath and cyanosis. Check vital signs, check skin color and temperature. Check wound size and location. Check for the paradoxical chest movements, distended neck vein, tracheal deviation, and respiratory stridor, bilateral breath sounds. Look for epigastric and supraclavicular in drawing, listen to hear sounds.

Intervention-maintain airway, ensure adequate air movement, administer oxygen, cover any chest wound, frequent recheck vitals, get X-ray, monitor for dysrhythmia.

How will you manage traumatic injury like motor vehicle crashes? Ask certain questions like were you the driver or the passenger? Were you wearing a seatbelt? Did you hit the steering wheel or the dash board, if so, with what part of your body? Did you loose consciousness, if so, how long/how fast was the vehicle going? What did the vehicle hit-moving object or non moving object? Where is your pain? How far were you throw? What is the condition of other passengers?

After head injury observe increased drowsiness or confusion, inability to be awakened, vomiting, convulsions, bleeding or drainage from the nose or ear, weakness in either arm or leg, blurring of vision, slurring of speech, enlargement or shrinkage of one pupil.

Because of the complexity of brain disorders and neurologic nursing is one of the most challenging areas of practice. Prevention and early intervention are key to patient outcome. Advice to wear helmets, avoid overuse of alcohol, illicit drug use, avoid driving when drinking.

How you Manage Hemorrhage as a Nurse?

Hemorrhage is internal and external may prove fatal due to excessive loss of blood. When external arterial bleeding takes place it is bright red, comes with high pressure, occurs due to deep cut/injury and takes time to stop. Pressure need to apply on main trunk of the artery. Venous hemorrhage is dark red, blood escapes as a continuous flow with low pressure stops automatically. In capillary bleeding is bright red, oozes from the surface, sometimes oozing causes heavy loss of blood? To stop bleeding apply digital pressure with index finger for 5-10 minutes. With this if bleeding does not stop pad press it by palm of your hand 5-10 minutes. Tourniquets used on limbs to stop circulation of blood. Sign and symptoms of bleeding due to stab/injury, crush accidents shock may follow-pallor/sweating, rapid pulse restlessness, cold and calming skin, fall of pressure. Put patient to absolute rest, elevation of limbs, restoration of blood volume, blood transfusion, plasma given as doctor's orders.

Bleeding from internal organs such as fracture rib, pelvis, skull, stomach, lung, and lower bowels, kidneys which is visible in vomit, cough, stool and urine. Liver, spleen, pancreas collect blood in abdomen cavity which is difficult to detect.

Sign and symptoms- giddiness, faintness, collapse, pallor face and lips, cold and clammy skin, profuse sweating thirsty, shallow breathing weak and faster pulse, restless, excitable and talkative, low BP. Head low , not to move, cover patient with blankets and do not give anything to drink.

How will you Manage a Violent Patient?

Violent and aggressive patient lose control when intoxicated with alcohol or drugs. Adapt a calm, non-critical approach. Help patient to aim control and confidence. Listen to patients crisis with attitude of interest acknowledge his state of agitation, give him opportunity to express feelings verbally. Try to hear what he is saying. If uncontrollable doctor order give sedation.

What Special Care will you Take with Patient who Undergoes Radiation?

For diagnosis and treatment of radioactive radium needless substances are used in hospital. Which has effect on biological tissue in excess exposure they are harmful. The intensity of radiation the penetrating power the time exposure to, the rate the general health condition influence radiation hazards. The nurse is required to wear protective apron and gloves, before handling such patient with implantation read all protective instructions and employ distance and speed technique while handling such patient. Nursing care of such patient is shared by all nurses and not only one nurse all the time such patient is treated in separate room. The radium needle/container never be handled by naked hand, for transportation of needle the special lead box container be used. Radio active iodine is used in cancer of thyroid gland. When a patient is receiving radio active iodine by mouth, some iodine is excreted in urine. Nurse dealing with bedpan/urinals use protective gloves. The urine should not be thrown into normal drains. Radiotherapy deep X-ray site of cancer is exposed. Demarcation of area should not apply soap or antiseptics. Hot and cold applications avoided. Adhesive tape not applied. A special cream provided for the area. Shaving should not be done, encourage good nutritional food.

The organism has diverse pattern of behavior, how they enter the body and how they spread infection from person-to-person. The knowledge of microbiology is very essential for nurses to take precautions to avoid preventing spread of infection in hospital. Therefore the practice of nursing should be based on a sincere application of sound microbiological knowledge which is valuable science.

Each organism is a part of a community of living thing and connects with each other like the meshes of a 'giant spider's web'. Mans entire life is spent in contact with microorganism, and his body at the end decomposed by them after death. His health and well-being is influenced by the presence or absence of it in environment. When all the organs in the body is function at there best level in perfect balance you have health. Diseases are lack of ease and comfort, an abnormal condition of body. The nurse represents the hospital to patient and he feels that she is responsible for his well-being. She needs continuously strive for improvement in-patient care.

How do you Understand the Suicidal Tendencies Patient?

Tendencies are those who have suffered the recent loss of a loved one, of body integrity or status, failed in extra, in love, unemployed try to commit suicide. History of previous suicidal attempts, patient with psychic illness, lack of resources and those who express hopelessness.

WHAT IS POISONING? TYPES OF POISONING AND NURSING CARE

Poisoning is a substance which when taken into the system producing ill health disease or death. Medicines if taken in excessive do acts as poisons. Nurse's duty is to maintain the anti-poison tray in the ward for emergency use for stomach wash. She should know basic management of poison case. She has to take history of poisoning time, type, quantity. For elimination of poison absorbed into system use antidotes and attempt for removal of unabsorbed poison from body, treat for shock and keep the patient warm. If inhaled poison in a gas, remove patient to fresh air, artificial respiration, oxygen therapy. Antidotes are remedies which neutralize effects of poison.

If poison is swallowed in stomach, does gastric lavage by stomach wash. Never introduce stomach tube in corrosive poisoning except carbolic acid. Corrosive destroys or burns the tissue like acid and alkalis. Signs and symptoms of corrosive acid from mouth to stomach there is intense burning pain, intense thirst, vomiting, fall, blood pressure. Excoriation of lips and angles of mouth; hoarse voice, mind remains clear till death.

To induce vomiting, a table spoonful of grounded mustard seeds or two table spoonful of common salt. Half drachms of zinc sulphate in a glass of warm water repeated at 15 minutes interval.

Elimination of Poison by Giving Intravenous Fluids for Excretion by Kidney

Peritoneal dialysis can be done in acute cases of snake bite. Diuresis can be promoted by diuretics infusions/injections. Elevate the foot-end nine inch block till blood pressure reaches a point 106/60 mm Hg, clean airway; give artificial respiration, oxygen to conscious patient.

Washing soda/sodium carbonate— Neutralize alkali by vinegar, orange to lemon juice, white of egg, olive oil, milk for soothing effect.

Tic-20 and other agriculture insecticides— Signs and symptoms of headache, nausea, vomiting, giddiness, tightness over chest, dimness of vision, constricted pupils, profuse frothing convulsion, twitching mental confusion, diarrhea, delirium.

Treatment—Atropine sulphate IV/IM 2 mg/10-30 minutes till pupil dilate. Stomach washes 2% potassium solution, oxygen inhalation artificial respiration IV fluid.

Opium—Barbiturates depressants valium symptoms—mental excitement, restlessness, hallucination, flushing of face, nausea, vomiting, giddiness, lethargic condition, drowsiness, pupils are contracted, desire to sleep, deep coma.

Treatment—Wash stomach with potassium permanganate, administer Mag-suph, do not allow patient to sleep, IV fluid and antidote like Nalorphine hydrochloride IM can be given. Strong tea, black coffee, awake by constant talking, fresh air, and leave lights on, empty the bladder to prevent reabsorption of drug from bladder.

Kerosene poisoning—Burning pain in stomach, throat and chest, cough, thirst, nausea, vomiting, colic's, diarrhea, giddiness, heaviness in head, drowsiness, stupor, coma. Pupils are first constricted but later dilated in coma, convulsion may occur.

Treatment—Stomach wash, head low to avoid aspiration to lungs, purgatives and stimulants, artificial aspirations, penicillin injection, IV fluid, high carbohydrates and B-complex to protect liver. Do not give oils or fats.

DDT—Nausea, vomiting, cough, excitability, vertigo, weakness, muscular tremors, and convulsions, paralysis of legs, unconsciousness and collapse- treatment wash stomach with tap water, hypodermal injection atropine IV calcium gluconate, and paraldehyde for convulsions, oxygen and artificial respirations.

Mercury/irritants—Sign metallic taste in mouth, bloody vomiting, bloody diarrhea, severe abdominal pain, scanty urine, convulsions, and unconsciousness.

Treatment—Give antidote, give emetic or gastric levage, give egg albumin and castor oil, milk and egg is normal. Opium may be given by doctor orders. Keep the patient warm. Cleaning and dusting patients unit. Basic nursing activities are care of the patients unit. Maintain personal hygiene, making patient comfortable caring for patient's spiritual needs, caring for elimination needs. Follow-up and advice to patient after discharge from hospital, prevention and control of infection, sterilization of articles.

What is Rigor; When is it Cause Rigor in Patient?

Rigor is a sudden disturbance of heat regulating system of the body. This condition occurs in malaria, pneumonia, filarial, intravenous drip, blood transfusion, drug reaction. Observe cold, hot, perspiration stage. Stop infusion, provide blanket in cold sage, hot water bottle, hot drink. Hot stage takes away blanket, cold drink, cold sponge. Sweating wipes sweating with warm damp cloth, do not expose, give tea or coffee inform doctor.

What is Shock?

Shock is classified as hypovolemic, carcinogenic and distributive. Shock is a critical condition with a high mortality rate. Shock is the effects of a threat to existence. Signs of fainting, cold and calmly skin, weak and rapid pulse, fall in pressure and temperatures, shallow respiration, relaxed muscles, thirst, cyanosis, pallor, some time restlessness, etc. put patient in comfortable place and reassure if conscious, raise foot end, loosen tight clothes, shoes and belt, message limbs for return of blood supply, keep patient warm with blanket and hot bottle, oxygen if cyanosed, intravenous fluid, blood transfusion etc.

Potential nursing diagnoses for patient in shock- ineffective airway clearance, ineffective breathing pattern, impaired gas exchange, altered tissue perfusion, cerebral, cardiopulmonary, renal, gastrointestinal, peripheral, decreased cardiac output, fluid volume deficit, altered nutrition less then body requirements, constipation, activity intolerance, impaired physical immobility, sleep pattern disturbances, self care deficit etc.

How will you Cope up Emergencies as a Nurse?

Emergencies is a sudden development in the condition of a patient, that is likely to endanger his life, and calls for immediate constant observation and nursing care such as collapse, cardiac arrest, asphyxia, pulmonary embolism. Sudden hemorrhagic shock, attempted suicide, fire hazards, etc. are put in ICU where kept for specialized medical and nursing care.

To provide prompt and best management to critically ill patients. To prevent deterioration of condition before specific treatment are given. Here all life saving equipments are available here with best services of technically competent staff handling the sophisticated machines and equipments to provide quality care personnel who are professionally prepared to work. Nurse must observe very carefully to the actual condition of the patient such as general appearance, nose, ear mouth for bleeding or discharge of any fluid, smell of breath, skin dry/cold and clammy. Recording every 15 minutes vital signs and reported to the doctor. Pupils of the eye whether equal dilated or contracted.

Types of critically ill patient who need ICU care- coma, severe burn, acute poisoning, cerebra vascular accident, respiratory failure, kidney failure, pneumonia, hear failure, severe accidents with multiple injuries, major surgery, hemorrhage from gastrointestinal tracts, myocardial infection, premature babies, shock, etc.

Equipments—ECG tube and BP apparatus, ventilators, defibrillators, oxygen suction, emergency tray and necessary life saving drugs, infusion and transfusion sets, bedside monitors, portable X-ray machines, pacemakers to regulate heart beats. Blood gas measuring instrument, measurements of oxygen and carbon-dioxide levels in the blood, incubator suction machine, hypothermic box, cardiac monitor and cardiac board, equipments of gastric lavage and gauge, sterile supplies such as- drum and dressing materials, drum with sterile tools and aprons, tracheotomy set, ray with LP, with manometer, catheterization set and drainage tube, Ryles tube/N/G tube, drum with gloves of different sizes, disposable syringes with needle, trolleys, rubber goods like hot water bottles, ice caps, tubes, mackintosh, enamel wares like bowls, basins, buckets, jugs, pint measures, urinals, bedpans, kidney tray, linen.

Constant observation of respiration, pulse, blood pressure, maintenances and fluid and electrolyte balance vital signs, recording temperature, input output chart, position change, passive and active exercise, breathing exercise, etc. cocking, chills, observe, protect hurt or injury, blood drainage, vomit us.

In what Conditions in which Input and Output Chart is to be Maintained?

Sever diarrhea, vomiting, fever, heart case, kidney disease, unconscious patient, burn cases, patient receiving certain drugs, e.g. digitals, diuretics, patient with intravenous infusion of blood transfusion, etc. check diagnosis of the patient whose intake and output chart has to be maintained. Because in some cases the doctor may restrict the fluids and in other it may be to force fluids.

Neonatal intensive care unit—An increasing number of babies who require immediate attention and emergency treatment; to eliminate inconvenient to parents and to manage sick newborn to enhance the health care a well-equipped NICU- unit needs facilities like—

NICU set up has servo controlled neonatal warmers; radiant heat warmers, recovery beds, infusion pumps, bear cup 720 neonatal ventilator, multipara monitors, centralized oxygen/ suction, infant high intensity phototherapy systems, neonatal resuscitation trolley, infant intensive care incubator, neonatal ventilator, pulse oximeter, infant care trolley, oxygen hoods, silicone manual resuscitators, resuscitation kits, digital weighing scales, aqua thermo matt are the neonatal and pediatric intensive care equipment needs. Round the clock availability of a pediatrician and qualified staff is must.

Doctors—We care, he cures- it is all about doing service to humanity- very often people find it difficult when they are sick which doctor to go. They need to go to the doctor according to their illness involves to a particular specialist, many do not know this and so it is the duty of a nurse to educate the public for awareness of the services available in the particular areas and the different services given by specialist. Facilities available in hospitals are:- residential MO–medical officer, RMO–residential medical officer, doctors in all faculties are general physician, chest physician, cardiologist, nephrologists, gastroenterology, dermatology, psychiatric, pediatric, general surgeon, oncology, plastic surgeon for cosmetic, urologist, endocrinologist, orthopedic surgeon, maxillofacial surgeon, ophthalmology, ENT, gynecologist, neurosurgeon, physiotherapy, audiologist, dietician, radiologist, echocardiologist, pathologist, anesthesiologist, counselor.

Facilities available in hospital—Also the nurse have to make known to the public so that they can benefit and without wasting time get the treatment in appropriate hospital. Therefore, that nurse helps to nurture respect for human dignity and life with compassion irrespective of cast, creed or religion. Well equipped ICU, causality department, operation theatres, computerized Lab, X-ray, ECG, sonography-2D Echo, color Doppler, endoscope, gastroscopy, colonoscopy, sigmoidoscopy, audiometric, PFT-Test, uroflometry, stress test, CT scan, dialysis, dental treatment, physiotherapy, dieticians guidance, medical store, ambulance service, mortuary-air conditioned, A.A. meetings service, health check-up schemes. Diagnostic and other facilities like pathological laboratory, speech therapy, pastoral care, clinical counseling, medical social worker and community health center.

Remember do not be afraid to admit when you know you are wrong. Always do the right things. Never compromise your values and beliefs. Be true to yourself. Refuse to run away from the things that scare you, over come fears.

Today even in India so many machines are equipped in the hospitals. Nurses are 8 hours in and around patient. It is imperative that she comprehens the severity and improves the quality of life by emergency action.

The angel asked God anything stronger than Rocks. Yes IRON- iron can break rocks; anything stronger than iron yes fire because fire can melt the iron. Anything stronger then fire yes water because water can quenched by water, anything stronger then water –wind because wind can scatter water, anything stronger than water yes sympathy and compassion. And this is the virtue a nurse should develop towards patient while caring ill.

We nurses play a vital role in reducing the pain of a patient. The first thing we have to do is to smile at a patient to be delicate, sensitive, warm towards the patient. While talking to a patient we can hold there hand, just by this gesture we can feel how much the patient suffering. Likewise we can communicate healing and courage.

To give the patient hope and respect, no matter how serious the illness is. The illness of patient does not make her less human. Not to scold the patient when they are sick, they tend to be more sensitive. Understand their feelings. The person includes body-mind-spirit, the sick person needs not only our Medicines but loving care, kind words and attention. Every sickness is unique because every person is unique. Hence it is not possible to find two identical ways of reacting to suffering. Sometimes our experience of a person who is known to be a very strong,- worry about any minor indisposition, while other person who seems to be weak is able to bear great pain with admirable courage. Besides physical sickness there are suppressed, internal, moral, spiritual sufferings, Death, separation of a person we love, to feel despised and rejected by others, etc. sometimes extreme sickness has caused to loose very meaning of life and existence of God, our role here is of value.

Real healing takes place only when the person is brought back to the purpose for which God created her. Human life is significant and it is dear to us. It is universal truth that failure in health systems hit the poor people the hardest. They are forced to live in the vicious circle of poverty, indebted and ill health. The sign of the times are frightening further hardships for the poor who are living below the magical line.

The private sector in the medical care and diagnostic services has mushroomed in large cities giving rise to unethical practices and negligence.

The major share of progress in our country is passed on to the cities. 75% of our population lives in the villages which are still in underdeveloped or semi-developed. When we serve with love and begin to see God in the faces of those who suffer. Then we are transforming the entire working environment and giving power to the poor. To have concern for the person rather than the sickness.

To help patient to integrate there sufferings and instill Hope in their lives. Liberate the patient from forces of evil in order to give fuller life. To heal the unhealthy tendencies that hide in our human condition such as selfishness, ego, ambitions, individualism, and lack of solidarity.

Nursing is a helping profession contributes health and well-being of people. Nursing is not simply a collection of specific skills and the nurse is not simply a person trained to profession specific tasks. Nursing is a profession. A profession requires an extended education of its members, as well as a basic liberal function. A profession has a theoretical body of knowledge leading to defined skill, abilities and norms. A profession provides a specific service. Member of profession have autonomy in decision making and practice. The profession as a whole has a code of ethics for practice.

The nurse systematically evaluates the quality and effectiveness and nursing practice. Nurse acquires and maintains current knowledge and competency in nursing practice. She interacts with and contributes to the professional development and uses reaches findings in practice to fulfill professional responsibilities. She plays major role in determining and implementing desirable standards and nursing practice and nursing education.

Her attitudes and personal qualities- caring, commitment, compassion, perseverance, assistive, acceptance, fairness, self-esteem, tolerance, sensitivity, self discipline, consideration, humaneness, integrity, morality, accountability, honesty, rationality.

Doctor and Patient Relationship

Whenever a patient comes to a doctor for treatment there is a contract established between the doctor and the patient.

Medicolegal Purpose

1. Any medical record may become evidence in accordance with Indian evidence Act
2. Insurance and other claims settlements
3. Medical certificates such as fitness for employment sickness certificates etc
4. Workmen's compensation Act
   The clinical data recorded by medical practitioner to indicate the extent of injury and the degree of disability of the individual is taken as documentary evidence to settle the claims for payment by certain claimers of employers to give there workmen, some compensation for injury arising out of and in the course of his employment under the workmen's compensation Act.
5. *Patients will*—Medical record gives the day today progress of the patient and is indicative whenever the patient was of normal mental state or not at the time of making his will
6. For the settlement of personal injury suit-it is used to obtain the required the length of treatment given in order to settle the claim by an individual damage as a result of injury
7. *Malpractice suit*—It protects doctor and the hospital if action for dangers be brought against hospital by demonstrating that these was no negligence involved with treatment, was scientific, adequate, proper and prompt.
8. *Criminal cases*—Medical records play important role in the investigation of murder cases, assault cases, rape cases and dowry deaths.
9. *Authorization for operation*—Consent is required for operation. Incase of children, parents or guardian, in case of persons of unsound mind, the person in whose custody and in case of the patients has been lawfully committed have to give necessary consent. The consent of husband is required in case of a proposed operation on his wife the operation may result in sterility.

DUTIES OF RMP (REGISTERED MEDICAL PRACTITIONERS)

Compulsory Duties

To report births, deaths and cases of food poisoning to inform police all cases of crime and homicide: To respond during war and national emergencies.

Fundamental Duties

Maintain good character
Treat patient using maximum knowledge care and skill
Patient becomes alright
Patient does not refuse treatment
Patient gives consent for treatment
Patient does not consult another doctor without his knowledge
Patient is cooperative
Patient pays his fees.

Other Duties

Not to involve in unethical practice to professional misconduct
Maintain professional secrecy
Attain the patient regularly
Keep the patient well informed of his condition
A substitute can be appointed only after information and consultation with the patient
All investigation and treatments to be done after proper consent
All medical certificates and medicolegal reports issued should be based on facts and observation
Encourage second opinions
While referring a patient to another specialist send all the details of the patient
Use clean instruments
Should strive to improve his knowledge
Should take precautions not to spread infections
Should use standard drugs, instruments and procedures
Should maintain proper medical records
Should not do illegal operations
Should not do sex determination test in pregnancy

Second opinion when patient requires

When patient does not respond to treatment
When patient can not be diagnosed
When patient becomes serious
Any operation in emergency
Any operation that is dangerous to life
Mutilating, e.g. amputation, breast removal
Any operation that can interfere with intellectual capacity

Any operation that can interfere with reproductive capacity
Homicidal injury, homicidal poisoning, homicidal burns
Criminal abortions
MTP beyond 12 weeks
Declaring a person as dead, if organ transplantation is to be done from his dead body
Removing organs from living for organ transplantation
Declaring a person as a insane
Postmortem on dead body of a newly married girl (within seven years of marriage or her age being less then 30 years)
When complications of treatment not informed to patient/therapeutic privilege

Rights of a RMP

A RMP can choose his patient; he can refuse treatment a patient provided it is not unethical
Provided patient is not in emergency
However a public hospital he has to treat all the patients.
He can practice medicines
He can practice drugs including dangerous drugs
He can remove organs for transplantation
He can administer anesthasia, he can perform PM (Postmortem)
He can issue medical certificate

Rights of a Patient

Proper medical attention required at earliest by qualified medical staff. Humane treatment by the doctor
Considerate behavior from the hospital staff
That the doctor will take all the decisions in good faith and for the benefit of the patient's health
Detailed information of his condition that is dangerous treatment
To refuse treatment or experimentation on his body
To know the prognosis
Proper follow-up and necessary instructions
That no procedure ill be done without his consent
Not to be left unattained when in emergency or in labor
To know details of how to avoid recurrence

Duties of a Patient

To be polite and sober to the hospital staff
To be neat and clean
To give correct and full history
To allow the doctor to examine
To follow instruction in relation to treatment and drug, food
To preserve all medical records given by the doctor
To pay professional fees.

CHAPTER 12

Obesity

He who has heath has hope. Moreover, he who has hope has everything. Obesity is no longer a laughing matter. It is a high time we recognize that obesity is not a cosmetic problem but a kaleidoscope of deadly disease, which warrants treatment like any other disease in the world.

What is Obesity?

Obesity is described as the excessive accumulation of fat. If your weight is more than 20% of your ideal body weight, then you are obese.

What is the Ideal Body Weight?

Your body weight is based on age, sex and height.

How do I Know if I am Obese?

Overweight and obesity both are defined in terms of BMI (body mass index).

$$BMI = \frac{\text{Weight in kg}}{\text{Height in meter square}}$$

If your BMI is more than 23.5, you are overweight. If your BMI is more than 27, you are obese. Moreover, if your BMI more than 37 you are morbidly obese. Morbidly obese person is susceptible to serious disease like hypertension, diabetes, high cholesterol, sleep apnea/snoring, joint pains, chronic heart disease, polycystic ovarian disease/PCOD and infertility. These conditions are called co-morbidities, which may result in either significant physical disability or even death. It is a chronic disease, which increases morbidity and shortens your life.

What are the Types of Obesity?

There are basically two types of obesity. Android/apple shape; Gynoid/pear shape

Apple shape obesity where the excess fat is primarily in the abdominal region, is common among males, and is linked to chronic ailments such as type 2 diabetics because of insulin resistance, hyperlipidemia and hypertension.

Pear shaped obesity where excess fat is accumulated in the thighs and buttocks, females are more susceptible to this kind of obesity.

What are the Causes of Obesity?

Various factors contribute to obesity, which includes: hormonal causes such as hypothyroidism lead to modest weight gain maximum 6-10 kgs.

Genetic factors can also lead to obesity.

Certain medicines have weight gain as a side effect

Psychological causes like depression wherein patients tends to heal the symptoms by eating leading to weight gain and obesity.

However, life style accounts for more than 80% of the current causes of the obesity epidemic because of an increased in the caloric intake, food symptoms, and an increased portion size coupled with sedentary lifestyle and decreased physical activity due to modernization and industrialization.

Obesity affects the quality of life. You have two options nonsurgical and surgical. Diet and exercise form the cornerstone therapy. Medications are an adjunct to lifestyle modification, not a replacement. The key to lose weight is to maintain a balance between your caloric intake and caloric expenditure. Eat fruits, vegetables, grains. Limit your fat and sugar intake. Avoid fried foods, bakery products. Be active, a healthy diet improves your energy and feeling of well-being while reducing your risk of many disease. Adding regular physical activity and exercise will make any healthy eating plan work better. Establish new food habits listen to your body and savor your food. Ask yourself if you are really hunger, and stop eating when you feel full. So eat slowly, chew your food, practice modification.

Exercises are important not only from a weight loss perspective but to keep you healthier and fitter for life. Set aside at least 45 minutes a day for moderate exercise like walking, swimming, jogging, etc.

Who has the slimes waist? Fiber takes one feel full longer, it seems to inhibit fat absorption eat fiber reach food.

Surgery to help *lose weight*.

What is Sleeve Gastrectomy?

Sleeve Gastrectomy—The vertical sleeve Gastrectomy is a restrictive form of weight loss surgery in which approximately 85% of the stomach is removed leaving a cylindrical sleeve shaped stomach with a capacity ranging from about 60 to 150 cc. As the new stomach continues the foods, which patient can consume after surgery quantity of food eaten will be reduced. The removal of the majority of the stomach results in the virtual elimination of Ghrelin hormones produced within the stomach, which stimulates hunger. 2/3 of the stomach is completely removed laproscopically, the stomach thus takes a shape of 'sleeve' effectively turning what is a big bag into a small tube. The part of the stomach secretes Ghrelin a hormone that plays a major role in determining how hungry we get is removed. The patients have a greatly – reduced appetite and as they lose weight they do not suffer the hunger pains experienced by dieters. This option surgery is suitable for most morbidly obese patients.

It is performed laproscopically, with fast recovery and short hospital stay. It is effective short to midterm weight loss with average of 60% excess weight out in 5 yrs. It is not reversible and no long-term effort known.

Gastric banding involves tying of a band around the stomach to section off a small portion called as stomach pouch, creating an hourglass effect. It works by reducing the amount of food consumed at one time. The net result is a reduction in daily caloric intake without a feeling of deprivation.

Gastric by pass involves creation of a small stomach pouch with the help of stapes, which restrict the food intake. In addition, the initial part of the small intestine is bypassed. This procedure alters digestion so that the body absorbs fewer calories. Patients have to be on liquid diet for two weeks after the surgery and gradually progress to semisolid and then solid foods. These surgeries are highly specialized. The approximate costs range around 2.5 lakhs and above.

Instant sliming lose inches instantly without cuts, stitches, pain or injections with non-surgical sliming technology is ultrasonic Lipolysis. What is ultrasonic Lipolysis? A non-surgical procedure helps to get rid of unwanted fat from abdomen, thighs and hips. It is similar to the lithotripsy treatment used to break kidney stones. Ultrasound waves are focused on the fat cells through a transducer. These high intensity focalized ultrasound/ HIFU waves target fat cells up to 1.5 cm below the skin and typical UL session takes one hour. Patient lies down and can read, watch TV or chat. It is painless with no burns, scars or redness. Patient can walk out immediately after the treatment and carry on with daily routine. It is safe without side effects. Choose the area of target abdomen, thigh etc. UL reduces the number of fat cells in body permanently. It is called precise body contouring obesity management. Keep fit consistency, discipline self in terms of schedules is the key, it takes time to get back your shape. It is important to keep appointment for yourself.

Liposuction improves appearance and problem areas that are resistant to diet and exercise can often be dramatically improved, eliminated unwanted pockets of fat that accumulates disproportionately in various areas of the body. This helps one to get a perfectly contoured body. It helps celulin removal eating proper and balanced meals for your age and activity level. Side effect- such as bruising, swelling, temporary numbness and discomfort in the surgically treated area, blood clot, infection. Your doctor will talk and discuss possible side effect with you.

Endobarrier plastic bag-like device may help curb obesity, diabetes. A removable device that lines the gut and shape the body from sucking in calories may soon offer hopes for people who are dangerouslyn obese.

Inserted into the gut through the mouth, the Endobarrier developed by US-based GI Dynamics - is an impermeable sleeve that lines the first 60 centimeters of the small intestine.

But unlike a gastric band, the sleeve can be inserted in less than half an hour-without the need for surgery. Nothing is done to the stomach. Patient can eat normally, it helps to reduce weight and brings type II diabetes under control.

Using an endoscope, the device enclosed in a capsule is inserted via the mouth. Once place below the base of the stomach, the capsule releases a small ball that, with the help of the catheter, pulls a flexible polymeter sleeve through the intestine. The ball is then chucked out and the sleeve is fixed in place by releasing a spiked attachment. Cost Rs 3.66 lakh.

The moment you restrict yourself from having any particular food, your body automatically triggers a craving for the same. Eating less the formula for extending human life span up to 5 years has now been accepted by leading researchers. Eating less could add years to your life. caloric restriction found to cut risks of many age related diseases such as cancer, heart diseases and allows us to row more gracefully and healthy.

Kept your calorie count in check and yet ended up piling on kilos? This could be why

Lack of sleep—Many a times, we end up compromising on our sleep. However, when we do not get enough sleep, the body goes through physiological stress. As a result, it ends up storing fat more effectively than ever. In the process, we stock for more calories than we require, resulting in weight gains. Symptoms that indicate lack of sleep and inadequate rest are fatigue and low energy levels. Always make sure you meet your daily sleep requirement if you want to keep your weight under check.

Stress for a prolonged period triggers a biochemical process in our body wherein our metabolism slows down. Such stress causes weight gain especially around the waist.

Medication some drugs deal with depression, migraines and blood pressure and even those taken during hormone replacement therapy may lead to weight gain.

Medical condition—A deficiency of the thyroid hormone, known as hypothyroidism is a common medical condition that leads to weight gain. The medical condition decreases metabolism, causes appetite loss and leads to weight gain. Feeling lethargic or sleeping too much are symptoms of hypothyroidism.

Offering a spectrum of aesthetic and *cosmetic surgery* option, right from the non-invasive methods like lasers to surgical procedures like tummy tucks in a day.

Liposuction and body contouring is among the most popular surgeries performed currently. It can be used to remove excess fat from the tummy, arms, thigh, hips, chest, breast and the face.

Tummy tucks are also quiet common and are done to remove excess skin and fat around the lower tummy, giving a sleeker appearance. It is also often done after childbirth, when the skin does not shrink back to its previous condition.

Which is the most commonly performed barbaric surgery? Is it different from liposuction? Can it be done in cosmetic purpose? At what age can it be performed? What are the risk/complications involved in this surgery/how safe is pregnancy after the surgery? How does it improve the quality of life/does surgery cures type-2 diabetes? How soon can one loose weight after the surgery/does one need to be on nutritional supplements after surgery? How much the weight loss can one expect after the surgery? Does insurance cover the surgery? These and other doubts your doctor will be able to tell you in detail.

According to figures available, 50 percent of people in USA and Australia and 15 percent in Europe are either overweight or obese. At present, there are about 10 million obese people in India and this figure is on increase at an alarming rate. 43 percent of the adults in big towns are overweight, 17 percent of the adolescent population is overweight and 6 percent is obese. These are some of the startling figures. Obesity and diabetes are twin diseases with the risk of diabetes increasing with increasing of fat content. India is already is the diabetics capital in the world. Healthy eating and exercise is to overcome obesity is very vital. World obesity day was observed on 24/10/2008- making of a slim and healthy nation.

Do not overeat—Eating fast and full can make you fat. Wolfing down meals disrupt signals to brain to stop, doubling risk of being overweight. Do not let yourself get too hungry, too angry, too frustrated, too lonely, too tired or too boarded. All these states are powerful, watch for it. How many gadgets modern technology blessed us with yet, they only seem to add to the stress and tension of our lives, people walk with earphones completely shutting out the world of beauty around them. Possession and acquisitions may seem marvelous. However, after a while you do not own them, they own you. When our life becomes complicated with power and possession, we move farther and farther away from the simple joys and pleasures of life. We fail to notice the green grass and the fresh morning flowers. We do not have time to hear bids singing or watch our little ones smiling, childlike innocence, and simple joy, which is our basic nature.

Simplicity is not self-denial. It is a return to those values that matter most in life. It emphasizes spontaneity and intuition. It helps us to rediscover the feeling of wonder of joy that we have lost as adult. Getting they may give you momentary happiness. However, not being able to get them often makes you miserable. It is a stormy and stressful period filled with inner turmoil.

Yoga—Easy breathing exercise can restore the energy, it is all together different feeling. It is a great way to de-stress. It teaches us the healthy living.

Exercise—You need water when you work out- before, during and after. The more water, the better if you do not drink enough water your head can ache, or you can get cramps and tire without knowing why. You should take plenty of fluids to prevent dehydration.

Some older people tend to think that it is too late to start an exercise routine if they did not work out when they were younger. Studies have showed that it is never too late to start working out; you can reap benefits at any age. As we age, exercise can help reduce that risk of bone and muscle diseases and help enhance daily functions. The benefits of exercises are not age related but health related.

The best time for exercise is the time that appeals to you and fits into your schedule. Lifting weight or doing strengthening activities like push-ups and crunches on a regular basis can actually help you maintain or lose weight. These activities can help you build muscle, and muscle burns more calories than body fat. Therefore, if you have more muscle, you burn more calories even sitting still. Doing strengthening activities 2 to 3 days a week will not bulk you up. Only intense strength training, combined with a certain genetic background, can build very large muscles.

Studies show that a half hour walk three or more times a week significantly reduces your risk of heart attack and stroke, lowers blood pressure, relives stress and boosts your energy and immune system.

Warm up raise the heart rate so that the body is prepared for physical exertion. They speed up nerve impulses so that reflexes are enhanced, reduce muscle tension, send oxygenated blood to the muscle groups, reduce the risk of injury, particularly to connective tissues like tendons and increase flexibility and joint mobility.

Getting fit physically and mentally is a process that takes time and patience, fitness depends on the amount of calories burnt, and any type of exercise with which you are comfortable is beneficial for your body.

Nurse Connecting Herself to Institution and Community or Transferring Technology from Hospital to Rural Field

Community Procedures and Minor Illness

Community health—It is people oriented. Our approach, our focus is group, people's movement, issues related to peoples needs. It was the community and not the individual patient who came to be considered as the entity for which health services are needed. Therefore, the individual who is a part of a family, which in turn is a part of a community, were required to be healthy as a healthy individual is a part of economical resources to the nation. With this outlook, importance was given to the community health.

Community health nursing is science of caring. The first nurse on this earth must have been the mother with her motherly instinct. She nursed her baby, with her maternal cum nurse like feelings to the sick and ailing. Nursing and medicine go together. Medicine is the science of curing while nursing is the science of caring.

India is a vast country with varieties of culture, variation in geographical factors, such as climate, people, their eating and clothing habits, the dialect of language, religion, custom, traditions, cast and creed. India is second largest country in the world having the largest population with such a vast variation found everywhere she has large problems to deal with in all aspects of life.

For example, there is significant relationship with this with health. Economic point of view grim facts- every 100 children born in India today.

26 will weigh less than 2500 gms at birth

25 will not be immunized against any disease

10 will die before their 5th birthday

47 will suffer from malnutrition first 3rd year of their life

15 will never go to school

30 will never complete 5th grade

16 will have no access to clean drinking water.

The nurse has varied roles and functions. 80% population live in rural communities and due to shortage of doctors nurse in this area will be involved both in caring for patients with serious and fatal infectious diseases and in helping to develop public health programmes for their control. Nurses important function in child health, high birth rate, high IMR, fetal diseases being diarrhea, pneumonia and protein or calorie malnutrition in early childhood. Nurse builds up a relationship by altering the behavior patterns and convincing people to build trust for positive health, infant welfare for under five, and immunization. Family planning involves the nurse in helping parents to avoid too large families, which over extend their financial resources and burden the mother with the care of too many children and constant pregnancies may ultimately affect the mother's health.

Nursing today has all the hallmarks of a profession; it mirrors their diverse roles and new tasks, which are more complex. With use of computer, clinical investigation advanced in scientific knowledge the role and function has been extended. Techniques which were formally regarded as the doctors province may now be cried out by the nurse like dialysis the doctors relies on the nurse to report any change in patients condition or any adverse treatment she has observed which may lead him to alter his line of treatment.

A community nurse must have wider knowledge of social services. Unique functions of the nurse are to assist the sick or well, in the performance of those activities contributing to health or its recovery or to peaceful death. Develop pride in their profession besides keeping abreast with current knowledge and professional trends for a successful career ahead.

Functions as efficient member of the health team, to keep pace with latest professional and technical developments and use these for providing nursing care services. Use of ethical values in personal and professional life.

Without health can you think of happiness? NO. The secret of happiness in life is well-being.

When health is a way of life, well-being follows.

Holistic living

Health is considered to be superior to wealth. Health itself is wealth. If you know how to live healthy life half of your sickness will disappear. If you know the signs of your body alarm 80% of disease can be prevented. Respect the law of nature.

In today's world of fast forward ultramodern life, globalization, privatization, and liberalization, fast food modernization, unhealthy competition, tensions of heavy responsibilities, unhealthy living has increased disease like diabetic, heart problem, cancer. So one has to invest in health.

As some one said that people first run after money and lose health and then lose money to get back health when it becomes too late.

Today health is considered as one of the fundamental rights of man. To protect and promote the health of its citizens is a primary duty. It has been observed that in countries and regions where better public health action took place health level went up.

There is a significant relationship between poverty and the poor health status. For example, on an economic point of view the develop country like America; they take great care of people's health. They have so many schemes for the welfare of health system. Their people are very healthy because government takes care of them. Old, crippled, handicapped, widows, are very well looked after by government.

Now take the example of developing countries like India, Africa, health care is determined by poverty. Tropical countries have neither money nor resources, people die of hunger, starvation, and no basic needs are provided. Poverty and lack of food first hits the women and children. Government is responsible to provide universal education, safe drinking water. Poor people cannot afford to pay the health services so government has to have a budget higher for the free services. This is the paradox of hunger and over eating of rich and poor countries.

Doctors trained at huge public cost are not available to serve the rural areas. Modern health services are generally urban based and elite orientated. Majority of people in this country after independence have no meaningful form of health care. Inspire of progress made by modern medicines, millions of people in India are deprived of the most basic form of health care.

The problem of disease, malnutrition; High IMR, psychological oppression and waste of human potential and resources are linked with the socioeconomic reality where poverty and malnutrition, low wages, bonded labors, exploitation exist where health system is a part. The distribution of health care is unjust and uneven. No quality services. The many who suffer chiefly from poverty and poverty related diseases in the rural areas and urban slims are the marginalized people. We need to focus on basic factors like health education, nutrition, clean water, sanitation and environment as foundations of health care. That which is holistic and affordable.

In order to make people aware of their health, community health nursing is very important and is taught in nursing schools.

CARE OF THE EYES

A common problem of the eye is secretions that dry on the lashes as crust. This mat is soft ended and wiped away under sterile conditions. In newborns the eyes are treated soon after the baby is born to prevent ophthalmia neonatorum which is caused by gonococcus.

Cleaning the eyes using antiseptic technique is called eye care.

Purposes

- To clean the eye
- To remove the irritating discharge from the eyes
- To prevent infection
- To prevent 'ophthalmic neonatorum' in the newborn.

Procedure

Explain the procedure to the patient and assess general condition
  Wash hands
  Pour sterile saline into the bowel, to wet the cotton swabs
  Stand in front of the patient
  Pick up the wet cotton swab with the thumb forceps, transfer it to the hands and squeeze the excessive water from the swab without touching the part which will come in direct contact with the eye.

Repeat the same for the other eye
No pressure on the eyeball
Wipe gently
Discard the used swab in the paper bag
Wash and replace the articles in proper place

Articles

Plastic sheet prepared as a sterile field
    A sterile bowl with sterile cotton swabs
    Sterile normal saline
    Thumb forceps
    A gauze piece
    A paper bag and a kidney tray
    A clean face towel

Instructions

Clean the eye from inner canthus to outer canthus
    Use a separate swab for each stroke.

If eye is infected and there is more pus formation more than one stork can be done with fresh separate swab each time until eye is clean. Less infected eye clean first before the infected eye.

For crusted secretion place a wet warm gauze piece or cotton swab over closed eye. Leave it in place until the crust become soft
    Instill if any medicine ordered

State the Disease Condition of the Eyes

The eye is delicate. That is why we have a cover or eyelids to protect it. In addition, the fine hairs on the edge of the lid help to keep away the dust from going into the eye. In the eye, there is a tube in the corner near the nose. Salty water, which we call, tears come through this tube and washes the eye when any dirt or germs enter. When germs enter and are not washed out, the eye becomes red and swollen. Thick yellow pus forms in the corner of the eye. Daily eyes must be washed with plenty of soap and water.

Eyes are important organs which require care in daily life. Hygienic care of the eyes prevents infection and helps to maintain the functions. A common problem of the eyes is secretions that dry on the lashes as crusts. This may need to be softened and wiped away under sterile conditions. In newborns, the eyes are treated soon after the baby is born to prevent ophthalmia neonatorum. Eyes are cleansed from the inner to the outer can thus. This prevents the particles and fluid from draining into the nasolacrimal duct. Each eye is cleansed with separate swabs, swabbing each eye once only. This prevents spread of infection from one eye to another and to avoid possible recontamination of the same eye. No pressure on the eyeball to be given. For crusted secretions place a wet warm gauze piece or cotton swab over the closed eye. Level it in the place until the crest becomes soft. So it can be removed without traumatizing the mucus. After care instill medication that is ordered. Wash hands thoroughly and record the observations made.

Sore eyes have chance to spread. Do not rub eyes. Conjunctivitis is a virus infection with sudden onset of pain or the sensation of a foreign body in the eye. The diseases rapidly progress to the full clinical pictures of swollen eyelids. It is common in tropical and warm climate. Health education is essential, especially personal hygiene, environmental hygiene, and sterilization of clothes, utensils, formites.

Blindness is avoidable, it can be improved nutrition controlling organism which causes infection and improving safety conditions. Conditions acute conjunctivitis, ophthalmic Neonatorum, foreign bodies, can be treated at grass root level by locally trained person, personal hygiene, sanitation, good dietary habits and safety at the community level. It needs community participation and adequate follow up and evaluation. Occupational eye health done by education by use of protective devices in some occupations is essential. The key to the prevention of accidents in factories is to improve the safety features of machines, to have proper illumination of the working area. Motivate community to accept total eye care program.

Eye injuries do not dig, handle gently and try to flush.

Blindness means darkness forever in life. Eye is the complex organ. It is composed of more than two million working parts.

Can process 36,000 bits of information every hour

Contribute towards 85% of total knowledge.

Utilizes 65% pathways of the brain.

In normal life span will bring you almost 24 million images of the world around you. The eye is the only part of the human body that can function at 100% ability at any moment, day or night without rest.

Eye donation—India has 40-50 corer blind patients. With death, eyes get finished by cremation or burial. With eye donation, two blind people can see. Any age group people, cataract, spectacles any healthy person can give it, any religion, cast, heredity, it can be given to any blind person within one to 3 hours eyes are removed.

Vision screening—Quick detection of several vision defects, using a single instrument for; Visual acuity impairment- nearsightedness, farsightedness, binocularity, double vision, color vision, muscle balance, squint, peripheral vision, etc.

A large number of the visually impaired are either unaware of their visual defects, if treated early stage 80-85% blindness can be located and prevented. Ignorance and malnutrition also leads to blindness. Childhood blindness causes are measles, retinopathy of pre-maturity, and rubella during pregnancy, cataract, glaucoma and diabetic retinopathy.

Trachoma is a disease of poor hygiene.

Xerophthalmia is a disease of poor nutrition

Glaucoma when detected early and treated can save the vision. Its early stages have no symptoms but one of the earliest symptoms is visual field loss, which is usually associated with increased intraocular pressure. Glaucoma is a group of ocular disorders in which damage to the optic nerve and loss of peripheral vision takes place. It is a leading case of blindness. If it is detected early and if due care is taken it is treatable.

Refractive errors, lazy eye syndrome, cataract treatable.

Color blindness is not treatable or preventable.

In cataract, opacification of lens takes place impeding the transmission of light rays to the retina.

Myopia/nearsightedness distant objects not being seen clearly.

Presbyopia is a naturally occurring process of aging whereby changes in ocular tissues result in loss of accommodation and thus near vision. It is more common in those above the age of 40 years.

Binocularity conveys the working of both eyes together with completely fused to separate images of the two eyes being termed as normal when the object is seen very clearly and the person does not complain of double vision. Binocular vision is a way of expressing the manner in which the two eyes work together. Has a grade 1, 2, 3, that is simultaneous perception, fusion and stereopsis.

Stereopsis abnormality is not easily treatable but being forewarned and is a difficult situation, when required.

Peripheral vision represents perception of objects in the outer areas of the field of view. Most people can see objects within an area of 170 degrees with both eyes open.

Specific conditions of phoria are called hetrophoria. Phoria always caused by muscle imbalance between two eyes. Strabismus surgery and corrective procedures.

Amblyopia impaired vision- few can be treated, few cannot be treated.

Lazy eye syndrome conditions seen in children. The binocular reflexes are much weaker in children. If one eye is diseased, then the image from the eye is blurred. The brain may not be able to join this blurred image with the normal image from the healthy eye. There is no stimulus for the diseased eye to remain pointing in the same direction as healthy eye and so the diseased eye develops squint. It may even lead to Amblyopia. When the squint first begins, the person sees everything double. In early stage, it can be corrected.

NURSE AND MINOR ILLNESS

Health care now comprises the third largest business industry in US. Diagnostic possibilities have increased, concern for health for the poor grows, need for comprehensive health education are widely recognized. Yet today health services are fragmented, duplicative, uncoordinated. As a result health care delivery system has been an acceleration of confrontation on the part of consumer.

What is Constipation?

It is the body's way of disposing of waste material, like all its functions, is a marvel of design. After food has been digested, the colon muscles contract in a wave action called peristalsis, which carries its content toward the rectum. On the way, the colon absorbs excess liquid from the mass of substance that comes from the small intestine. If you have not drunk enough fluids, the stool becomes dry and difficult to evacuate.

It is a disease in frequency of bowl movements, accompanied by prolonged or difficult passage of hard, dry stools, straining during defecation is an associated sign. When intestinal motility slows, the faecal mass becomes exposed over time to the intestinal walls and most of the faecal water content is absorbed. Little water is left to soften and lubricate stool, passage of dry stool may cause rectal pain.

Constipation can arise from organic causes, such as narrowing of the bowel and obstruction of the growths. In majority it is caused by a diet lacking in fiber or fluids, lack of regular exercise, older adults, gastrointestinal abnormalities, spinal cord injury, tumor, paralytic illus., negative emotional states, such as nervous tension, worry and anxiety, relaxation of anal sphincters, journey, ignoring the signal to move the bowels.

To avoid constipation change the above habits. If repeated you need laxative over a long period, you are not curing constipation, merely reliving it, and you need constitutional treatment. Avoid chronic use of laxatives, weather herbal to synthetic are habit forming.

Nursing Care

Encourage adequate intake of diet
   Intake of roughage in the diet, food containing a high fibrous
   The quantity and quality of breakfast is more important
   Establish a habit pattern regular time
   Health education to be given
A better understanding of the different aspects of *documentation* can motivate *nurses to* become better documenters. Clear and accurate documentation stands out as a defense in a court of law in case of a malpractice suit. Documentation is necessary to help verify quality of care, to assist in the coordination of care, to seek reimbursements, to comply with regulations of the government and accrediting organizations, to provide evidence in the court of law, and to generate data for research. A clear, unambiguous, accurate, and complete record of client care is authentic. Quality of care simply means accountability, responsibility, professionalism, and survival.

What is Alcoholism?

Alcohol—is a colorless liquid. It is usually prepared by the fermentation of carbohydrate. It is derived from cellulose and it's toxic. Addiction is excessive consumption on regular basis, which results in health endangerment.

Men often start dinking in order to forget the miseries and problems of life. Alcohol serves temporary escape. Many men take up drinking because of occupational factor, physical exhaustion to get temporary boost of energy and relives fatigue, e.g. truck drivers, labourers, manual workers indulge in heavy drinking. Friendship drawn into this habit just for company and get addicted. Living in unhealthy environment slums where surrounded by addictions. Due to ignorance, labourers feel it gives additional strength and vigor's. Weak personality with weak moral fabric who gets easily temptated. Not able to face hard realities of life, just to escape and forget such anxieties and tensions of life. Sudden losses and frustration in love life, life is ambitions fall loss of business leads to drinking. People who became rich over night, fast money inn, have tendency to talk drink to feel elited grouped and feel it is a additional statues to improve the standards.

Effect—Alcohol stimulates the secretion of gastric juice. If taken concentrated form it increases gastric acidity and produces gastritis. In skin, it produces sense of warmth and flushing due to dilatation of peripheral vessels. Produces toxic effect on bone marrow leading to the thrombocytopenia and anemia. It inhibits glucose formation from lactate and from amino acids and during starvation, it produces hypoglycemia. It depresses the nervous system which actually produces false sense of well being. It causes intellectual impairment and brain damage. It also leads to peripheral neuritis and myopathy. It has a direct destructive effect on heart muscle. So irregular pulse, fibrillation, cardiomyopathy leading to congestive cardiac failure, Liver enlargement/cirrhosis fatty liver hepatitis. Pancreatitis common in chronic alcoholism.

Consequences—Crime, murder, prostitution, neglect of families, malnutrition, diseases, unemployment, child delinquency, loss of friends, property, money. It affects socioeconomic, biologic problem.

Losses self respect, short life, does not enjoy life.

Alcoholism is a root cause of family unhappiness.

Ten percent of people drink enough to become intoxicated. Drunken drivers have accidental death in highway. Alcoholism is one of the countries most serious problems. Alcohol induced diseases, the social consequence of alcohol are extremely serious. Alcohol is rapidly absorbed from an empty stomach and its effect on CNS can often be felt very quickly. Blood alcohol level may reach a peak within 20 minutes. Food tends to dilute the alcohol specially taken with milk and fat contain foods. The rate at which the body tissues burn up alcohol varies from person to person The metabolic breakdown of alcohol that passes through the liver is oxidized by the same enzyme system that also metabolizes many other drugs.

Continued heavy drinking leads almost inevitably to organic damage. The failure to eat occurs because of the high caloric value of it when it is metabolized in the tissues. Every gram of alcohol that is oxidized produces seven calories. Thus, heavy drinker can satisfy a large part of his daily energy requirements by his alcohol intake alone. He fails to eat more nutritious foods containing proteins and vitamins, as a result develops deficiency of B- complex.

High concentration of alcohol is directly irritating to the mucosal lining of the stomach thus gastric health problem is common in heavy drinkers. Other digestive disorders found such as constipation or diarrhea, pancreatitis, gastric bleeding is common, liver disorder, fatty liver and cirrhosis. Nervous system disorder occurs, muscle paralysis ataxia and mental confusion peculiar intellectual impairment called Korsakoff's psychosis disturbance in memory, inability to learn new material, heart muscle damage.

People who have been drinking heavily need emergency treatment in hospital for acute pathological intoxication. Alcoholic stupor or coma or acute withdrawal Recovery from alcoholic addiction requires long-term treatment.

Do not lose hope for the eventual recovery of patient who relapses repeatedly to avoid negative effect of the care given. Keep hyperactivity patient from hurting and exhausting himself. Set firm limits on his behavior if he becomes destructive. In dealing with a delirious patient, help him orient himself to his surrounding by telling them repeatedly and slowly where he is in concrete. If the patient is not fully awake, keep in his room dim light at night to help prevent time disorientation. Do not leave him alone. Counsel the patient and his family when problem arise during the period of rehabilitation. Advice on good nutrition, adequate fluid intake and personal hygiene.

Disaffirm Therapy—Action and Indication

This drug is used as an aid to psychotherapy or other supportive measures in the treatment of chronic alcoholism. It is not cure, it helps patient to stay sober, do not even take a cough mixture. If he takes any alcohol while this drug is still in the system, he will suffer the anterior or anti-abuse alcohol reaction. This is marked by such a discomfort as a throbbing headache, nausea and vomiting, breathing difficulty and heart palpation. Causes occasional skin rashes or mild drowsiness. Drug is contraindicated in heart disease. It is never given without patient's knowledge.

Dosage begun with a single daily dose of 0.5 gm in the morning; after a week dose is reduced and 0.125 gm maintained this level for a month or for a year.

Is the patient free of physical conditions if not it is contraindicate the use of this drug?

Is the patient strongly motivated, cooperative and intelligent enough to follow instructions for the safe use of this drug?

Psychotherapy and support from family, that person who takes daily does and warn patient to avoid other medications such as cough, cold, asthma remedies including mouth wash and after shave lotions.

Alcohol is a drug and may be classified as a sedative, tranquilizer, hypnotic or anesthetic depending upon the quantity consumed. Alcohol is rapidly absorbed from the stomach and small intestine within 2-3 minutes of consumption; it can be defected in the blood the maximum concentration is usually reached about one hour after consumption.

Today, increasing number of young people has started to drink alcoholic beverages, with increased quantity and frequency, because of this road accidents have increased. The health problems for which alcohol is responsible and social damage, which includes family disorganization, crime and loss of productivity. Alcohol abuse is universal problem. More the alcohol thinner the brain. The size of your total brain volume gets smaller as you drink.

Understanding and its effect on health on tobacco smoking causes about 3 million premature deaths a year. Tobacco is responsible for about 30% of all cancers deaths. More people die from tobacco related diseases other than cancer such as stroke, myocardial infection, aortic aneurysm and peptic ulcer. Young people who take up smoking have been shown to experience an early onset of cough, phlegm production and shortness of breath on exertion. There is evidence that the earlier a person begins to smoke, the greater is the risk of life, threatening diseases such as chronic bronchitis, emphysema, and cardiovascular disease and lung cancer.

Experimentation of smoking as a symbol of adult behavior is common in adolescence smoking also harms the health of others. Among non-smokers, exposure to environmental tobacco smock increases the risk of lung cancer. The babies of mothers who smoke weight less than those of non-smokers.

Because of the long delay between the cause and full effect, people tend to misjudge the hazards of tobacco. When young generation adults begin to smock, the risk felt at reach middle age.

The withdrawal symptoms include irritability anxiety, craving, sleep problems, headaches, tremors and lethargy. Its symptoms may continue for 4-6 weeks and craving may continue for many months.

October 2-10-2008, a law is passes clearing the air for our children- on guard against the ill effects of passive smoking can have on kids. Passive smoking has negative impact on the child health. Every child has right to smoke free environment. Children and youth are influenced when they see celebrity's smoke. They should stop smoking in public. Passive smoke can cause cancer and coronary heart disease. It leads to sudden infant death syndrome. It leads to low birth weight babies.

Hotel, restaurants, airport, non-smoking area, A nationwide ban on smoking in public places with Supreme Court, backing the ban and the state government yet to implement it. Public places includes railway station, government offices, all workplaces, educational institution, libraries, courts, amusement centers like cinema hall, hospitals, shopping malls, public conveyance like buses, trains, taxis, autos, open space surrounding, refreshment rooms, canteens, private clinics etc.

Nicotine is addictive, making it difficult for people to quit smoking. However, it is not impossible to quit. Will power alone can do the trick; throw away all ashtrays, cigarette stocks and so on. Avoid bars, a visit to smock cessation clinic where psychologist and counsel how to quit.

Diarrhea is an increase in the number of stools and the passage of liquid, unformed Faeces. It is a symptom of disorders affecting digestion, absorption and secretion in the gastrointestinal tract. Intestinal contents pass through the small intestinal and colon too quickly to allow the usual absorption of fluid. As a result, faces become watery, so the patient may be unable to control the urge to defecate.

Conditions that Cause Diarrhea

Emotional stress increases intestinal motility.

Intestinal infections increases mucus secretion in colon

Food allergies reduce digestion of food elements

Food intolerance increases intestinal mobility

Medications like iron and antibiotics cause irritation of intestinal mucosa and supra infection allowing overgrowth of normal flora, inflammation and irritation of mucosa

Laxative causes increase intestinal motility leading to diarrhea

Colon diseases, e.g. colitis causes inflammation and ulceration of intestinal walls, reduced absorption of fluids, increased intestinal motility

Surgical procedures like Gastrectomy, colon resection lead to improper absorption and diarrhea.

Nursing Care

The fluid lost from the body should be replaced immediately to prevent shock and collapse of the patient. This is done by ORS fluids.

Small and frequent feeding of nutrition

A balanced diet

Avoid hot or cold spices
Care of the skin
Adequate rest
Psychological support
Medication like anti-diarrhea, antiseptic, antispamindone, etc.

ORT—Oral Rehydration Therapy

It is the cheap, simple and effective way to treat dehydration cased by diarrhea; essential fluids and salts are lost from the body and must be quickly replaced. Extra fluids at home such as tea, soup, rice water, fruit juice.

What is ORT?

It is fluid by mouth with special drink.
Formula—3.5 gms sodium chloride
2.5 gms sodium bicarbonate
1.5 gms potassium chloride
20 gms glucose
Dissolve in one liter clean water

Preparation of ORS

Hands should be washed
Clean drinking water should be taken
Exactly one liter of clean water/boil should be measured in clean container
One entire packed of ORS should be then added to this one liter clean drinking water mixed and then kept covered
One teaspoons/2 minutes to child less then 2 years
Older child made to sip frequently from cup
Dose given according to age like
4 months-200-400 ml or 1-2 glasses
14-15 years 1200 ml-2200 ml, 6-11, 6-11 glasses, each glass measures about 200 ml.

How does ORT Works?

It does not stop diarrhea, it replaces the lost fluid.
Can ORS be used for every one? All who are dehydrated can take.
How to asses the degree of dehydration
What should be done if child vomits?
Should feeding continue at the same time as ORT?
What sorts of foods are good during diarrhea?
Can the solution be made with daily water?
Can ORS solution be stored?

What is Dehydration?

It is dryness of mouth and thirst, sunken fontanelle, fast, weak pulse, fast breathing, and loss of skin elasticity, sunken dry eyes and reduced amount of urine. Rehydration is correction of dehydration.

Accidents

Accidents do not just happen, they are caused; they are caused by thoughtlessness, carelessness, neglect and momentary lack of concentration. Unfortunately, it is not always the person who causes the accident who suffers very often is the innocent.

Tiredness, stress, illness, worry, anger, drinks, bad or good news are the few reasons of accident. The very old and the very young are at risk of accidents because of lack of physical inadequacy or lack of judgment.

Highways to death-blood on road- no lights, narrow roads, no phone link with the world in a nightmarish experience. To avoid accidents do not drive continuously through the night. Get adequate sleep if you are planning to start early. Try not to listen to music; it may reduce your level of alertness. Chew something in mouth and talk to someone on long journey to help you remain awake. Never drink and drive; do not talk on cell phone while driving. Always signal before change lanes. Do not give a lift to strangers. Always wear a seat belt. Check before you drive treys, air pressure, fuel and engine, radiator must have enough water. Engine must be well serviced, ownership documents, driving license and insurance documents before you set on a journey. Keep list of hospital and phone numbers to meet with an emergency, drive more responsibly.

A child below five is prone for the following accidents.

- Asphyxia during breastfeeding due to pressure of breast on the child's nose.
- Covering the baby's face with blanket out of ignorance
- Injury to cervical ligaments due to failure to support the baby's head below the age of 5 months
- Fall from cradle or with the cradle if the support of the cradle breaks swallowing of the foreign body
    - Accidental falls poisoning due to ingestion of poisons substances
    - Foreign bodies in eye, nose, ear and airway
    - Burns while playing with fire, or due to accident in kitchen
    - Electrical shock while playing with faulty electrical appliances
- If the child is mentally subnormal, or suffers from conditions such as cerebral palsy, epilepsy it is more prone for accidents.

Electricity can be a Killer; to Avoid Accidents due to Electric Shock

Do not have unnecessarily long, short circuit causing fire. Have three pin plugs for all appliances, so that the appliance is earthen via the wall socket and not via ones body during accidental contact. Do not touch electric switches with wet hands. Disconnect plugs from sockets after switching off. Leaking water can soak through electrical equipment to cause short circuit and fire.

Some of the coal gas, natural gas and cylinder gases are poisons and can cause death if inhaled. All of them are explosive when mixed with air.

To avoid dangers associated with fuse gases- turn off all the gas taps properly when not in use. Do not turn on a gas tap until you have a lighter or matches in your hand. Turn off at main before leaving the house empty for a period. Do not light a match if you smell gas. Immediately turn off gas flames, heaters, cigarettes, open all the windows and doors and switch on fans to disperse the gas.

Open fire can prove dangerous young and old may fall in the fire. Smokers can burn themselves when they fall asleep while smoking and the cigarette falls on bed.

Kitchen knives can cause accidental cuts. Toddlers can fall on burning stoves. Bath water make sure not too hot, keep petrol and paraffin away from children. Do not store inflammable or poisonous materials in bottles of cold drinks or fruit juices, because children may accidentally drink.

Know and obey traffic rules. Walk on road on right side. Do not operate machines without adequate training; when sleepy, tired. Parents allowing their under aged minor children to get behind the wheel in such incident parents must face the consequence. Parents by their negligence make accidents or crimes happen, they should be made accountable. They are guilty of criminal negligence.

Food adulteration—Means mixing of other substances intentionally to the food, in order to increase the quantity of food. Adulteration of food consists of a large number of practices. Mixing substitutions, abstraction concealing the quality, putting up decomposed food for sale Misbranding or giving false labels and addition of poison. Some forms of adulterations are injuries to health. For example, mustard oil with argemone oil Most adulteration have only economic significance, e.g. adding water to milk, removal of fat and add starch to make milk thicker. For example, ghee add dalda or vanaspati pig and animal fat, rice wheat mixed up with chips and mud to increase bulk, wheat flower mixed with stone power and maize flower mixed, pulses chemical added to old stocks to improve the appearance. Tea and coffee with old used tealeaves, coffee with chicory, honey with jaggery.

1986 Act purpose is to protect the health consumer and assure foods of honest nutritive values. Prevent malpractice and do not get cheated. Report to consumer protection act and can take legal action.

Food is a potential source of infection; bacteria and other microorganism and parasites at any point can contaminate it during its journeys from the producer to the consumed. Producing, handling, distribution, serving is important. Food handler connected with cooking, unhygienic habits, handlers with skin disease, typhoid history, chronic dysentery, infected wounds not permitted. Specific hand washing, hair covered, and food fresh, see color, touch, odor, prolonged storage.

The body needs many kinds of foods.

Some foods build the body, e.g. milk, egg, fish, meat, nuts, deal and pulses.

Some foods give the body energy, e.g. potatoes, bread, rice, sugar, jaggery, ghee and oil.

Some foods help to preserve health by protecting the body from illness, e.g. fruits, green leafy vegetables and other vegetables.

During the first five years of the Childs life, growth is very rapid. The child is developing physically as well as mentally. In order that growth and development may be normal, the child requires the right type of food in the right quantity.

When the body does not get the right type of food in the right quantity the child suffers from malnutrition. In India, out of every ten pre-school children below five years of age eight suffer from some degree of malnutrition. Malnutrition can be different types.

MALNUTRITION IN THE PRE-SCHOOL

Kwashiorkor—There is welling of the feet and legs and peeling of the skin. The hair is light reddish in color and is very brittle. The condition is caused by talking a diet, which is deficient in proteins. It can be prevented by giving the child plenty of protein rich foods such as milk, eggs, meat, fish, dals, pulses or nuts.

Marasmus—Child is very thin with the bones showing. The skin is wrinkled and loose, the abdomen is bloated and the child has a wizened expression on the face like that of an old man. This condition can be caused by giving the child too little to eat or by starving the child. It can be prevented by feeding the child with sufficient amounts of food. Diet includes carbohydrate, protein and fat that is chapatti, milk, deal, green leafy and yellow vegetables, oil, ghee and fruits.

Rickets—Child has a potbelly and bony deformities such as bowing of the legs, knock knees, bulging of the bones of the forehead, and knob-like swelling or beading of the ribs. It can be prevented by exposure of the child to sunlight, which is plentiful in our country and is rich in vitamin D. certain foods are also rich in vitamin D such as ghee, egg and fish liver oil.

Vitamin A deficiency—Certain foods like yellow vegetables and fruits such as pumpkin, carrot, papaya and mango, and green leafy vegetables, ghee and butter are rich in vitamin A. This vitamin is necessary for keeping the eyes and skin healthy. If there is less vitamin A in the diet, the whites of the eyes become dry and wrinkled, the child cannot see in the dark that is night blindness, and if the condition is not treated with vitamin A, the eyes become ulcerated and the child may become totally blind.

Anemia—Iron is very essential for the body. This element is found in foods like green leafy vegetables such as spinach, amaranth, methi and the tops of turnips, beetroot, etc. if food rich in iron are not given, the child suffers from anemia. The inner lining of the lips and eyelids look pale, the skin, and the nails are pale. The child lacks interest in play, is listless and tires easily.

It is, therefore, very important to give every child the right type of food in the right quantities. Give nutritional supplements iron and folic acid, vitamin A solution.

You are nursing human beings and not disease. Your attitude, dignity of patient, supportive care will help in speedy recovery. Take care of cleanliness, orderliness, neatness, ventilation; lightening, spiritual needs are important aspects.

Dietary services—Food sufficient calorie value with all nutrients in correct amounts, type of food, methods of preparation habit of eating, taste, appetite, serving meals, hot food, dietician calculate diets, plan menus, supervises preparation, special diet.

Different Types of Fever

Diseases on this earth have been present ever since the birth of living beings. It has been problem of human beings. To animals it is the instincts that make them eat herbs for cure. Man has been able to find out causes for diseases and their cure through research which has been in operation even today and will continue to be in action in times to come. As the civilization made progress, the theories also changed. The bacteriological era gave rise and new avenues of modern concept. The root causes of disease were the core factor for research.

Bird flu or avian influenza -lethal virus- is a contagious disease of animals caused by viruses. The bird flu virus is normally found in the intestines and nasal secretions and saliva of wild migratory bird. It is a deadly virus. The wild birds shed the virus and domestic birds contract it through water, contaminated feed or soil. Domestics poultry are especially valuable to infections that can rapidly reach epidemic proportions. Infection to human beings is currently limited to bird to person infection through nasal secretions, saliva or Faeces of an infected bird. Avoid undercooked or raw poultry dishes. Try not to eat raw eggs and meat. Use gloves when in direct contact with wild birds and poultry.

Chikungunya fever is a vector borne viral disease transmitted to humans by the bite of infected AEDES, CULEX mosquitoes. Its clinical manifestation is fever, severe arthralgia with chills, headache, photophobia, anorexia, nausea, vomiting, abdominal pain, small joint pains. Diagnoses and treatment to be done in time Prevention measures to control mosquitoes.

Dengue fever—Dengue also called backbone fever because it sometimes causes severe joint and muscle pain that feels as if bones are breaking. Dengue virus is transmitted to human through mosquito bites, a specific species of mosquito biting an infected person and then someone else.

Symptoms—It starts with chills, headache, pain upon moving the eyes and low backache. Painful aching in the legs and joints occurs during the first hours of illness. The temperature rises quickly as high as 104°F with relative low heart rate/Bradycardia and low blood pressure. Theses become reddened. A flushing or pale pink rash comes over the face and then disappears. The glands/lymph nodes in the neck and groin are often swollen.

Fever and other sings of dengue last for two to four days, followed by a rapid drop in temperature with profuse sweating. This precedes a period with normal temperature and a sense of well being that lasts about a day. A second rapid rise in temperature follows. A characteristic rash appears along with the fever and spreads from the extremities to cover the entire body except the face. The palms and soles may be bright red and swollen. Nevertheless, to save ourselves from these deadly diseases, we can take certain prevention measures like—

Wearing Light Colored Clothes

Wearing long sleeved and full length garments to avoid skin exposure.

Avoiding eating bananas during rainy season because mosquitoes love bananas

Spraying insecticides on the walls and roof of the home to kill adult mosquitoes

Empty stagnant water from old tiers, trashcans, flowerpots and coolers

Cover the utensils containing water in the kitchen properly.

Sleeping under bed nets is must.

Wearing insect repellent if outdoors at night

Cleansing bath tubs daily and avoid storing water bathrooms.

Planting marigold around works great as bug repellent because the flowers give off a fragrance bugs do not like. Mosquitoes are not merely irritating insects that bite into your precious sleep hours, they also carriers of lethal diseases that claim millions of lives around the world. Keep your family safe from their bites.

As a precaution against dengue, limit the exposure to mosquitoes by staying indoors two hour's after sunset. The aedes aegypti mosquito is a daytime biter with peak periods of biting around sunrise and sunset. It may bite at any time of the day and is often hidden inside homes or other dwellings, especially in urban areas. Is an acute fever caused by a virus? It occurs in two forms. Dengue fever and dengue hemorrhagic fever-DHF. It is marked by the onset of sudden high fever, severe headache and pain behind the eyes, muscles and joins pains. DHF is a more severe form, in which bleeding and sometimes shock occur leading to death. The high fever continues for six days, the patient feels much discomfort and is very weak after the illness. Early treatment can relive the symptoms and prevent complications and death. Aspirin and brufen should be avoided in dengue fever, as it known to increase the bleeding tendency. It is spread by the bite of an infected mosquito Aedes aegypti, 5-7 days time symptoms appear. The mosquito live in dark places, in stored exposed water collections such as barrels, drums, jars, pots, buckets, flower vase, plant saucers, tanks, discarded bottles, tins, tires, water cooler ect. And a lot more places where rain water collects or is stored. The female mosquito lays her eggs in water in and around homes, and these eggs become adult in about 10 days. Remember always that dengue is a serious viral disease transmitted by mosquito, so prevent mosquito bites. One thing that makes Aedes aegypti the mosquito that spread the fever virus is its egg laying habits. Female will deposit their eggs in just about anything that holds water and many of these things are found in and around dwellings-flowerpots, vases, cans, tires. Researchers have shown, for instance, that they are attracted to water that has leaves in it.

Malaria

August 20 was celebrated as World Mosquito Day. Fight against malaria. It was in august, 1867, that Dr. Ronald Ross, a renowned physician, begun dissecting mosquitoes that fed on malarious patients. On august 20, while dissecting a mosquito, he found many cells on the stomach wall of the mosquito and concluded that these were the malaria parasite stages in the mosquito. This research was quite significant because until then, no one had any idea of how parasites in the blood of malarious patients were transmitted via mosquitoes.

Mosquitoes cause more human suffering than any other organism. Over one million people die from mosquito born diseases every year. Mosquito bit can cause diseases such as malaria, dengue, chikungunya etc.

Malaria is caused by a tiny parasite called plasmodium. The parasite grows in liver of a person for few days and then enters the bloodstream where it invades the red blood cells. There are three types of malaria depending upon the parasite, which causes it.

The symptoms characteristic of malaria include flu-like illness, with fever, chills, muscle aches and headache. Some patient develops nausea, vomiting, cough and diarrhea. Cycles of chills, fever and sweating that repeat everyone; two or three days are typical. There can sometime be vomiting, diarrhea, coughing and jaundice of the skin yellowing and whites of the eyes due to destruction of red blood cells and liver cells.

Common malaria now a deadly killer patient with vivax malaria now land up in an ICU while a decade ago they needed only conventional choroquine treatment. 10-20% in ICU, 70-80 needs admission in hospital. The research shows that the strain has led to 50,000 deaths a year in Asia. This highlights vivax causes organ failure. Malaria has become resurgent in the last two years, with cases increasing drastically. Floods and the resulting change and other reason in the unfettered construction boom in the city. Vivax is now causing multi organ failure among patient. They come with lung injury or bleeding in the lungs there have also been cases of kidney and liver being affected. These complications had earlier been associated with falciparum malaria. What are the reasons for this new virulence of the vivax causing malaria? Doctors blame the emerging drug resistance to patient.

Diabetics is a chronic disease that occurs when the pancreas does not produce enough insulin or when the body cannot effectively use the insulin it produces insulin is the hormone that regulates blood sugar.

Diabetes can affect your heart, blood pressure, nervous system, eyesight and kidneys. It is a high mortality disease. The symptoms include excessive urination, thirst, constant hunger, weight loss, vision changes and constant fatigue. Blood tests can help in early diagnosis. Type-1 diabetes often called insulin dependent or childhood onset diabetes is characterized by a lack of insulin production in the body, so patients have to take daily shots of insulin. Type-2 diabetes also called non-insulin dependent or adult onset diabetes results from the body's inability to use insulin effectively; excess body weight and physical inactivity can result in this type of diabetes. Counter diabetes a healthy lifestyle can prevent type 2 diabetes. Avoid becoming overweight. Be physically active, you should be doing at least 30 minutes of moderate intensity activity regularly.

India is on its way to becoming the diabetes capital of the world. What is diabetes? It is a condition in which the body's mechanism for breaking down glucose is hampered. Thus the blood level of glucose rises. It is commonly referred to as sugar problem. long uncontrolled diabetes lead to kidney damage. India in 2007 had 4065 core people with diabetes; the diabetic's incidence rate is predicted to increase by 73% by 2oxygen5 to reach 8 cores.

Combating to diabetes epidemic needs an innovative grassroots approach that vibes with mass mobilization model.

Eye—Sutures retinal surgery gets new breath of life where Mumbai doctors shows the way

Less than five babies in one million are struck by heart outside the body born. Most babies die from diseases before birth.

Food—Fined the hidden salt in your food. Pizzas and burgers contain over a gram of salt per serving.

You may be a diabetic and do not even know it; 10 percent of the city to be diabetic. Now we are seeing more of the diseases than ever before. Metabolic syndrome is emerging as one of the risk factors for diabetes. Figures India is home to 40 million diabetes patients, accounting for 20% of the world diabetic population. The number of diabetic's ill increase to 80 million by 2030. Most people with dainties in low and middle income communities are middle aged 45/ 65 and not the elderly say WHO date.

CARE OF NOSE AND EAR

Excessive accumulation of secretions makes the patient sniff or blows the *nose*. The secretions becomes crusted and obstructed the airway.

For patient who cannot remove the secretion, assistance is necessary to clean the congestion and protect nasal mucosa. External crusts can be removed with a wet wash cloth or a cotton applicator moistened with oil, normal saline or water for babies a wipe cotton moist with oil, introduced into the anteriorly and rotated gently cleansing nostrils.

When there is poor hygiene the *ears* debris may accumulate behind the ear and in the anterior aspect of the external ear. This may lead to ulceration of the skin. A common problem of the ear is the collection of cerumen or ear wax in the external auditory canal. This may cause difficulty in hearing warm liquid paraffin or vegetable oil instilled into the ear can soften wax and it can be easily removed. When it cannot removed, consult ENT surgeon.

TEST FOR URINE SUGAR

Procedure

Pour 5 ml of benedict solution into a test tube

Heat it over the spirit lamp to check the purity of the solution.

If there is no color change in the Benedict solution, add 7 to 8 drops of urine to it with a dropper

Boil it again

Allow the test tube to cool

Record the result as follows:

Blue liquids with no deposits-sugar Nil

Greenish deposits in a greenish liquid-sugar 1%

Yellow deposits-sugar 2%

Orange deposits with the colorless liquid-sugar 3%

Brick red- sugar 5%

Articles

Test tube with test tube holder
Spirit lamp
Benedict solution
Match box
Urine sample bottle with urine
Paper bag
Pipette/dropper
Record book

URINE TESTING FOR ALBUMIN

Cold Test

Pour half inch of nitric acid 2% into a test tube then pour urine about two inch from the sides of the test tube.

If albumin is present a white opaque ring will appear at the junction of urine and nitric acid.

Discard the urine and clean the test tube.

Hot Test

Take three fourth part of urine in a test tube

Holding the test tube from bottom, heat the upper part of the urine over the flame of the spirit lamp

Rotate the test tube constantly, so that it will not break

If a cloudy layer appears in the hot urine, it may be due to protein or phosphates

Add nitric acid to it with the dropper

If the cloud disappears it was due to phosphates

If the cloud still remains, it indicates the presence of albumin

If will not disappear with acetic acid

Discard the urine and clean the test tube

The result will depend upon the cloudiness in the urine

Record the result

STEAM INHALATION

Inhalation is the deep breathing of vapour or gas into the lungs for a local effect on the air passages or for systematic effect. For example, relief of bronchial spasms.

Purpose

To relieve inflammation of the mucus membrane in acute cold and in a sinusitis

It produces symptomatic relief

It softens thick mucus and relieves coughing

It provides antiseptic effect on the upper respiratory tract

HOT APPLICATION

Heat is applied in either a moist or dry form, e.g. giving hot water bags, infrared rays.

COLD APPLICATION

Cold applications are also moist or dry. Moist application includes cold compresses, packs, sponge bath, and ice bag.

Purpose

To reduce fever

To relieve pain and inflammation

For treatment of sprain and epitaxis

ORAL MEDICATION

Drugs are given by mouth in the form of liquids, oils, water solutions

In solid forms tablets, power, capsules, pills.

Oral medication route is the most common and most convenient route

Observe five right patient, right drug, right dose, right time and right method.

PEDICULOSIS

Pediculosis is a state of being infected with lice. Pediculi or lice is a small blood sucking parasites. Pediculosis is associated with poor personal hygiene. It can be acquired in over crowed, unsanitary conditions and exposure to infected person.

To prevent it proper personal hygiene should be maintained by every person. Daily hair combing and frequent washing it. If the patient complains of itching or scratches the head examine head and scalp thoroughly.

Treatment

DDT powder one part and nine part of talcum powder

It kills the lice in two hours, but it does not destroy nits.

Kerosene mixed with equal parts of sweet oil destroys both

Carbolic lotion 1:40

Readymade available listrill

GBH Gama benzene hex chloride can be used

Apply vascelln to the skin, the hair line to prevent irritation, and then apply the medicine to every part of the scalp and hair. Roll-up the long hair on the top of the head, and cover the hair with triangular bandage to prevent the spread of lice to the other area of the body. Give thorough head bath on the next day. Hair should be fine combed daily for a week, repeat the treatment after a week.

Do not touch that portion of the cotton swab which will come in direct contact with the eyes.

Physical Assessment

It helps to gather data regarding the patient's health status

To identify normal and deviation

It offers an opportunity for health teaching

It is indicated during home visits and health camps

Specific Examination Like

Eye-torch; ear-torch and tuning fork; nose nasal speculum; throat tongue depressor, torch, throat swab and paper bag.

Chest and abdomen-stethoscope and measuring tape

Virginal examination-gloves and vaginal speculum

Neurological-a percussion hammer, safety pins, cotton swab

Practical Evaluation of Students in the Field

Students are posted for urban slums and rural field experience where they visit families, do the surveys, attain emergencies, give treatment for minor illness, give health education, ect. Where they have to learn the concept of community health nursing and the actual situation of people living in that areas and assess there needs and there problems. They also have to do physical assessment of different groups of people? Attain deliveries, immunization programmes and know PHC set up. Adopt family and do the family care plans. Educate the people on different issues on health with role play and exhibition.

- Define eligible couple.
- What are the different methods of family planning?
- What are the objectives of family welfare program?
- List the national health program in India.
- Role of a nurse in malaria, blindness programs.
- What are the objectives of MCH programme?
- Functions of a nurse in school health program.
- How will you maintain records and reports?
- Importance of health education?
- List the activities carried out in antenatal clinic?
- What is the staffing pattern of PHC?
- What are the functions of CHN?
- How will you maintain cold chain?
- What is meant by midday school meal?
- How will you identify malnutrition?

- What is dug well latrine/what is bore hole latrine?
- Importance of kitchen garden.
- What is the water born diseases?
- Which are the fly born diseases?
- What are the purposes and principles of home visit?
- Household methods of water purification.
- What is sanitary well?
- Methods and purpose of sewage purification.
- Methods of food preservation.
- Food and personal hygiene.
- What is the soakage pits?
- What are three triage systems?
- Define health.
- How will you give health education on weaning, malnutrition, and balance diet.
- How do you understand environmental sanitation?
- How will you prevent worm infestation?
- Importance of personal hygiene.
- Food hygiene/methods of cooking.
- Open air defecation and its effect on health.
- What are the causes of air born diseases?
- Define safe water, immunity, ventilation, disinfection.
- What is the difference between community nursing and hospital nursing?
- How will you identify anemia, its sign symptoms and prevention, diet?
- Source of carbohydrate; protein, fat and its functions.
- Deficiency of vitamins and the diseases caused by lack of them.
- Shallow well, deep well.
- Types of family.
- Aims and purpose of AV aids.
- Purpose of home visit.
- Methods of chlorination process.
- Pasteurization of milk.
- Methods of food preservation.
- Method and purpose of sewage purification.
- Household methods of water purification.
- School health services and its importance.
- Aims of antenatal care, MCH.
- Examination to be carried during pregnancy. Detection of high-risk cases.
- Objectives of immunization- how will you protect various childhood diseases?
- Objectives and elements of cold chain.
- Dimension of health.
- Indicators of health.
- Levels of health—what do you mean by health for all by 2000AD?

- Physical health assessment- define anthropometry.
- Triage system, reference slip, categories of referral.
- Steps of nursing process.
- Job responsibilities of female health worker, community health nurse, dai, village health guide, anganwadi worker, multipurpose worker.
- Family welfare services.
- Role and functions of community health nurse.
- Nurse's day celebrated on ___________.
- WHO day celebrated on ___________.
- Records, reports, and its importance.
- Content of the bag.
- Bag technique and bag principles and functions.
- Procedures and minor ailments.
- Qualities of a nurse.
- The role of a nurse in primary health care.
- Define eligible couple.
- Anganwadi, ICDS, baby friendly hospital.
- List the national health programs in India.
- Health problems due to industrialization.
- Methods of AV aids.
- Demography, causes of population growth and its effect on nation.
- Indigenous system of medicine.
- Voluntary health services.
- Five-year plan.
- National health policy.
- What is meant by term RCH?
- Common geriatric problems you noted in your home visits.
- Care of handicapped.
- Rehabilitation.
- Nutritional problem you noticed in family members and what advice and suggestions you gave.
- Communicable disease mention the types and the preventive measures.
- Population problem-explain.

CHAPTER 14

Nurses' Role in Female Health

A happy home should be the heritage of every person who comes in this world. A happy home is never an accident. A true center of every home is the *mother*. No one else ever can take her place. Every girl should be given trough training in the principles of health, childcare and home skills. The success of the family, the community, the nation depends on the young woman of today and the kind of homes they establish. There is no greater responsibility than this. Happy parents create happy homes. Happy homes produce happy children. Happy children make happy community, and happy communities make a happier world.

The changing decades: Every human being is the author of his own health or disease. In the course of a lifetime, a women's body undergoes striking changes, from puberty to pregnancy to menopause. While these changes are natural, each stage of life may raise special health concern. Knowing how your body works can save you from unnecessary worry. Understanding your body's functions will alert you to potential problem. The series of bodily changes, the reproductive system transforms young girls into a woman, prepares her for childbearing, and supports her through *pregnancy*.

Fertility period from 14 to 45 is actual bearing of children. A woman married at 15 and living till 45 with her husband is exposed to risk of pregnancy for 30 years and may give birth to 15 children. But this maximum is rarely achieved. An average woman gives birth to 6 to 7 children. If married after 22 years, the number of births would decreases by 20 to 30%. Early marriage is a long established custom in India. Therefore, fertility depends on age, duration of married life, spacing of children, education, economic status, caste and religion, nutrition, family planning adopted, widow remarriage, breast-feeding, urbanization etc still births, foetal deaths and abortions are not included in this.

The journey to womanhood: You are about to experience a change that nature has planned for you. If you understand why this change takes place, you will know it is the most natural and exciting thing in life. A challenge to be met with confidence the nature equips your body to function as a grown woman as you approach your teens. At the base of your brain, there is a tiny gland called the pituitary gland. This gland is responsible for sending out messages to different parts of your body to grow and develop to full maturity. This gland starts sending chemical messengers called hormones to the reproductive organs to develop and prepare for motherhood.

Being a woman means being a complete person- independent, caring and beautiful. Moreover, beauty starts from within you. Nature meant woman to be her masterpiece. In addition, as you grow and mature into the woman you are meant to be, you will find few treasures every day, within yourself and in the outside world. Moreover, you will be proud to be a woman.

Every developing society has built inequalities—These can only removed by education, by reaching out and opening the doors to equality, by helping to bring about a change in the level of technology that is used in the daily lives of our people at every level. The education policy must give a new momentum to our society, enable it to shed superstition, instill a sprit of freedom and attitude of independence, spread a national integration, of tolerance and defend against violence and other methods which adopted by certain sections. A society can be judged by how well half of our society progresses and if they are to progress, half the talent and energy cannot be ignored, women should be allowed to full freedom and action.

Women stand at the pinnacle of a new era where prosperity is a reality. From rural landscape to throbbing cities, the women undergoing major transformation, blend rich cultural heritage and modern development, spell hope for women. Last few years, women's education is a hallmark approach in its socio political economical development, initiatives women's self help group programmed, efforts for economic upliftment of women.

Ending violence against women and girls—India has the world's largest number of working women than any other country in the world. Still there are alarming statistics, that 20% of married women experience violence. Every six hour, a married woman is burnt, beaten to death or driven to commit suicide.

She works in fields. She works in her home. She works for her children. She works for the man in her life. She works from dawn until dusk, making life better for everyone. However, as for herself, nothing seems to get better. Her rights stand violated every day. Her voice stiffed, never to be heard. While the quality of her health turns from bad to worse why? Why such neglect? Why the complacency? Why the ignorance of the fact that without her, we would be nowhere. Show you care, because only with her well being can a nation stay alive and thrive.

It needs still strong actions to end the violence against women and girls; and eliminations of all evils. To mobilize in facing this great challenge. Do women need reservation in parliament/the government introduced the bill in the Rajya sabha to reserve one third of seats for women in parliament and state legislation. We are living in a male dominant society where women are deemed to be fit only as housewives. This bill will definitely empower women. They are equal to men and are able competing with them in every field. More rights need to be given to women.

With technology leveling the field, women today have more opportunities than even before. When physical strength was a major factor determining life, the masculine would dominate. Now enabled by technology anyone can get empowered. Women need to unburden themselves of the cultural baggage that they have come to bear for themselves of years. You are so much more than you can see or think.

Importance of respecting and protecting our women- Men and women think differently. It is a basic psychological difference. They bring in different perspectives. House is incomplete without a woman, their talents need to be given wings even though women have proved themselves in every field, we still have long way to go. Female infanticides talking place, low girl literacy, dowry etc. no social work can be complete until women are empowered. We refer to our country mother India but hardly allow her to have any daughter. Swami Vivekananda said-educate a girl child and the nation will awaken.

The nurse as a midwife—The birth of a baby is a marvel, a miracle, far greater than the most intricate nuclear device or most elaborate machine. Planning for a baby is such a lovely experience for both the parents. It is the part of the real fulfillment of marriage. Caring for and feeding a young baby is a responsibility and a privilege. Every young woman should realize that her future is largely governed by her own attitude toward life. Any normal girl has one basic goal in life- to become a successful mother. Setting up a home is a great adventure and thrilling privilege.

Nurse as a midwife must be able to give the necessary supervision, care and advice to woman during pregnancy, labour and the postpartum period, to conduct deliveries on her own responsibilities and to care for the newborn and the infant. This care includes preventive measures, the detection of abnormal conditions in mother and child, the procurement of medical assistance and the execution of emergency measures in the absence of medical help. She has an important task in health counselling and education, not only for patients but also within the family and the community. The work should involve antenatal education and preparation for parenthood and extend to certain areas of gynecology, family planning and childcare. She may practice in hospitals, clinics, health units, domiciliary conditions or in any other service.

Mother and child health is a vital aspect of community health. It promotes and ensures healthy infant to every pregnant mother. They are entitling to special MCH care as they are in vulnerable group. By improving the health of a mother and child, many deaths can be prevented if we give high priority for MCH services in the development of health services in India. It is utmost important to emphasis safe motherhood and child survival.

Under the ICDS scheme, MCH work rendered in health checkup, immunization, supplementary nutrition, health education and referral services. Antenatal care during pregnancy is to promote and maintain nutritional status. To detect high risk and to reduce maternal and infant mortality and morbidity.

Provide to antenatal mothers regular examination, health education and advice special attention to elderly prime mother, identify high risk and pay special attention to them by home visit, referral services, record keeping, giving antenatal cards.

Motivate them for the importance of atleast minimum three visits at 20 weeks, 32 weeks, and 36 weeks of pregnancy. Special advice for diet, personal hygiene, rest and sleep, care of breast, importance of breastfeeding. Give clear cut instruction on warning signs incase of swelling of feet, fits, headache, blurring of vision, bleeding or discharge per vagina and any other unusual symptoms.

Any danger signals such as severe bleeding, cord prolapsed, signs of toxemia, mal presentation, meucanium stained discharge, fetal distress, prolonged labor.

Neonatal after birth note general condition, colour, congenital abnormalities, temperature, birth injury, pallor, jaundice, low birth weight, cyanosis ect should be immediately reported to medical officer.

Abnormalities of pregnancy—Entopic pregnancy, hydatidiform mole, uterine malformations and displacements, ovarian cysts, malpresentations like breach, cord, face, transverse lie, pre-eclampsia, placenta previa noted. Pregnancy associated with cardiac diseases, diabetes, pulmonary tuberculosis, anemia, STD, should be reported at once to medical officer.

Serious neonatal disorders—Such as asphyxia where baby does not breathe due to blockage of airway with mucus, maternal cyanosis, intracranial damage, hemorrhage, should be promptly responded.

Hydrous fetal is is the serious form of Rh hemolytic disease.

Icterus gravis neonatrum severe form of jaundice cleft palate, cleft lip and palate, double-headed monster, baby with Amelia, i.e. no arms, long born absent. Setting sun eyes of hydrocephalic baby, epencephalic a crania, maningocele cervical, anencephaly with spina bifida, achondroplasia condition the limbs short due to failure in the ossification of the long bones during early fatal life. Downs syndrome- the nurses role in dealing with the parents of the handicapped child and assurance and emotional support to be given.

Goals of MCH Care Includes

Family planning that is crude birth rate, total fertility rate, couple protection rate.

Collection of vital statistics- Maternal mortality, infant and neonatal mortality

Treatment of minor ailments and health education and immunization coverage

Prophylaxis against nutritional anemia, vitamin A deficiency

Maternal health services included a pre-marriage counseling; to improve the health states of young women. It takes many years for a girl to become a healthy mature woman. If she is healthy, she can give a healthy child to family and society. Young age pregnancies are dangerous for both mother and the baby.

Through the MCH to reduce the rates of babies born with low birth weight,

To reduce the deaths due to diarrhea,

To teach mother craft and responsibility of motherhood,

Family health history to find out hereditary diseases History of socioeconomic, cultural practices, living standards of the family.

24 hours delivery services at PHC, to promote institutional deliveries, to promote safe delivery practices, essential newborn care, so that we have healthy mother and bouncing baby, by making motherhood safe, as each pregnancy represents a journey into the unknown journey from which too many women never return. Health care at critical time of birth can help ensure that childbirth is a joyful event.

More than 27 million pregnancies occur in our country; MCH programmed can bring down population and ensure future generations of healthy citizens. To make MCH successful joint efforts at grassroot levels is necessary. MCH is pillar of the community health. MCH services can give healthy children to healthy mother thus healthy community and productive citizens.

During pregnancy, nurse supervises and teaches the expectant mother; throughout labour, she observes, examines on MCH wellbeing; having delivered the baby, she attends to mother and child during the postnatal period. Should a complication arise she gives emergency treatment pending the arrival of the doctor.

She has to receive a comprehensive, sound, professional education, deep knowledge of the physiological processes of human reproduction being an essential foundation for MCH. With adequate clinical experience to enable her to carry out various examination skills associated with childbirth.

Learn to use of the electronic monitoring equipment, which can add a new dimension to the management of labour by improving the quality of fetal life and the safety of mother and child; in order to keep space with the scientific advances. To meet the needs of the community with improved socio-economic standards applied to client and family. Delivery in the hospital is strongly advocated during mothers prenatal visits.

Working in the team with collaboration expert and nurse is an efficient member of a team in motivating and encouraging with supportive role and caring attitude; comforting mother with assurance, prudent judgment and behavioral insight. Teaching expectant mothers on nutrition, preparation for childbirth, baby care and counseling them.

She is economic practicing in the homes of the socially less privileged community who cannot afford doctors fees. Provide more advance scientific approach and to incorporate the preventive, social and supportive aspects and providing family center, high-quality MCH service. When socioeconomic standards improve, the community becomes receptive to health education and more interested in MCH and child welfare. She has to register and notify the baby's birth.

Some diagnosis she makes is period of gestation, screening for high-risk conditions, e.g. pre-eclampsia, asses the onset and progress of labour. Some congenital abnormalities and complications diagnosed; and deal with asphyxia, intracranial injury. Prevention and management of emergencies fetal distress, prolapsed cord, rupture of the uterus. Urgent immediate action to be taken to support or save life.

Traditional birth attendants (TBA) helping woman be educated and equipped for home delivery. Extending teaching in the homes will help to eradicate the causes of anemia and infectious diseases the undermine MCH grow grass root level upward. For rich or poor, in every sphere, professional nurses are needed.

The family center MCH care, e.g. health education, nutrition, keeping fit, baby care, breast-feeding, immunization, family planning, accidents in the home. She should be concerned with the wider features of family life that is childbearing and child rearing, establish happy home by giving sensible advice.

She studies the physiological changes due to pregnancy is the uterus enlargement to give nourishment and protection to the growing fetus, so it increases in weight and size. Food requirements are increased during pregnancy. It provides need of the growing child, maintains the maternal health, and physical strength and vitality during labour and successful lactation. To ensure a mature, live, healthy infant, prevention of congenital abnormalities due to viral infection, drug, alcohol and other causes. To detect early high-risk conditions that would endanger the life or impair the health of mother or baby.

First pregnancy produces a certain degree of emotional turmoil in the mind of mother. Not all women are well balanced or emotionally mature, and their reactions to pregnancy will depend on such factors as temperament, intelligence and education, health, age and the marital situation. Weather the child is wanted or not dominates almost everything else in that period of time. All babies are not planned or wanted at the time of conception but the majority of married women adjust to the situation and when baby is born is welcomed. The attitude of husband is he should exercise forbearance and respond with understanding and kindness rather than logical argument.

Nurse to be sensitive to the expectant mother and tell her that childbearing is a natural event and try to foster a cheerful outlook. Nurse must also be aware of the conflict and fear that can be so disturbing to the expectant mothers peace of mind, her willingness to listen and give sympathetic advice will help her to overcome difficulties. Nurse's valuable contribution is to bring a woman into labour in a serene, courageous frame of mind.

Even a woman is delighted at the prospect of motherhood and eagerly awaiting the birth of her baby, upset by vague fears, some real, and some imaginary. She dreads the unknown experience. Fear of death no doubt crosses the mind of every pregnant woman at some time. The expectant mother should be reminded that thousands of women give birth to babies, simply and easily, every day, and focus on the baby's birthday- happier thought.

Everything possible would be done for her comfort and no harm will be done to both physically and psychologically secure and team is interested in her welfare. she is in receptive frame of mind ,once she builds a confidence she is ready to cope with the situation.

Pregnant women are advice to avoid contact with infectious diseases particularly rubella and viral infections. To refrain from talking drug, stop smoking and to take foods rich in body-builders, minerals and vitamins.

Promote mental health and emotional stability. They should be encouraged to ask questions and to express their points of view, wrong conceptions should be clarified. Some mothers prefer their babies to be born at home familiar surrounding and the doctor and midwife she knows. Nurses have to have theoretical knowledge, expertise, and manual skill, vast experience with scientific point to make delivery safer, shorter and easier, is the aim and goal of MCH services.

The kangaroo mother care was designed to reduce hypothermia which poses a serious risk to newborns even in the warmest climate. When a baby is born, its temperature drops. It is a universally available and biologically sound method of care for all newborns, but in particular premature and low birth weight babies, with three components that is **skin to skin contact, exclusive breastfeeding, support to the mother infant**. The kangaroo mother care programme shows mothers how to keep their newborns warm with continuous skin to skin contact.

By keeping mother and newborn together. It has encourages mother and child to bond emotionally and enables the baby to breastfeed at will, giving the baby the energy to produce its own body heat. In many cases, the need for incubators, which are prohibitively expensive in developing countries?

Making motherhood safe at home—MMR continues to be an area of concern despite advances in science and technology. The tragedy of MMR represents a major source of suffering and injustice in our societies. Pregnancy and childbirth are special events in women's lives and the lives of their families. This can be a time of great hope and joyful anticipation. It can be also a time of fear, suffering and even death.

Although pregnancy is not a disease but a normal physiological process- It is associated with certain risks to health and survival both for the women and the infant she bears. These risks are present in every society and in every setting. Due to access to special care during pregnancy and childbirth, developed countries have overcome such problem but it is not the case of our under developed countries where each pregnancy represents a journey into the unknown from which too many women never return.

India MMR ratio as high as of 540/100,000 and NMR34 per/1000 live births comprising 60% of all infant deaths.

About 65% of all births occur at home, of which 35% are attended by dais, 11% by nurses, and 30% by doctors. Worldwide every minute of every day one woman dies of pregnancy related complications. The reality of home birth in rural villages and urban slum-nearly 600,000 women die each year of these 99% of death occurs in developing countries. For every single woman who dies, 30 women develop lifelong illness and injuries. MMR according to RCH- in India in every 5 minutes one woman dies from complications related to MCH- this adds up to total of 121,000 women per year. Every pregnancy faces a risk 15%. Women develop life-threatening complications. 65% of women have skilled attendants; 28% women have complication during labour or after childbirth.

We need to focus on strengthening universal provision of preventive quality care, identifying high risk cases based on clinical criteria and advising them on institutional delivery. Increasing knowledge about high-risk conditions and promoting clean delivery practices at home.

Through primary care and with less sophisticated, less expensive cost-effective strategies be made available to prevent MMR and have safe motherhood. The risks the women face in bringing life into the world are to be taken up as social justice and duty of the society to remedy.

The system of *home deliveries* would continue for many more years to come. Therefore, need to improve socioeconomic condition of Dai.

Responsibility of government to provide better infrastructure and technical support in rural area. Give importance to midwife's, provide transport to reach urgent cases on time to hospitals. In most of remote area Dai is only person available. She is comprehensive health care provider, a Counsellor and an opinion maker, a mediator. If she does not attend delivery, MMR would increase. Safe motherhood is a fundamental right to life.

Role of families and communities during pregnancy is vital. To treat pregnant mother with particular care community must know danger sings, give good nutrition.

To make dialogue and make decision about the place and condition for delivery in advance.

Establish confidence between woman and health care provider. Problems may arise at different times of pregnancy; it is an on going process. Help the family to cope with emergency and danger signal is responsibility of community. Promote clean hands, clean surface, clean sheet, clean perineal area, clean cord stump, clean blade/clean cutting cord. Cost of maternal death has serious consequences in the family, she plays crucial role in the child's health and welfare.

Institutional deliveries—Find the last menstrual period date, and get the expected delivery date in the visits. Find out the gravid a, period of gestation. Find membranes intact, leaking, and ruptured. Find the fundal height and presentation/stations of presentation that is position of an infant head engaged or not engaged. Take fetal heart sounds and do the per virginal examination to find the dilatation of the OS in cms effacement of cervix, any edema, varicose veins, state of pelvis, perineum and molding.

Clinical chart of the puerperium, temperature, pulse, respiration, blood pressure, lochia, urine, motion observe and mark in the chart.

Labour record in that dilatation of cervix, membranes ruptured spontaneous/artificial. Baby born at and the condition of a baby; baby active/asphyxiated.

Placental expelled spontaneous, manually removed, complete/incomplete, observation of placenta.

Type, weight, cord length

Condition of perineum, any tear, intact, lacerated, repair, episiotomy/suture.

Vaginal bleeding normal or heavy, condition of mother after delivery, genetic/psychiatric disorder etc note in the chart.

Clinical charts of *baby* temperature, heart rate, respiration, urine, stool, vomit, jaundice, weight, type of feeding, congenital abnormalities.

Anemia is a major health problem, which requires careful management including investigation to determine the underlying care. Reduction in the concentration of hemoglobin in the blood, poses problem during pregnancy. Each mother should be tested for its level. WHO- says if she has 10 gm/dl hemoglobin she is mildly anemic, 4-7 gm/dl moderately and below 4 gm/dl severely anemic. Nearly 8 out of 10 from poorer population suffer with this.

In physical examination, clinical sings could be noted- pallor, severe fatigue, malaise, weakness, light headedness, fever, dyspoea, headache, vertigo, weight loss, dry skin, brittle nails, spoon shaped, tachycardia, palpitation.

Anemia is a condition that results from an insufficient supply of healthy red blood cells to oxygenate the body's tissues adequately resulted in hypoxia. It is caused due to decreased production of healthy RBC and increased destruction of RBC. Pale eyes, lips, tongue, nails and palm can suggest the presence of anemia. 100 mg iron, 0.5 mg folic consumed for 100 days. Diet green leafy vegetables, sprouts, animal source is good source of iron, with it include lemon and guava. Note that mother does not have hookworm and malaria, which too can bring down counts down and make her anemic.

Diet advised such as apricots, beef, beets, cabbage, dates, mushrooms, oranges, radish, raisins, guava, apple, green leafy vegetables.

Birth weight is one of the indicators that the babies are healthy and well nourished in most parts of India the birth weight is between 2700 to 2900 gm. A birth weight of less than 2500 gm/ cut off point is considered less favorable for the survival and well-being of a new born. The birth weight should be taken within the first hour of life. The naked baby placed on a clean towel on the scale pan/beam balance scales. Low birth weight is a major health problem in India. 30-40% low birth weight in India estimated. Due to home delivery no record of this is kept. It connects to iron deficiency, iodine disorder, antenatal care, early marriage, and ICDS-is only hope to remedy the problem. We need to make this as people movement.

India 5/1000 MMR; 68/1000 IMR; the young who die could be avoided Illiteracy, poverty, inadequate medical aid, repeated frequent pregnancy too cause this problem. Effort to improve birth weight should start long before mother actually becomes pregnancy. Help mother to gain 10 kg weight, marry after year of 21 and her weight at least 45 kg.

For MCH to improve need cleanliness and waste disposal, poor condition of labour rooms and lack of privacy in many places, inadequate new born care, quality of services lacking, early discharge after delivery is a problem, need to prepare facilities for in patient care, sharp increase in institutional deliveries, and shortage of staff nurses.

A *call center* has been established by ministry of health and family welfare under the integrated disease surveillance project to receive alert/information for outbreaks and epidemic disease. Call from anywhere in the country 1075 toll frees. Thrust on difficult areas and vulnerable social group.

- *Cervicograph*—Done when weak dilatation.
- *Fetal blood sampling*—Done when fetal heart rate pattern deviates from normal.
- *Cardiotocograph apparatus*—Simultaneously measures and records uterine activity and fetal heart frequency and relative uterine activity. These readings are indicated by meters on the front panel of the instrument and simultaneously by the recorder.

  An endocervical swab for bacterial culture.

Instruments and Drug

Towel clip, fine toothed dissecting forceps, non-toothed dissecting forceps; mosquito artery forceps; no.2 me silk suture size 2; cutting needle; ethic on 503; 1% lignocaine 10 ml; IV cannula, galipot/bowl, Hollister umbilical cord clamp; draping sheets; baby wrap; mayo forceps/mayo scissors 15 cm; mucus extractors, cord ligature, baby identification bands.

Drug—syntometrine, ergometrine, syntocinon

Doptone ultrasonic fetal heart monitor

Ultrasound module record, FHS Fetal ECG, from scalp electrode

Mp40 infusion pump which administers dose of Oxytocin, Rubber wedge to insert when convulsion, perennials pad, swab holding forceps, stiles, electric vacuum pump for evacuation of uterus, Sims speculum, cervical dilator no. 8, blunt and sharp aneurysm needle, stitch scissors, needle holder, leggings, obstetric forceps, wool swabs, gauze swabs, swab holding forceps, uterine sound, body bath linen and equipment for rooming in, removal of perennial sutures using stitch cutter blade, Allis's tissue forceps, chromic catgut no. 20, no; linen thread no. 60, me silk no. 0.

Pediatrics

Transfer to hospital baby in heated incubator wrapped in silver swaddler.

Model 79 servo incubator provides continuous monitoring of temperature of preterm/sick babies, automatically alters the environmental temperature adjusting infants changes, audible and visual alarms for over heating power supply or air circulation failure.

Nasogastric feed given by gravity drip.

Naso jejunal feed given by slow continuous infusion pump.

Intravenous alimentation using slow syringe pump Apnoea and cardiac monitors in use.

Transcutaneous Doppler electronic blood pressure apparatus with stereo head phones used for babies with cardiac disease, respiratory distress syndrome and when have intravenous nutrition.

Oscilloscope for visual recording blood pressure

Cardio vision introducing intravenous umbilical catheter proximal to the right arterial chamber by radiological control for intravenous alimentation

Baby receiving partial pressure of oxygen recorded via an indwelling umbilical arterial catheter

Electrodyne contact less Apnoea monitor

Phototherapy unit

Dextrostix test

Oxygen analyzer

Gurhrie test (toe blood sample)

Temperature recorded per rectum

Radiant heat shield to conserve heat round the infant

Ambu bag with end tracheal tube

Ventilation-humidifier and oxygen analyzer electrode on right arm attached to cardiac monitor baby lying on Apnoea alarm mattress.

Servo heat control, oxygen head box,

Bilirubinometer- newborn bilirubin assessment

Not just a tiny issue- do not overlook your bodily sings; *watch out for these warning signals.*

Anemia

Anemia occurs due to an iron and folic acids deficiency and can impair oxygen supply to the placenta and cause complications like shock, thrombosis or excessive bleeding after birth. Sings of anemia includes poor appetite, breathlessness, extreme lethargy, rapid pulse and palpitations, dizziness and fainting.

Decrease fetal movement—Babies differ in how much they move. 10-12 movements a day from about fourth month is considered normal. The movements decreases close to due date.

However, if there is dramatic change in baby's movements could indicate placental problems, too little or too much amniotic fluid or high blood pressure in the mother.

Contractions—The uterus contracts mildly throughout pregnancy. Most women become aware of contraction in the second half of pregnancy and you may get them after a busy day on your feet. If they become intense, it could mean the start of labour. Do not delay in contacting your caregiver.

Pain and burning when passing urine—This may be accompanied by cloudy urine with a strong odour and could be the sign of bladder infection. Other signs are sudden abdominal pain or tenderness on the right side. Treat it early.

Pale fluid from vagina could be sign of a tear in the amniotic sac, allowing the amniotic fluid to escape. If this occurs close to your due date, it could indicate the beginning of labour. If it occurs earlier, it may be start of premature labor.

Excessive vomiting—Vomiting beyond limits can cause electrolyte imbalances. In serious cases, need admission.

Severe abdominal pain—Seek medical help if you had a fall, an accident, or simply have such pain, which does not improve with rest. It may indicate preeclampsia, severe urinary tract infection; start of labour, a strained round ligament felt more in the side of the abdomen.

Swelling—About 40% of all pregnant women experience swelling in the third trimester Contact doctor if it does not go down with rest or is accompanied by more than normal weight gain, blurred or disturbed vision, severe and sudden headaches, and abdominal pain. It could be sign of preeclampsia which could be life threatening to both of you.

Vaginal bleeding is not normal at all in pregnancy. Beware, overlooking this can end up your baby's life.

Bacterial infections are common in clinical practice, causing infections of various organs. Both gram positive and gram-negative bacteria and cocci produce a variety of infections like bronchitis, tonsillitis, pneumonia, ear infection. Most infections need use of chemotherapeutic agents, to control them, with the help of defense mechanism of the body.

Human care—Animal and birds may get sanctuaries but there is none for humans. Reality unfolds worse situation of deprived set of old aged, neglected women and unprotected children. Industrialization, westernization, urbanization and migration have considerably changed the value system and structure of families. Modernization and globalization has added to negligence. Malnutrition, disable, destitute, illiteracy, child labour, no safe drinking water, urban areas lack drainage facilities, rivers polluted we can go on describing heart breaking situations.

Breastfeeding: Key to Child Health

Several studies on child nutrition undertaken in different locations have established that the mother's milk contains all the ingredients essential for proper growth and good health of children. That is also nature has way to feed our young ones. Global strategy for infant and young child feeding as well as national guidelines strongly call for initiating breastfeeding within an hour of birth, exclusive breastfeeding for the first six months and then complementary feeding along with breastfeeding for two years. The practice establishes a strong emotional bond between the mother and child and also helps in cognitive development of the latter.

Breast milk is a fascinating fluid that supplies babies with more than just nutrition; it actively helps the new born to avoid diseases in a variety of ways. There is scientific evidence that some factors in human milk may induce an infants immune system, antibodies are called immunoglobulin.

During pregnancy, the mother passes antibodies to the foetus through the placenta. These proteins circulate in the infant's blood for weeks to months after birth, fighting the invading organism. Breastfed infants gain extra protection from antibodies other proteins and immune cells in human milk.

Infants who are bottle fed do not posses the strength to cope up with ingested pathogens until they begin making. Besides there are other protections materials the breastfeed milk has.

Lactating mothers face multi-faceted constraints and difficulties in breastfeeding. They require support from various quarters- from family, society, workplace and the government. The problem is more acute, for working women who go out for work, as the environment at work place is hardly supportive. Misleading publicity of baby foods industry allures many women to avoid breastfeeding, depriving their progeny of the benefits of mother's milk.

It is unfortunate that most of the 1.4 million infant deaths apparently due to diarrhea, pneumonia and newborn infections are basically attributed to the absence of breastfeeding. Breastfeeding is a key strategy for child survival as well as reproductive health by supporting baby friendly hospitals envisioned.

All infant formulas are inadequate attempts to duplicate mother's milk, and none is as good as original breast milk. Every mother will be able to breastfeed successfully if she suckles he baby early enough. The best way to promote the milk flow is to encourage the baby to nurse immediately after cutting the cord. To nurse as often as possible during the first few days until the milk supply comes in. If despite diet and enough rest, your milk supply not adequate may be due to emotional strain and mental stress connected with disappointment or distress. It could be due to plugged milk duct, soreness, breast infection, breast engorged, tender. To keep nipples soft, rinse off babies saliva after each feeding, and apply olive oil or vitamin E oil. Toughen tender nipples by exposing them to the air.

Do not stop nursing your baby. Breast milk is the best and most appropriate food. It fully meets the nutritional requirements it protects the baby from infections. It is always clean and sterile. It is available 24 hors in at correct temperature. It creates bonding and is natural food. Breast milk is a fascinating fluid and should be initiated within the first half hour after birth.

Exclusive breast feeding is when a baby receives only breast milk and no other food or drink, not even water. WHO, UNICEF, recommends it to continue upto 6 months. Just after baby is born it is given breast milk because colostrums yellowish secretion is ideal, is like vaccine, it promotes emotional bonding. Mother's milk is available on demand and supply principle. Mothers who work outside home expressing milk can be given. Bottle feeding is an important cause of diarrhea in infants.

Continued breastfeeding after 6 months of age the child is given complementary food along with breastfeeding, gradually family food is given.

Complementary food is pulses, cereals, mashed vegetables, meat, egg, and fish.

Infant Weaning

Mother's milk is the best for the newborn baby. It usually remains the main food for the baby in the first few years of life.

During the first year of life, growth is very rapid. *A newborn* infant weighs about *3 kg*. By *4 months,* the weight generally doubles, i.e. *6 kgs,* and by *one year,* the weight should be about *9 kgs.*

The length of the newborn infant is about 50 cm and by one year, the child reaches a height of 75 cm, that is on and half times its length of birth.

The rate of growth in the infant is much faster than in the older child

For normal growth to take place, the baby must have sufficient nourishment.

Many mothers do not know that for this rapid growth to take place the baby needs sufficient nourishment.

At times, they give the baby foods such as thin gruel or a piece of chapatti to keep the child from being hungry. However, these foods are not enough to meet the needs of the growing child. As a result, the baby becomes weak, it tends to fall ill, and its growth is stunted.

Illiteracy, ignorance and improper food habits lead to malnutrition and infants stunted growth.

Breast milk is the best food for infants because-

It is clean and safe

It contains all the necessary nutrients for the newborn infant

It is easy to digest

It protects the child from disease and infection

However, after 4 months mother's milk alone is not sufficient to meet the needs of the infant

From this age, it is necessary to supplement breast milk by giving the baby milk from other animal sources such as cow's milk, buffalo's milk or goat's milk. Milk substitutes can also be prepared from vegetable source such as ragi, groundnut or soybeans.

These different kinds of milk also contain the nutrients which are present in mother's milk and which are required for normal growth of the baby.

The milk must be well boiled and cooled before giving it to the baby. Use a clean cup and spoon or feeder to feed the baby.

Avoid using a feeding bottle, as it is difficult to keep it clean. A dirty bottle breeds germs and will make to baby sick. If a feeding bottle has to be used, it must be washed well and boiled before use.

From the age of four months, the baby should be given green leafy vegetables made into a soup, or fruit juice. These foods contain vitamins and minerals, which are necessary for keeping the baby healthy.

By the fifth month, boiled mashed potato and mashed banana can be added to the baby's diet. This will ensure that the baby gets a sufficient amount of food.

By the seventh month, the baby can digest semisolid food such as khichadi or Dalia. This can be made as follows- roast the cereal and grind it. Mix it with deal and water and cook well. This food contains proteins, which are important for growth.

Fruits and vegetables should be made soft and easily digestible before giving them to the baby. This can be done b-cooking them well, mashing to remove lumps; straining to remove sin and seeds.

From age of six or seven months, the baby can be given eggs. Eggs are rich in protein, which is necessary for bodybuilding.

The egg should be hard-boiled. A first only give a small portion of the mashed yolk yellow part. Gradually increased the amount by one year, the baby can be given the whole egg.

Other sources of protein are meat. Fish and pulses. These help bodybuilding and growth. The meat should be finely chopped and cooked well without spices, or the bones can be cooked in the soup.

The fish should be steamed or boiled. Be careful to remove the born and mash the fish before giving it to the baby. Different kinds of deal, beans, and groundnuts are cheap and rich sources of protein. Some pulses can be sprouted and eaten raw. Others can be cooked as soft deal or khichadi.

Do not give the baby solid foods in the beginning. Weaning foods should be introduced gradually. First, give the baby liquid foods, then semisolid foods and then solid foods.

At first, give the baby only a spoonful of the new food. Increase the quantity gradually. Do not force the baby to take more than he accepts.

Do not add spices to the food prepared for the baby.

Wash your hands well before preparing food for the baby and use clean utensils.

Serve the baby with food, which has been freshly prepared.

Protect the food from dust and flies by keeping it covered. Otherwise, the baby will get diarrhea and other infections.

Water is essential for the baby. This is especially so in the hot weather and when the baby has diarrhea or fever. Otherwise, the baby can become dehydrated. The water given to the baby must be clean and safe to drink. Therefore, boil the water and keep it in a clean covered container. Give it to the baby several times during the day.

If weaning foods are gradually introduced, by one year the child can be given the food, which is normally taken by the rest of the family. However, the child's portion should not contain hot spices.

At one year, the child is ready to take the normal diet of the family. A variety of foods must be given every day.

Community Nursing

COMMUNITY NURSING—CARE PLAN - I

Date	Assessment	Needs/problems	Objective	Plan of action	Implementation	Rational	Evaluation
	Poor environmental sanitation due to lack of Knowledge about the environmental sanitation. Family getting affected by uncovered gutters and open drainage giving smell and breeding mosquitoes and potential hazards like communicable diseases related to the presence of insects and rodents Family members are practicing open air defecations	Awareness about impotence of environmental sanitation There is an open drainage in front of the house so there is chance of health hazards like cholera, diarrhea, and malaria. Since there are mosquitoes, flies, rats the chance of communicable diseases open air defecation due to inappropriate toilet facility	To explain about the importance of environmental sanitation To prevent diseases like malaria and communicable disease to explain disadvantages of open air defecation	*To advice the family about avoiding collection of garbage around the house *To advice the family to sweep the house daily *To advice the family members regarding burning of waste products *To advise the family the importance of growing plantation *To explain the family members about the importance of lighting and ventilation not to dump any household garbage into gutter and clean the gutter line to avoid blockage and inform municipality to cover to gutters Advise them to use mosquito nets and coils and observe breeding place and sprinkle DDT. To advise the family to use public toilets that are available in the community to avoid defecation near any water source to wash hands properly after defecation	*Advice the family members about avoiding collection of garbage around the house *Advised the family to sweep the house *Advised family to burn the waste products *Explained family the importance of growing plantation *Explained family the importance of ventilation Observe the drainage for smell, stagnant water. Advise them to disinfect the drainage and avoid water to stagnate Advised family to use public toilet, not to defecate near water source and wash hands after defecation	*To reduce disease condition due to unclean environment * To keep the house clean * Aids to protect the environment from contamination of micro-organism '*Helps for proper ventilation to prevent infection. Prevent diseases like malaria, filarial. Potential health hazards will be prevented to give knowledge regarding ill effects of open air defecation	The family members understood about environmental sanitation The family members learned the disadvantage of open air defecation

COMMUNITY NURSING—CARE PLAN - II

Date	Assessment	Needs/problems	Objective	Plan of action	Implementation	Rational	Evaluation
	Family members are not maintaining proper personal hygiene	Poor personal hygiene due to lack of knowledge	To explain the family members about importance of personal hygiene	*To advice the family to take bath every day. *To advice the family members to wear clean clothes and comb the hair and wash hair twice a week. *To advice family to wash and change clothes everyday. Wash hands before and after the meal and keep nails shortcut	*Advised the family to take bath *Advised to wear clean cloths and comb hair *Advised to wash hands and wash clothes everyday	*To reduce skin infection caused by unhygienic condition like scabies to prevent infection while eating food to avoid contamination	The family understood the importance of personal hygiene and were taught to practice it

COMMUNITY NURSING—CARE PLAN - III

Date	Assessment	Needs/problems	Objective	Plan of action	Implementation	Rational	Evaluation
	*Patient has fever 100 F *Patient is having hypertension BP 150/100 mm of Hg*	Alteration in body temperature related to fever*. Alteration of blood flow due to hypertension	*Assess fever and provide tepid sponge *To provide blankets provide adequate fluids and water *To provide antipyretics to provide adequate rest, and restricted food. To check vital signs 3a. to maintain BP	*Patient has feverprovided tepid sponge provided blankets taught to avoid oily foods *Provided adequate liquids provided antipyretics Vital signs are checked that is temperature 100, pulse 82 and respirations 20. minutes, * Assess condition of patient, to have restricted salt free diet, check the pressure regularly	To reduce fever and provide comfort to patient *Assessed the condition, oil and salt restricted diet, checked BP	*To know the condition of patient to reduce fever to prevent chills *To prevent dehydration and provide hydration *To reduce fever to know the condition and provide comfort, to know the variation in body temperature to know the patients condition and the variation of BP	Patient feels better and the fever is reducing*the pressure came to 140/90 mm of Hg by following doctors advice and treatment

COMMUNITY NURSING—CARE PLAN - IV

Date	Assessment	Needs/problems	Objective	Plan of action	Implementation	Rational	Evaluation
	Family members are not knowing about the maintainer of food hygiene vessel containing food items are kept open	Lack the knowledge regarding food hygiene	To educate family about food hygiene	To advice family to wash the grains and vegetables before cooking*to advice the family to cover the food items advice them to avoid growing of nails	Advised them to wash grains and vegetables before cooking *Advised the family to cover the food items advised family to avoid growing nails	To maintain hygiene of food and vegetables *To prevent food poisoning to prevent infection caused by such unhygienic condition	The family members understood the impotence of food hygiene and able to practice it

COMMUNITY NURSING—CARE PLAN - V

Date	Assessment	Needs/problems	Objective	Plan of action	Implementation	Rational	Evaluation
	Potential problem of water born disease/ family members say they get contaminated water to drink	Using raw, unclean and un-boiled water	Explain family to practice household methods of water purification	Advise to boil water, cool it, strain it in clean vessel, cover it and wash hands before talking water	Advised to boil and cool water and drink advised to strain and store in clean vessels cover the water with a lead advised that wash hands before talking water	To kill the micro-organism which are present in raw un-boiled water By straining help to remove dust particles. To prevent recontamina-tion of water	The family understood about the household practical easy way of water purification to avoid water born disease.

COMMUNITY NURSING—CARE PLAN - VI

Date	Assessment	Needs/problems	Objective	Plan of action	Implementation	Rational	Evaluation
	Presence of anemia in the family members *potential problem of infection due to unhealthy cooking practices and malnourishment	Alteration in blood hemoglobin level due to presence of anemia *Potential problem of malnourishment due to unhygienic and unhealthy cooking practices	To prevent anemia and anemia related problems *To improve nutritional pattern and to improve cooking practices	Advised to include green leafy vegetables like drumstick leaves spinach in diet encouraged them to eat beetroot, carrot, brinjal etc encouraged them to consume and add jiggery advised family to drink adequate liquids and water *Increase diet rich in protein, vitamins and add fruits and green leafy vegetables to daily meal	Advised family to include green leafy vegetables like drumstick, spinach, jiggery, carrot, brinjal, etc. Advised to take medication of folic acid and iron, calcium from PHC *Eat pulses, sprouts, fruits in daily meal	To improve blood hemoglobin level. * To get proper treatment	The family members are advised to have good nutritive food to prevent anemia. *Family to have balance healthy diet that is cheep and within there limit which also contains nutrition to prevent malnourishment

OBJECTIVE DATA OF NURSING CARE PLAN

A. Mother Complains of Frequent Loose Stools Since Morning

Mother complains that the child is usually warm today
Mother complains that child has running nose
That child gains weight poorly
That appearance of the child looks thin and weak for the age

B. Nursing Diagnosis

Alteration in bowel pattern/diarrhea related to GI infection
Alteration in body temperature/pyrexia related to infection
Alteration in breathing pattern related to respiratory infection
Alteration in body mass/under weight due to faulty feeding practices/worm infestation/delayed milestone

C. Objective

Restore hydration status
Prevent further episodes of diarrhea
Attain normal body temperature
Prevent further episodes of fever
Achieve normal breathing patterns
Prevent further episodes of ARI
Treat for worm infestation/correct feeding practices

D. Interventions

Assess the level of dehydration and assess TPR
Assess the stool color and consistency, frequency, odor
Enquire on the food intake previous 24 hours
Administer ORS if mild dehydration is present
Advocate home available fluids like rich water
Advice feed
Advice soft solid carbohydrate based diet
Avoid wheat and protein diets, roughage diet
Administer antibiotics
Advice cleanliness, disposal of stools, hygiene of napkins, discourage bottle feeds
Demonstrate specific diet preparation rice fried channa conjee, arraroot canjee
Assess TPR every 2 hours as required
Administer anti pyretic and antibiotic if required
Assess the bowel pattern
Encourage mother to administer plenty of fluids at frequent intervals
Continue breastfeeding

Advice soft solid, non greasy and non-oily diet
Encourage the mother to dress the child with loose cotton
Advice mother to keep the room, house ventilated
Advocate tepid sponge, ice pack if required
Health education
Not to take child in crowded place, not to allow people with infection to handle the child

E. Rationale Fever

Assessment helps to manage the case appropriately
Reduces body temperature
Sometimes GI infections may accompany with signs of fever
Helps in maintaining hydration, as water is lost in elevated temperature
Raise of temperature is often a prodromal sign for ARI/diarrhea
Rational for diarrhea
Corrects dehydration
Organisms
Helps in Apt management and in preventing further episodes of diarrhea

F. Evaluation/Outcomes for Fever/Diarrhea

The child is hydrated adequately
Mother verbalizes the importance of cleanliness, cause, spread and prevention
Mother demonstrate the preparation of conjee
The child is able to breathe freely following the steam inhalation
Child exhibits 4 to 5 episodes on infection in a year
Child passed worms in the stool
Mother promises to monitor the weight of child

A Model of Nursing Process Plan

Nursing process is a logical framework/sequence on which nursing care is based, a systematic problem solving approach. As orderly way of identifying the patient's problems, akin plans to solve them. Each step flows on to the next step. It is outcome oriented.

Assessment—Irritating cough makes me breathless

Diagnosis—Ineffective airway clearance and discomfort

Goal—The patient maintains a patient airway removal of secretions by effective cough which can reduce discomfort

Intervention—Assess cough pattern, consistency and amount of secretions, breath sounds to remove secretion
Give patient 8 to 10 glasses of warm fluids daily
Two hourly encourage diaphragmatic breathing and coughing exercise

Administer humidifier oxygen
Tree time a steam inhalation
Avoid smock dust and clod atmosphere
Administer prescribed antibiotics, e.g. Cap. Mox 500 mg tds

Rational—Systemic hydration moisten airway
These help improve ventilation; keeps airway and secretions wet/loose and easier to cough out
To prevent possible respiratory infections

Implementation—Encouraged using diaphragmatic breathing and coughing exercise
Humidified oxygen administered
Instructed to avoid bronchial irritate like cigarette, smock, dust, cold atmosphere
Cap. Mox 500 mg tds administered

Assessment—I feel so tired to get up and bathe. I become breathless if I move around

Diagnosis—Activity intolerance and constant fatigue

Goal—Reduced fatigue and dyspnea on exertion

Intervention—Encourage patient the importance of regular daily exercise –plan for it
First sitting on bed, then dandling feet, standing, walking around bed and so on
Advice rest period
Administer oxygen as needed

Rational—With daily exercise the weak and spastic muscles including the respiratory muscles gain strength and work of breathing reduces
Prevents unnecessary exertion on the patient which promotes well-being by reducing fatigue and dyspnea on exertion

Evaluation—Looks less tired
Performs activities of daily living with less assistance
Less dyspnea, less complaint of fatigue.

Nurse and Health Education Model

HEALTH TALK ON CARE OF THE AGED

Subject—Care of geriatric group

Group—Above 60 years of age

Date:

Place:

Time:

Aim—To provide knowledge about care of geriatric

Specific Objectives

1. To define concept of geriatrics nursing
2. To gain knowledge regarding the various body changes
3. To follow-up with different health examination
4. To maintain personal hygiene
5. To follow appropriate diet
6. To realize the importance of rest, sleep and exercise
7. To make adjustment with family members and society
8. Explain the various factors that help for a successful aging process
9. To deal with the physiology of aging and the diagnosis and treatment of diseases affecting aging
10. Prevention and health teaching

Self and topic introduction—Here I introduce myself and would like to explain the different ways of talking care of the aged. How can we make the lives of the aged safe for the rest of their life? The modern rush has taken toll of our day today life. Our parents who give up their entire life time to raise us, to make us successful need to be taken care in their old age. That will give them inner contentment and satisfaction. Money does not compensate for love. It is our duty to look after them when they need us the most. Life is a precious gift. So do not abandon them when they need your company the most. Value your elders; our elders deserve our love and protection. With these sentiments let us understand old age why and how it happens and how it can be prevented by care and safety.

Subject Objectives	Subjective Matter	Method of Teaching	AV Aids	Evaluation
To explain the term of healthy aging	Growing old is an inevitable process in everyone's life. Aging is a normal process of human development. Aging is not disease, nor it causes diseases, but the old people are susceptible to certain disease, disorders and accidents. Care of the aged deals with the assessment of needs, psychological and biological support to be given to the elders.	Group discussion and oral questions on aging	Flash cards and sharing of personal experiences	Group understood and showed interest about the aging by active sharing
Knowledge regarding various bodily changes	The aging process is a complex. How a person ages, it depends on his life experiences, available support system, and previous coping skills. Many continue to live healthy and happy life in there home.	What is old age? What, when, how it happens?	Flash card showing the bodily changes	People understood the bodily changes that occur
Some myths about aging——— ———	*Old age begins at 65 years of age. *Most older adults live in nursing home *Most older people are senile and demented *Most older people feel miserable and depressed *Older people cannot work as effectively as younger people *Older people experience a decline in intellectual ability and cannot learn new skills *Most older people are sick and need help for daily activities *Older people are set in their ways and cannot change *Older people do not care about their looks and appearance *Majority of older are isolate and are lonely	Can you share the myths you or others in society hold about aging?———	flash cards showing the myths———	Group understood the myths and common misconception of aging———
To safeguard and increase health to the extent possible thus provide comfort	*Certain physical changes* occur in everyone, as age advances. All the systems of the body are affected directly or indirectly. Biological Body changes as person grows in age- this leads to diseases such as diabetes mellitus, rheumatic heart diseases and arthritis. Body cells, structures and functions wear out, and degenerative changes take place in body.	Can you in short explain about the body changes that occur in aged people?	Flash card showing bodily changes	The group followed the importance of normal biological changes
Explain skin, graying, muscle shrink, sleep, slow reflexes, changes	*Skin-* skin becomes less elastic. Fatty tissue layer is lost which makes the skin thin and sagging. This also makes the person more sensitive to cold. Folds, lines and wrinkles appear. There is decrease secretion from oil and sweat glands leading to dry skin. Skin is fragile and easily damaged. Skin breakdown and pressure sores develop. Nails become thick and tough. Feet usually have poor circulation. *Graying/whitening of hair* occurs; they loose a lot of hair. Hair gets thin and hair tends to be more dry due to decreased production of scalp oils. *Muscles shrink* and decrease in strength. One mass decreases, calcium is lost from the bone, causing brittleness and easy break ability. Joints become stiff and painful. Hip and knee become slightly bent decrease in mobility. Changes in *sleep* pattern occur. Loss of energy and decreased blood flow cause fatigue. *Reduction in nerve cells*, leads to nerve conduction slower, reflexes are slower causing slow response	How do we maintain healthy skin	Flash cards explaining Care of skin	Group understood the reason of skin and graying changes

Contd...

Contd...

Objectives	Content	Question	AV Aids	Evaluation
	to stimuli. There is decrease blood flow to the brain causing dizziness and increased risk for fall. There is a progressive loss of brain cells, thus forgetfulness increases, confusion, fatigue occur.			
To remove the fear of aging	*The sense* of touch, smell, tast, sight affected. The ability to feel heat and cold reduced, making the elderly susceptible to injury. Smell and tast decreased causing decrease appetite.			Peoples fear was removed and there was acceptance of normal changes of aging
Impaired of vision leading to difficulty in reading	*Vision*-eyelids become thinner and wrinkled. Tear secretion lessens. This can cause irritation by dust or air pollution. The pupils become smaller endless responsive to light, which causes decreased vision at	What is the importance of vision	Flash card showing impaired vision	
Impaired hearing leading to lose of hearing	Night or in dark room. muscular degeneration and partial lost of sight that is central blind spot which makes a person difficult to read and recognize faces			
Importance of medical check ups	*Hearing-* there is atrophy of ear drums. The capacity for hearing high pitched sound is lost. As these progresses, severe hearing loss occurs. Secretion of the wax decreases and it becomes harder and thicker with age. *Circulatory system* -efficiency of the heart muscle decreases and the force of contraction of the heart reduces. Elasticity of blood vessels reduces. A weakened heart has to work harder in order to pump blood through the narrowed arteries. *Respiratory* muscles weaken so dyspoea may occur with activity *Digestion-* there is less production of saliva causing difficulty in swallowing, decrease secretion of digestive juices, loss of teeth cause chewing difficulty. Decrease peristalsis causing delayed emptying of the stomach, constipation occurs. *Urine-*lack of adequate fluid intake and weakening bladder muscle can lead to incontinence of urine. *Good Personal and environmental hygiene-*avoid bed body odour, sores, rashes, soiled clothing	Importance of hearing What is importance of personal hygiene?	hearing	People understood the importance of early Diagnosis and importance of medical check ups People understood how to maintain personal hygiene and
Prevention of illness with important tips for Regular physical examination	To maintain *regular medial check ups*, BP, ECG, and blood test for early diagnosis of diabetes, cancer, HBP, infections, short or long sightedness, glaucoma, cataract if neglected may lead to visual blindness.	Healthy balance and specific diet in elderly	different various diet to be included in diet	Importance of vision, hearing diet, rest and sleep, and exercise and family and society adjustment People understood the disease condition
Alzheimer's disease increases greatly with increasing age	*Alzheimer's disease* is a disease of the brain. Alzheimer's disease is a form of dementia. It involves progressive decline in two or more areas of cognition, usually memory, language, calculation, judgment, perception, he forgets to eat, he forgets he has to go to toilet. If he goes to, he can not remember his home address, etc.	What are Alzheimer's diseases?	Flash cards	
Purpose of treatment/medications,	The cause not found, although several risk factors are found. Person does well in familiar surrounding and lack ability to adapt new challenges, can follow well-established routines.			

Contd...

Contd...

what to observe and report to the physician	Second stage impaired word finding speech becomes empty words used in wrong context. Repeat words and phrases, difficulty in using everyday object such as toothbrush, comb, razor and utensils. It creates safely problems. He may leave burner on in the kitchen to forget to extinguish a cigarette. Talking everything in the mouth to suck, chew or taste, sees bugs crawling on bed or throughout the house wandering at night in common.			
Regular examination of vision, hearing, teeth, cancer sites	*Prevention*-There is no cure to enhance memory as brain continues to atrophy. Speak only single word or short phrases; speak slowly with low pitch tone of voice. Reach him by touching, holding hand, and putting an arm around waist. Intervention to enhance memory, reorient by placing a calendar and clock.		Flash cards	
	Risk for injury- in home electrical devices, toxic substances, loose rugs, hot water tap, unlocked door and dangerous object should be kept out of reach. Cooking should be supervised, driving skill should be evaluated a regular intervals. Remove furniture with sharp corners.		Flash cards	People understood the importance of medical check up and early diagnosis and treatment
Importance of diet and nutrition	Boost his confidence and self respect, constant encouragement. Assist family in understanding symptoms related to memory loss, nature of illness, symptoms and stages of diseases, progression and behaviour manifestation.			
Good health habits exercise, practice of yoga	*Diet- adequate nutrition* daily die should contain necessary calories so as to get needed energy, to eat roughage, vegetables and fruits to stimulate peristalsis and relive constipation.	Why do elderly have digestive problems and what is the importance of diet	Flash cards showing balance diet	People understood the importance of preventive tips People understood diet importance
Safety measures- prevention of falls and accidents	*Regular exercise*, rest and sleep to maintain good health' daily walking, jogging as the health permits. Take part in social activates Adjust to the bodily changes and acceptance and adaptation to the Growing age.	Importance of exercise What is the important point of prevention?	Flash cards	Understood value of exercise and rest People understood the tips of prevention
Prevention of elder abuse	*Prevention* of accident- the floor should not be slippery. Use walker to assists in walking, do not takes bath in river or ponds. Have adequate lighting over the staircase. Use dim light burning in bedrooms and bathrooms all through night. Place furniture in a convenient place. Get the cleaning of the auditory canal for wax. Use well fitted shoes, use side rails and use low height cots to get in and out of cot easily. Use spectacles; check the temperatures of the water for bath. Take precautions while application of hot water bottles. Administer the prescribed medications by a member of the house, who will be responsible to prevent wrong administration. Teach the traffic rules to prevent road accidents while walking on the busy roads. Daily observation of the skin for its color, integrity. Check the gas leak.	How will you prevent aging problems	All the charts and flash cards once again exhibited	Revision of important points and feed back was good.

Contd...

Contd...

	Abuse of elderly persons can occur in there own homes, hospitals or homes for the aged. The abuses may be a family member or a care giver. There are different forms of abuse. Sometimes intentional harm may be done to the elderly. *Types of abuse-* physical abuse refers to any use of force resulting in bodily injury, physical pain or physical impairment. This may involve such acts of violence as striking, pushing, shaking, slapping, kicking, pinching and burning. It also mean use of medication, restrains, force feeding etc.Psychological or emotional abuse is the infliction of pain or distress through verbal or nonverbal acts. It includes verbal assaults, insults, threats, intimidation, humiliation and harassment.	People understood the types of elder abuse and its prevention
Financial resources	Abandonment or desertion of elderly, financial or material exploitation includes the illegal or improper use of an elders funds, property or assets without his permission, forging a signature, stealing possession, deceiving into signing documents and improper use of power of attorney or guardianship. Prevent physical, psychological, abuse, neglect, and violation of rights of elders. Focus on secure and safe comfortable environment. Help to prevent self neglect- inability to maintain activities of daily living such as personal care, shopping, mental preparation, obtain adequate food, poor hygienic practices etc. Inability to manage personal finances indicated by failure to pay bills, boarding or giving away money improperly. Failure to keep important business or medical appointments. In emergency get in touch with help line, day care center, home for the aged, police, layer, hospital, etc. keep all the important contact number. Arrange for part time job, pension, and contact funding agencies/social workers.HHHHow we	People understood self help and where to go in emergency

---

Sub: Worm Infestation - 2

Aim: To make the people understand about worm infestation and its prevention.

Date:

Time:

Place:

Self introduction-

Specific Objectives

1. To make the people to understand about what is meant by worm infestation
2. To make the people understand the causes of worm infestation
3. To make people understand the types of worm infestation
4. To make people understand the sign and symptoms of worm infestation
5. To make people understand the life cycle of worm infestation

6. To make people understand common ways of finding and investigation
7. To make people understand the treatment and complication of worm infestation
8. To make people aware of preventive method of worm infestation
9. Summery of man points with evaluation

Specific objectives	Subjective Matter	Method of Teaching	AV Aids	Evaluation
To make the group to understand about what is meant by worm infestation	The term "amoebiasis" has been defined by WHO as the condition of harboring the protozoan parasite entamoeba histolytica with or without clinical manifestations. The symptomatic disease occurs in less than 10% of infected individuals. The symptomatic group has been further subdivided into intestinal and extraintestinal amoebiasis only a small percentage of those having intestinal infection will develop invasive amoebiasis. The problem of helminthes infestation is common in all tropical countries due to prevalent methods defecation and disposal of excreta. Intestinal infestation adds to the burden of the rapidly growing children whose health status is already compromised by illness, malnutrition and unsanitary living conditions.	Lecture cum discussion Explanation and input on the topic in detailed	Awareness song A small skit play	After explanation and short discussions the group understood the meaning of worm infestation
To make the group understand the types of worm infestation	There are round worms, thread worms, Hook worms, Tape worms, pin worms, etc. Round worms otherwise called as 'ascariasis' it is more seen common in the children between the age of one to five year, in lower social economic status. Thread worms other wise called as pin worm or seat worms. It is commonly found in children. It is transmitted through soil, finger and linen. Hook worm or ancylostamiasis-they may occur as single or mixed infections in the same person found in all ages from 15 to 25 years	Questions and answers and discussion	Charts and flash cards Flash card	The group was able to tell the different types of worm infestation The group understood the causes of worm infestation
To educate the group causes of worm infestation	More common in children of 1 to 5 years and found also in low socio economic group *Thread worms* found in children, in unsanitary living conditions, e.g. school, hostels, institutions and families	One more awareness song	Flash card	The group understood the signs and symptoms that are caused by this problem. Of worm infestations.
To make them aware of the signs and symptoms of the worm infestation	Sign and symptoms of *round worms* is fever and eosinophilia due to larva Ascaris pneumonia due to larva n the lungs Abdominal pain Intestinal obstruction *General symptoms* like diarrhea and high fever, pica, abdominal distension, sleeplessness, irritability and loss of weight Ascaris encephalopathy may occur with other infection *Thread worms* sign and symptoms is asymptomatic children may not have any complains, lack of appetite, loss of weight, grinding of teeth and abdominal pain, purities at the anal region, nocturnal enuresis may occur.	Continued the topic with lecture	Flash card Flash cards	The group was made to understand through flash cards and explanation the life cycle of worm infestation

Contd...

Contd...

To educate people about the life cycle of roundworms	Sags and symptoms of *hook worm* is epigastric pain, fatigue and weakness, pica may be present, eosinophilia may be found *Life cycle of roundworms*-they live in the upper part of small intestine. It resembles on ordinary earth worm. It measures up to 20 cm to 45 cm in length. The female lays eggs in large number which are passed in the Faeces. They contaminate the soil or vegetables. Given optimal conditions, the eggs take about 10 days to become embryonated. When the infective eggs are ingested, they reach the intestine where they hatch into larvae. The larvae penetrate the intestine and migrate to liver and lungs and then travel up the human host. They reach the small intestine where they become sexually mature in about 6 to 10 weeks.	Repeated the same ideas in different terms	Flash cards of round worm	
To educate people about the lie cycle of hookworms.	There are two types of hook worms. They are found attached to the mucosa of the small intestine, particularly of the jejunum. Each worm measures about 8 to 10 mm in length. Adult are believed to survive for on an average of one to four years respectively. The worms are passed in the Faeces by infested persons.	Continued explanation	Flash card of hookworm	
Explained the group the importance and types of simple investigation done	The female parasite lays eggs which are passed in the Faeces. A single female may lay 10,000 to 20,000 eggs per day. The egg hatch into larvae outside the human body in the soil where they grow and develop into infective larvae. When a person walks bare foot on the contaminated soil the infective larvae penetrate the skin and enter the human host. They pass into the lymph and blood stream and reach the lungs; they travel up to trachea and the pharynx from where they are swallowed. The larvae finally reach the small intestine where they develop into sexually mature worms and start laying eggs in about 6 weeks.	Advised and practical demonstration of showing medicines available	Flash cards	Group understood the advice and the importance of investigation and diagnosis is done to trace the presence of worms to give appropriate treatment People understood the complication of such infestation could be grave and life-threatening
The common treatment	Stool examination for ova or worms and microscopic examination of stool Piprazin citrate or tablet mebendazole/mebex bd, tablet albendazone od a signal dose of 2.5 mg.kg	Explained severity if not acted the complication that may occur	Flash card	
Explained the group the complication caused by it	It is advisable to treat the entire family at a time Is given in health centers free of cost Iron deficiency anemia, oedema, heart failure, general fatigue, cardiac failure, appendicitis, lymphadenitis		Flash cards	
People were made to understand the prevention part	Use boil water for drinking Develop hygienic habits of eating and washing hands with soap before and after eating and defecation To prevent oral infections Proper disposal of excreta is essential Control of flies Wash vegetables and eatables well in running or plenty of water Keep the children's nail short	Taught different ways of prevention and control	Flash cards	People understood the preventive advise

Contd...

Contd...

	Use of long pajamas to prevent auto infestation of pin worms Antipruritic cream can be used to prevent itching Detection early treatment of all infected persons can reduce soil contamination			
Prevention and control	Use of sanitary latrines helps to control spread so promote it Efficient sewage disposal Habit of using foot wear which prevents contact with contaminated soil in open field Wearing shoos for personal prophylaxis Health education directed towards raising the standards of personal and domestic hygiene. Follow all sanitary measures as ascariasis is disappearing spontaneously in certain areas as a result of improved sanitation	All the points all over again summarized in short and got the feedback	All the flash cards number wise displayed to see the different type of worms that exist	People were enthusiastic and found it effect way of prevention and promised to improve there hygienic habits
Concluded the points in nut shell all over again	Mass treatment- periodic deworming at intervals of two to three months may be undertaken in a place where protein energy malnutrition is highly prevalent *Summary-* it has been estimated that about 45 million in India are infested with hookworm. The diseases are highly endemic. Round worms too are wide spread in India and 30 to 50 5 population are known to be infested. The parasite robs the human host of his nutrition especially in children. So let us take step to prevent control the ill effect of worm infestation. Each of us is responsible for our own health and so let us today count as number day one to make effort in practicing sanitary habits and get rid of this health problem and make our family free from worm infestation to enjoy health and well being. *Bibliography—*	Closed the health education with a common awareness song and continued one to one communication		

CHAPTER 17

Indigenous/Alternative System

Yoga transforms and liberates human being so that they can reach this unbounded state. To join mind and body for a happy, and healthy living.

Nurses too need to be aware or realize the therapeutic as well as the practical advantageous of yoga. Yoga practices are not for bodybuilding or muscle toning. It is more for mental and spiritual happiness, which in turn results in sound physical health and contentment.

It is compared to petal led rose, non-violence, body care, physical posture, breath control, mind control, meditation, concentration, and finally illumination and enlightenment. Physical well-being is a prime cause of yogic practice. The regular practice of its basic brings an amazing rejuvenation. It creates a positive frame of mind that is mental tranquility and internal cleanliness, there by rejuvenating our vital organs.

This in turn de-stresses the body and refreshes the mind, and there by removing the imbalance. The lifestyle and the rat race of our daily life induce unwanted stress at every stage. Sedentary lifestyle and over indulgence are a curse of modern times. The practice of yoga helps in negating these adverse effects and restoring sound health. Keep yourself mentally occupied and physically active and practice detachment from petty concerns and undue mental tensions, and enjoy all the good things of life.

A benefit of yoga brings down stress and enhances power of relaxation. In addition, it boosts physical strength, stamina and flexibility. Moreover, it bestows greater power of concentration and self control. Inculcates impulse control, intensifies tolerance to pain and enhancing mental clarity. Boosts functioning of the immune system, enhances posture and muscle tone, improves blood circulation which results in healthy, glowing skin; cleanses and improves over all organ functioning. Bestows peace of mind and a more positive outlook in life infuses a sense of balance and internal harmony. Yoga gives strengths of mind, body and soul. It tones up our body; it is highly therapeutic, the ailments proven to be relieved, reversed and even healed. Such as acidity, high blood pressure, kidney problems, so to enjoy better health, practice yoga everyday.

For example, your back has packed upto the pressures of busy life? All you need are a few minutes of yoga. The spine is the central axis of the body. It combines with the joints and muscles to make a supportive frame for the trunk to maintain an upright posture. It is made up of 33 small bones called vertebra with discs that acts as shock absorbers in between. Wear and tear of the backs supportive structures cause back pain, strain and injury. Why the back aches? Our lifestyles often give rise to poor posture, rounded shoulder and a hollow back. If the nature curves of the spine are overly arched or flattened for long periods of time, the spine gets stiff and weak. Where as say sitting all day in the office at the desk, traveling long distances on work and sedentary living long hours on sofa, etc. factors responsible for backache. Maintain good posture, sit and stand tall and keep your spine erect, but relaxed. Avoid sitting for long periods. Take frequent breaks to stretch and relax muscles. Sit on a chair that supports your lower back, the height of the seat should wear comfortable foot wear, exercise and maintain healthy weight.

The spinal cord comes through the spine and is connected by the waist. The spinal cord works on the direction given by the brain. Two spines are connected by a soft flexible disk, which absorbs the shocks coming to the spinal cord. Each spine is connected to another by spinal and cranial and meniges is made of vertebral columns, through which the spinal cord and other spinal nerves go through the legs. The body starts losing its vigor with advancing age. The bones start losing its strength.

Backache—The spinal cord is an important part of the human body. It does the work of providing support to the body and in important activities like turning the neck and bending is done with its help. Our lifestyles often give rise to poor posture, rounded shoulders, and a hollow back. If the natural curves of the spine are overly arched or flattered for long periods, the spine gets stiff and weak. Sitting all day in the office at the desk, traveling long distances on work, going back home and spending evenings sprawled on the sofa, sedentary.

Living is all factors responsible for backache. Maintain good posture, sit and stand tall and keep your spine erect, but relaxed. Avoid sitting for long periods, take frequent breaks to move and stretch your muscles. Sit on a chair that supports your lower back. The height of the seat should allow your feet to rest flat on the floor. Wear comfortable footwear with good arch supports, high heels cause backache excessively. Exercise regularly, maintain a healthy weight, and perform flexibility, yogaasanas work on flexing and extending different parts of the spine.

Meditation—Consciously directing your attention inward to a chosen focus includes stress reduction, strengthening of the immune system, more orderly thinking, improvement in powers of concentration and a slowing of the aging process. Engaging in self-examination and self-discipline is important in order to clear away any of the psychological conflicts that might pose a problem, so that they can live more effectively. Our relationship with God-why are we here and for what purpose? Endeavors to maintain a state of mental calmness and self-awareness.

Cultivates cheerfulness and optimism, maintain your emotional balance. Adhere to wholesome routines of activity and rest. Maintain a healthy lifestyle. Let all your thoughts, feelings and actions be wholesome and constructive. You will then be empowered to live enjoyably, effectively and successfully. A generous heart, kind speech and a life of service and compassion are the things, which renew humanity. The cure for all the illness of life is stored in the inner depth of life. Silence is the source of all language as words follow thoughts that come from mind. Silence is most eloquent language. It can be mighty weapon so nature has provided a clue to this by giving us two ears and one mouth.

Laugh away to good health—Laughter yoga to beat the blues and feel alive and zestful. Laughter is a gift that has been given to make us feel better. Believe in enjoying each moment to the fullest.

AYUSHYA is a center for healing and integration. *AYUSHYA* aims at wholeness and integration within persons, community and society through its various programs.

Integrated program focused on health as the right and responsibility of each person within the vision of promoting a new health culture. Emphasis is also on providing low cost health care utilizing the natural resources and promoting healthy life styles. Yoga, meditation, retreats, stress management, counselling, psychotherapy, integration program, non-drug therapies, herbal medicines and nutrition are included as part of an integrated approach to promote health and wholeness in persons.

The courses deal with the approaches in community health, dimensions of integrated approach to health. Analysis of the health situation in India, ecology, nutrition therapeutic massages etc.

Home medicines for acne—Apply lemon juice regularly to reduce pimples and acne. Rub with raw garlic several times a day. Garlic is known at cure the toughest of acne problems. The external use of garlic helps to clear the skin of spots, pimples and boils. Eat three seeds of raw garlic daily for one month. This purifies the blood stream and ensures basic cleaning of blood and keeps acne away.

Grated cucumber applied over the face, eyes, neck 15-20 minutes best tonic for complexions. Its regular use prevents pimples and black heads.

The term *pranic healing* originates from the Sanskrit word prana which refers to the vital energy of life force which keeps the body alive and healthy. It is a process of transforming the vital energy or life force from the healer to the patient. It requires no physical contact since the healer works on the bioplasmic body rather than on the physical body. Pranic healing can bring down abnormally high temperature due to fever in just a few hours, in most cases. It relives gas pain, toothache, headache, mild asthma, migraine, ulcer, wounds, muscle and back pain almost immediately.

Meditation is the greatest adventure the human mind can undertake. The ancient mystics have shown in various methods of meditation to move into our own original blissful state. The essential core the spirit of meditation is to learn how to witness our nature and be conscious of our day-to-day and learning techniques for higher concentrations, increase memory power which ultimately leads them to meditation.

The body mind connection science cannot explain. Medical science is now beginning to understand the ways in which the mind influences the body. The placebo effect demonstrates that people can at times cause a relief in medical symptoms or suffering by believing the cure to be effective, whether they are actually or not the body ability to heal itself is far more alarming than anything modern medicine could create. Near death experience reported mystical experience such as going into a tunnel and emerging in light. What causes near death experience. Psychic powers and extrasensory perception difficult to prove.

The real hindrance to *happiness* is that we have forgotten how to live content with what we have. Contentment is like a precious pearl. Whoever procures it at the expense of 10,000 desires makes a wise and happy purchase? The suffering and misery in life is direct cause is desire craving. Desires is unquenchable once desire is born, it knows not how to die. Desire, when transformed into aspiration, helps life soars into the highest liberation and supreme salvation can be reached. All people desire what they believe will make them happy. If person is fully content with self, he is happy that is called bliss.

Garlic can shoot down cancer, skin diseases, cholesterol and many more evils in one shot— garlic contains more than 100 biologically useful chemicals with health benefits. Historically it has been used around the world to treat conditions—hypertension, infections, and snake bites. It reduces bad cholesterol in the body. It improves blood circulation and helps prevent blood clots forming and regulates blood sugar, it is a natural antibiotic and has antifungal and antibacterial properties. Mashing 2-3 small cloves eating raw or boiled and take before going to bed, it can be taken with glass of milk or with water. Talking care of our health is a paramount importance.

Sleep minimize noise with earplugs and minimize light with window blinds, heavy curtains, or an eye mask. Do not turn on bright lights if you need to get up at night. Use a small night-light instead.

Avoid large meals within two hours of bed-time. If you are hungry, a glass of milk helps you to go to bed.

Regular exercise mat promote deeper sleep. Go to bed at regular time and avoid napping late in the afternoon. Stop working at any task an hour before bedtime to clam mental activity. At bedtime, keep your mind off worries or things that upset you and avoid discussing emotional issues in bed.

The pressures of life are so great that they begin to affect us physically and mentally. When we are angry or upset, the body releases hormones, deal with the problem, face the situation and not to keep the feelings bottled up. We need to find some acceptable way to overcome stress. Meditation brings about physical relaxation and mental well-being. Moreover, establish contact with your inner energy.

Avoid coffee, cola, tea, chocolate, alcohol. Learn a relaxation technique. If still you are having trouble in sleeping, tell your doctor about it.

What are Sports Medicines?

Athletic assistance—Sports medicines has a wider ambit in basic terms, it is fitness medicines or exercise medicines and it deals with any physical activity like a cardiologist deals with the heart. The professional deals with fitness guides you about physical activity. What is the scope for sports medicines—It is a multidiscipline physiological evaluation training control and counseling, looking after the health profiles, injury rehabilitation and diet. How we can best shape our human body to ensure best performance out of it. A team could have a physiotherapist, an osteopath specializing in muscular skeletal medicines, an orthopedic with a super specialization in only elbows or only knees and a physiotherapist assesses, evaluates and treats physical disability, pain resulting from injury, disease or other health related needs.

Golf helps burn calories, reduces cholesterol and stress. A single round of golf helps one burn around 1,000 calories. Eat healthy food to build stamina. When wake up drink bottle of water. The oxygen in water is good for the skin and helps to clear the system. Eating certain food could improve your mood, provide uplifting energy and make you feel fresh and alert walnuts and dark chocolate make you happy while apple keep you energetic. Fatigue is related to thirst so drink atleast 8 glasses of water per day.

Acupressure— your switch cannot always be on.

Stimulating certain acupressure points in your body starting with the top of your head and moving down to the soles of your feet.

You can tap the top of your heap; rub the back of your head where your skull meets your neck. Rub and message soles.

Your *dog can* cost you an arm literally. Infected dogs can infect you with a bug that caused hydrated. The disease can be fatal if not detected on time. Every petting is no good. Your pug can give you a bug that might send you to hospital, petting them, kissing them, sharing our beds with them, you are inviting bodily harm, touching them with your mouth infectious can be transmitted by the saliva. Diseases acquired fingers and toes get amputated another woman had to be operated upon for the removal of puss in her liver and kidney all due to this acquired infections.

Fever, rashes all over body, diseases carried by ticks, fleas, lice and mites.

One needs to be extremely careful with pets. Do not allow pets in areas where food is prepared or handled and do not bath your pet in kitchen sink: Wash your pets outdoors and control flea and tick problems. Dogs must be vaccinated to cover all diseases found in specific area, they must have balanced meals to help the fight infections, if they are healthy, and there are fewer chances of owners catching infections from them.

Mind—Pill popping may be the easiest and the most scientific way to treat everything from a headache to heartache, but practitioners of alternative healing techniques scoff at traditional medical science, as we know it. It focuses on treating the symptoms and not the cause. In addition, the medical science approach is external, where the patient has to take the medicines to cure a problem. Whereas in most alternative therapies, the focus is to turn inward, whereby the patients cure themselves, apparently with the power of their own mind.

Transliminal hypnotherapy—This technique uses special light and sound frequencies to penetrate deep into the subconscious mind, transporting the subject into a state similar to hypnosis, where the therapist gives suggestions for desired changes.

The premise of this technique stems from the fact that the human mind can be divided into the conscious and the subconscious. Whereas the conscious facilitates the day today functioning of life and living.

It is sad to be the subconscious, which serves as the storehouse of all past experiences and memories, which the individual generally cannot access. However, it is said that the information's stored in the subconscious subtly affects most of our conscious decisions and thought process.

Through this process, one is able to access ones subconscious. The suggestions given to the mind in this state are said to be very powerful, in that it stays embedded in a persons mind in a permanent state, functioning and decision making activities.

The mind believes the suffering to be real, under this technique, the filter between conscious and subconscious mind drops and one is capable of deeper insight with the help of the total mind, where the mind ceases to dwell upon the past and the future. Now the mind has nowhere to go, it is in the now- a timeless state. Harmony occurs automatically with this understanding.

Dang's technique involves strapping the subject with a pair of blinkers and headphones on a reclining chair. The gear is connected to a computerized device, which gives out a combination of special subliminal and transliminal sounds and Sanskrit mantras and psychedelic light wave patterns. The light and sound frequency are matched together, the combination of which helps one enter the subconscious mind. The therapist gives suggestions for desired change in behavior in that state.

The right frequency healing

This one's straight out of a sci-fi blockbuster.

Claiming to heal literally with the click of a mouse.

Tinkering with frequency machines for quite sometime now.

The subject is connected to the electronic device at five points with the help of special frequency reading bands one of each wrist and ankle and one on the forehead. The device is connected to computer software, which maps the entire physical, psychological and emotional profile of the individual through the frequency reading received. The machine does the reading of 7,000 parameters in 6 minutes flat.

The reading shows the minutes of anomalies, existing as well as potential, which is not possible allopathic diagnosis. It also has capability to read chromosomes and genes, so latent hereditary problem. Medical science announces the problem only once the damage is done or has reached a certain level of detection.

Silence calms your heart. It is a balm that heals the wounds of the soul. It strengthens the spirit and takes you to a world without sound where peace reigns. It allows us to remove all of the external and physical distractions in our lives and let us focus upon the essence of our being, the soul. Why are we embarrassed by silence, what comfort do we find in all the noise?

Beat the stress—Health determines the quality of life one leads. Stressful work, extended work hours, late night shifts, regular travel etc. have become an integral part of today's corporate world. With increased work pressure and global competition, the workforce is prone to move work related health disorder. Flexibility working can transform a business. Learn the art of relaxation. After a long run, sit under a tree, feel the miracle of your body, the dance of your heartbeat, the gentle kiss of the breeze being ease with oneself. Let your center be clam and silent and relax.

Contentment brings peace and satisfaction to ones soul leading one to believe in the grace of God. A content man accepts with all humility what he has been given by God. He leads a life of happiness and peace and finds the treasure of contentment. Such contented minds deserve to be called rich even though they may be literal sense be poor having meager worldly possession.

Disaster Management/ Natural Calamities

Disaster is a sudden, great misfortune where disruption arises in magnitude. You cannot take the clock back. Natural calamities in the vast cosmos human beings are like a speck. Essentially, there is no conflict between man and creation. Just as a child is entitled to enjoy milk from his mother and the bee is entitled to enjoy honey from flowers, there can be no objection to man enjoying the resources of nature. However, at a result of uncontrollable desires and reckless exploitation of natural resources, nature is exhibiting frightening disorders. Natural calamities like earthquake, volcanic eruptions, droughts and floods are the result of disturbances in the balance of nature; which causes disaster is the result of man by reckless exploitation of resources he does. Man wielding an axe at the branch of a tree on which he is sitting. Nature has proved to be kind parent or a merciless stepmother.

Scientists claim to have found a workable way of reducing carbon dioxide levels in the atmosphere to preindustrial levels by adding lime to seawater, which increases alkalinity. The oceans are already the world's largest carbon sink absorbing 2 billion tones of carbon dioxide every year.

Oceans death zones spread warming of seawater suffocating marine life, say scientists. Marine dead zones, where fish and other sea life suffocate from lack of oxygen, are spreading across the worlds tropical oceans, a study has warned. If global temperature keeps on rising consequences for marine life and for humans in communities that depend on the sea for living, organisms such as fish, crabs, lobsters and prawns will die in such a zones, the researchers say the change is closely linked to rising sea water temperature.

Global warming has led to expansion of low oxygen, underwater deserts in the tropical oceans. This means that organisms at the base of food chains do not get enough nutrients to survive. To combat global warming save the earth pack lighter suitcase, cut the weight of the baggage to below 20 kg, go jogging in a park rather than on an electrical treadmill, use a wind up alarm clock rather than an electrical new, dry clothes on a washing line rather than in a tumble dryer. Heat bread rolls in a toaster rather than in the oven for 15 minutes, reduce winter heating; our world is in the grip of a dangerous carbon habit. Canada is the first in the world to pass climate act. India to focus on solar power with a national action plan.

Shifting sea levels led to mass extinctions that wiped out to 90% of earths flora and fauna, many of the planets living organism rapidly die. Ebb and flow of sea levels and sediment tend to expansion and contraction of those environments has profound effects on life on earth. Researchers have warmed that climate change threatens and devastate coral reef fish population and increase the likelihood of fishery collapse. Mass die off corals because of warmer water, the fish have nowhere else to go.

Earths life we are paying too high a price for what we call progress- save the earth, secure life, pause and look back- continents drift across the oceans, jungles turn into deserts, dust storms and debilitating heat waves, high waves and storms and diva sting cyclone so give back to earth what is hers. Humankind has indeed despoiled the planet and we all heed urgently to clean up our act.

Stop cutting down forests, stop dumping industrial affluent into the earth, before it is too late. Why have temperature unarguably risen in certain areas? Because it could be of the urban island heat effect.

Mega cities with large population have become warmer, less populated town's heaven polar ice caps melting, galaxies calving. If nature becomes weak, we too are adversely affected. Strive for cosmic love in the cosmos all beings and power have deep connection with human; man has no alternative but to plant trees, save water, recycle resources and replenish environment.

We have so many examples of latest cyclone massive damage to property and infrastructure. The storm cut most electricity and telecommunication, the cyclone ripped down power lines, batters buildings and leaves uprooted trees and other debris scattered across the streets, the worst hit areas needs to be cleared up by special army and police to be deployed.

Myanmar aid trickles in, new cyclone fear discounted

The 1.5 million people left destitute by this devastating *cyclone*. May 08 storm that left up to 100,000 people dead or missing, 25, 00 remained buried and rescuer still searching for survivors as thousands remained trapped and the cries for help under the debris of a school. 2 million homeless, low-lying areas hampered by destruction of roads and communication Survivors desperately need medical help, food and water.

Losing your kin make, you feel the whole world around you has collapsed. However, you have to move on. Accidents, fires, building collapse lost kin in second losing several family members would be a tragedy beyond explicable proportion. It is important to learn to deal with death is a reality of life.

The pain of losing a loved one is similar to losing a part of our body. A part of the own self is missing and dead. It is simply, inconceivable to them that their loved ones simply do not exist. Reactions of shock, numbness and disbelief which all comes with catastrophic of disasters.

When you know someone going to die you are mentally prepared—Let it to go, make change and go on, to cope up with grief and talk to some one who can understand your need. As person go through major changes and a vacuum, social withdrawal felt.

Cyclone aftermath—Some villages destroyed with tidal waves, vast rice growing areas wiped out. There would be number of disease, air born and water born in a time when clean food, water and shelter is so scare, they would eat anything and stay anywhere. Piles of bodies begin rots in the disaster zone. Tsunami hit Indonesia and earthquake jolted Pakistan, terror- blasted terrify entire place chaos, people run screaming, jumping over dead bodies and severed limbs, skirting mangled; thousands feared dead in china quack. 80% of buildings flattened in are chuan country.

The magnitude of quack was 7.8, which hit the region the powerful earthquake tremors. Critical relief activities- forget politics, let help people who are dying. Military helicopters dropped food and water, and got assistance to people who are suffering and dying. Emergency declared; citizens have to become educated about their rights and assert themselves- a major step in using modern technology for the empowerment of the citizens and a new ray of hope where the website lodge where victims can lodge their complains.

Nature's clues to predicting an earthquake dogs erupted in wild hawing and barking hours before the quake struck. Mice and snakes skittered around crazily in the open. Horses and cows kicked at their stable walls. Water levels in local wells plunged in the weeks before, only to rise shapely in the hour preceding the quack. People are irritable and confused, geologist suggests a link to electromagnetic behavior is widely believed yet animal behavior is widely believed to hold the most promised in forecasting. One quack can trigger off another earthquake unexpected findings could one day help make better predictions about the frequency and intensity of after shocks.

Flooding is not a new phenomenon. It was a common feature even in the 1970s, over the years, work of widening the nullashs has not kept pace with the growing amount of constructions in the city and is a major cause for flooding, piled up garbage and debris have chocked the drains.

Take steps in your own private life to stop water wastage like closing tap when brushing your teeth, getting leaking pipes fixed immediately. If you see water wastage in public, places call the authority. We live in a nation where pure and safe drinking water is still a privilege for majority of our people. Problem located with local authority-solution lies with each individual. Do you want our future generation to go thirsty? How even most busy people can do his bit to save such a vital natural resources that water -a wake up call.

Downward social drift-God gives every bird its food but does not always drop it into the nest. So true with human being who needs to do conscious effort towards climatic changes.

Tsunami—It is wave train-series of waves generated in a body of water by an impulsive disturbance that vertically displaces the water column. Tsunami is a Japanese word, with the gash translation harbor wave. In deep water, it can travel at a speed of 700 km per hour. It can stoop coasts of sand, uproot trees and wipe out towns. It can travel hundreds of miles in land. The calamity caused on 26 December 2004 rendered lakhs of families homeless, lost everything, their near and dear ones, perished lakhs of lives, left hundreds of children orphaned. It can as unexpected, unprecedented in its suddenness and ferocity causing death the devastation all along our coats. The giant killer waves that swept, the economic losses might take years to compute. There were four earlier deadliest tsunamis that rocked the various countries in different parts of the world. On November 1, 1755, there was a terrible tsunami occurred in Lisbon, Portugal, killing more than 60000. Again on August 27, 1883, another horrible drowned 36000 in Jawa and Sumatra islands. Again, on June 15, 1896, a furious one caused the death of 27000 in the east coast of Japan.

Countdown to extinction—One hour from now, three species of life form will disappear off the face of the planet forever. In addition, the rate is accelerating. The cause is not natural, but fabricated, pollution, which is rampant, is actually eliminating three species every hour. Climate change and the loss of biodiversity are most alarming challenges. Failure to act on greenhouse gases and climate change could threaten food supplies and destroy the foundation of human life.

Nurses role in resources conservation—In today's world water, energy and cooking gas have become scarce and expensive. Water is a natural resource. Mother earth has blessed us with enough water for every one. Every living creature depends on water. Electricity is produced using water. For this, scarcity man alone is responsible for his injudicious waste of these resources. We need to educate people about scarce resources and how to save it. Sensitize people about its importance and its scarcity. Avoid wastage of water so that the less fortunate have enough water for their needs. Each one needs to shoulder the responsibility, water is precious, do not misuse it, use it wisely.

The nature shows the way to relief, all of life is maintained by the sun, air, water by the earth and its resources and sunlight as a gift freely given to all, a blue sky, white clouds, green leaves all is a miracle of nature God.

Warming may raise kidney stone cases, unwanted consequence hard deposits of minerals and salts that can form in the kidney tend to new more common in hot climates with dehydration key risk factor for such condition.

Hospitals disposing *biomedical waste* and carelessly dumping it

Used syringes, blood soaked dressings, vials of untreated urine and blood as well as stray animals foraging on medical waste, which is playing on lives of people. There are no safety precautions. They need to follow the biomedical waste rules.

Disposal rules—BMW shall not be mixed with other wastes. BMW shall be segregated into container bags at the point of generation in accountancies with schedule if prior to its storage, transportation, treatment and disposal. Untreated BMW shall be transported only in such vehicles as may be authorized for the purpose by the competent authority as specified by the government no untreated BMW shall be kept stored beyond a period of 48 hours.

Climate plan says India will not have eight national missions to reduce the emission of greenhouse gases in order to adapt to and mitigate climate changes. They include increasing the share of renewable energy, implementing fuel efficiency norms, creating on integrated water resources management system sustaining the Himalayan glacier and mountain ecosystem, creating and sustaining carbon sinks up and making agriculture sustainable to climate change.

New way to store solar energy for a rainy day—The US scientists have developed a new way of powering fuel cells that could make it practical for homeowners to store solar energy and produce electricity to run lights and appliances at night.

A new catalyst produces the oxygen and hydrogen that fuel cells use to generate electricity, while using far less energy than currant methods. With this catalyst, users could rely on electricity produced by photovoltaic solar cells to power the process that produce the fuel. If you can only have energy when the sun is shinning, you are in trouble. Solar has been growing as a power source in the US. Still it is a tiny power source, producing enough energy to meet the needs of about 600,000 typical homes, and only while the sun is shinning.

The ozone layer is important because it absorbs ultraviolet radiation from the sun, preventing most of it from reaching the earths surface. Ozone layer shields the planet from the radiations harmful effects. As health care providers, should be on the move, we need to have awareness of the problem, and introspect as to how we can contribute to the wellness of our planet.

Role of a nurse in the dealing psychological problems of disaster victims is vital. A wide spectrum of disaster plays havoc. Disaster are either natural, like floods, earthquakes, cyclones, and droughts or man made such as conflicts, refugee situations, firs, epidemics, environmental fall out, etc. disaster can significantly lead to degradation of social and economic progress achieved over decades of initiatives by the people.

The disadvantages of disasters like deaths, disabilities, destitution, as well as loss of livelihoods and property impose enormous social and economic losses.

Nurses play a vital role at times of disaster in handling the situation with competency. If the nurse is in the center of the disaster area, she may need to help with evacuation, rescue and first aid until the immediate needs are met. Hospital nurses will be needed to care for disaster victims as they are brought in for acute care problems.

Catastrophes always strain ones capacity to absorb shock; it brings about unimaginable and lasting psychological trauma. Immediate reactions are panic, fear and disbelief; difficulty in talking decisions, anger and blaming; disturbance in bodily functions. Feelings of being frustrated and feeling of powerlessness over ones own future. Nightmares, loss of personal possession that has high sentimental value.

Nurse should assess the victims at high risk for developing mental disturbances and needing crisis intervention.

Those who have lost family members; those who have suffered serious injuries.

Those who have lost their home or possessions.

Be efficient in observing verbal and nonverbal behavior. Keep families together, especially children and parents, remove the panic stricken persons from the main group and place them where they can help each other. Help them to occupy mind to reduce tension and increase sense of worth. Provide adequate shelter, food and rest. Teach coping strategies.

Protecting health from climate change is a challenging task. Throughout most human history, all climate changes were the direct results of natural forces. This has changed with the industrial revolution, when new industrial and agricultural practices began to alter the global climate. It is most important cause of worry in every aspect of life. The global warming is not unstoppable and human activities are to blame for the heat-trapping greenhouse gases that have caused global temperature to rise dramatically.

Main cause as we mentioned earlier is significant elevation of atmospheric carbon dioxide as major greenhouse gas, due to widespread use of the fossil fuels in the thermal power plants, industries and transport vehicles, deforestation, land use changes, chemical, agricultural and population growth also make a contribution.

Today global warming is progressing at an alarming pace, becoming too dangerous for the life on this planet. This climate change is looming as the biggest human catastrophe, threatening our ultimate survival. Global warming unleashes an unprecedented and widespread health hazards. 50 million environmental refugees, displaced by floods, droughts and rising sea levels are expected by 2010. Numbers may be doubled by 2030. Experts apprehend that global warming will kill billions in this century. Heat and heat related illness are on increase, vulnerable group, people who are not able to tolerate heat and cannot cope are not accustomed to hot weather as there house infrastructure is nor designed to cope up with hot climate.

Technological adaptation like installation of air-conditioners and construction of heat minimizing houses will save the rich but underdeveloped countries and the poor segment of society will be affected. Hot climate breeding of mosquitoes and spread of many infections mosquito born disease like malaria, dengue may take heavy tolled, as under changing environment, agents also are changing.

It is our duty as health providers and as responsible member of the society, to be conscious about the magnitude of this problem. We must, act now to save our earth planet, our civilization and our next generation.

Warming time bomb ticking in Arctic soil- release unexpectedly huge stores of carbon dioxide in Arctic soils.

Which would in turn fuel a vicious circle of global warming, a new study scientists have long known that organic carbon trapped inside a blanket of frozen permafrost covering one fifth of the worlds land mass would, if thawed, release greenhouse gases into atmosphere.

The increasing use of electrical and electronic devices including the rapid growth of tele-communication system, e.g. satellite system radio broadcasting television transmitters and radar installations have increased the possibility of human exposure to electromagnetic energy. Man is living today in a highly complicated environment, which is getting more complicated- if these trends continue, it is feared that the very quality of life we cherish may soon be in danger. The concept of environment is complex and all embracing; which in turn was causing even the hanging patterns in diseases.

Recycle grey water—Flushing and gardening grey water generated from domestic processes such as washing, bathing will be treated at societies and reused in an ecofriendly move.

Green guardians—Did you know trees could generate electricity? Scientists are now harnessing this energy to power wireless sensors fitted on tree trunks, to prevent forest fires from spreading. How it works- a charger inset harvests bi-energy created by reactions between a tree and soil and powers sensors fitted to the trunk. These sensors monitor temperature and humidity and wirelessly transmit the data to an existing weather station. The station in turn transmits the signal to a remote fire service monitoring stations.

Present day nurses role is getting more and more complex. The various electromedical gadgets and audiovisual monitoring devices call upon the ability of a nurse with very alert reflexes. She should be vigilant enough to a professional and competent manner to any eventuality such as disaster and natural calamities, and sudden emergencies of any unpredicted form.

If she is knee and enthusiastic, she is capable of overcoming almost any difficulty.

She can develops her qualities with skill in handling people with scientific base and adopting scientific approach. You cannot stop the rain, but you can open an umbrella. Noted astrophysicist Stephen hawking Galileo saw nature as a book whose author is God. Let us keep this sentiment in our mind when we deal with nature.

The climatic changes effects are immediate and delayed both. Total sanitation campaign- that is sanitation for all 2012. Sanitation is more important then independence Mahatma Gandhi had said. The day every one of us gets a toilet to use, I shall know that our country has reached the pinnacle of progress. J. Nehru. A sanitation revolution is one in the villages of India leading to dignity, health and prosperity through safe and sustainable sanitation. Unit cost of rural toilet 2500. Toilet model twin it pours flush contribution Rs.-300.56% have access to sanitation in rural India.

Disasters are man made ones and natural calamities. Man made such as riots, violence, terrorism, accidents, dam collapse, building collapse, food poisoning, fires, etc. which is caused by human failure. Traumatic experiences of helplessness and hopelessness, panic, nightmare, post-traumatic stress disorder. Physical as well as psychological consequences, loss of life, physical injuries and damage to property affects emotions. Plan of action is necessary because of lack of preparedness. Developing crisis team who are able to assemble quickly at any time of day or night, enhance linkages for referral system. So be prepare to meet the situation.

Healthy Aging/Value of Elders

Growing old is a natural inevitable process in every ones life. Aging is a biological process, which no one can avoid. As we grow old, the health needs also vary. You do not heal old age; you protect it, you promote it, you extend it. Our concern is to help the aged to live happy and dignified life to their satisfaction.

The aging process is complex. As it is a biological phenomenon; and as the years pass replacement of worn out cells slow down. Thus, the functions of each system of the body are impaired and give rise to disorders. The process of aging may also hastened by environment, disease, emotional stress, faulty lifestyle, malnutrition, etc.

The old age never causes a disease, but the old people are very susceptible to certain diseases, disorders and accidents. These include decline of vision and hearing, deterioration of teeth, loss of teeth may cause difficulty in chewing etc. Certain physical changes occur in everyone, as age advances all the systems of the body are affected directly or indirectly. The wear and tear of the living cells will leads to certain disorders such as arthritis; the bone will become brittle and tend to break more easily, weakening of the supportive tissues lead to hernia. Among the diseases that often affect the older people are atherosclerosis, cerebral-vascular accidents, stroke, diabetes mellitus, hypertension etc.

In addition, skin becomes less elastic. Fatty tissues layer is lost which makes the skin thin and sagging due to the folds, lines and wrinkles appear. There is decreased secretion from oil and sweat glands leading to the development of dry skin.

Nails becomes thick and tough, feet usually have poor circulation, hair gets thin and gray, muscles shrink and decrease in strength, joints becomes stiff and painful, hip and knee bent decrease in mobility.

Decrease of blood flow in brain causing dizziness adds increased risk for fall. The sense of touch, smell, taste is affected. There is reduced sensitivity to touch and pain. The number of taste buds decreases, sweet and salty tastes is lost first.

Decrease secretion of digestive juices causing difficulty in digestion of fried and fatty foods. Peristalsis decreases causing delayed emptying of stomach and colon constipation and flatulence.

There is a progressive loss of brain cells. All these affect the personality and mental function. In older people memory of the recent events declines, while the memory of the important events in the early life remains intact.

To help for the successful aging physical health needs regular medical checkups for adequate and appropriate treatment of diseases. Have adequate nutrition, good personal and environmental hygiene to be followed. Good personal appearance that is clean and appropriate dress, daily shaving, cutting of hair, proper rest and sleep to meet the daily activities of living. To keep physically healthy, do daily walking, jogging as per health permits; participate in the outdoor and indoor games, do household work.

Take part in social activities such as participating in meetings, birthday parties, and religious activities, to meet friends, watch TV, and get part time employment.

Prevent yourself from falls. use walker, have adequate lighting over the staircases, use low height cots, use well fitting shoes, prevent falls during acute illness, avoid unfamiliar environment, wear new spectacles, check the temperature of water before bath.

Follow traffic rules to prevent road accidents while walking on busy road, maintain oral hygiene, take balance food, do not smoke or drink, take adequate fluids, minimize sudden movements, have less salt and sugar free diet, as your immunity is reduced and are more prone and susceptible to infections have nutritious diet.

As we grow old, our health needs also vary. Many continue to live healthy and happy lives in their own homes. Each person ages in his own way. How a person ages, it depends on his life experience, available support systems and previous coping skills. The number of older persons is increasing everyday. People are living longer and healthier than before.

Society must be made aware of the values of aged people, their experience and wisdom, which can be great asset to the society. We must help the elders to make their final phase rewarding and meaningful. Therefore, plan for old age by saving, security and shelter. Nobody grows old by merely living a number of years. People grow old by deserting their ideals. You are as young as your self-confidence, as old as your fear, as young as your hope and as old as you despair.

Elders are our history, our heritage, and the very essence of whom we are. To get older and be left alone to die, or suffer a fate is worse than death. There is experienced feeling of frustrating emotional and social vacuum and insecurity. They feel their orphan hood despite offspring and their increasing medical and emotional needs being not meet.

Give a thought to old age in youth. This will serve as a cushion for personal needs in emergency. Travel light to enjoy the journey of life. We are all here on a spiritual journey. Along the way, we find several co-travelers who become part of our lives but they too have their own destination.

Things can never bring you happiness. You must have already experienced in your life one or more times that you wanted something desperately and once you have brought something, its value diminishes. It is one of the few truths in life. Actual happiness cannot be attained from anything external. Holding on to something does not give an ownership rights. So practice loving detachment.

Every spring season brings fresh growth flower while we still have season left in our lives to grow. Live unto the fullest way possible with optimistic outlook.

It is not safe, anywhere, in these days of greed, erosion of moral values. Today old are helpless to protect themselves in the event of mishap. Many of them have poor eyesight, ill and suffering from one or the other chronic disorders.

Parents living alone there children could do frequent phone calls, visits, financial assistance, ongoing help with shopping, home maintenance, payment of bills, health check ups to make sure they are safe and comfortable, healthy and happy, loved and wanted. That will give much more inner satisfaction and contentment to them than otherwise.

Money does not compensate for love and tolerance. How can we make the lives of the aged safe for the rest of their days? They should not fall 'put away' old be made secure by modern gadgets, door chains, peep eye, an intercom system, alarm bells ring and alert the neighbors, the security agency and the police, tight security to keep unwanted people at bay.

When someone wants to visit, the security guard at the gate connects the visitor with the people in the flat by the telecoms and lets the visitors in only after getting a clearance to ensure safety for the elderly.

Today's youth are hard pressed for time because they are engaged in a rat race to fulfill their aspirations. The modern rush has taken its toll on our day today life. Our parents who give up their entire lifetime to raise us, to make us successful and good citizens need to be taken care of in their old age. It is our duty to look after them when they need us the most.

In difficult circumstances get in touch with helpline and social support system, counseling, police help, legal help, and placement for retires who want to work second careers. Who are lonely and depressed to get professional advice and assistance as legal, financial, tax, investments, insurance problem, a day care center for seniors affected by dementia.

It is your life; your life is gift ; so get police verification for your domestic help, secure your flat with strong grills from all sides keep in touch with neighbors, do not open door without checking, do not make a display of cash and valuables at home in front of others. Keep phone number handy of those neighbors who would help in crisis, keep a diary of visitors with phone numbers. It is easier to find the culprit in unfortunate cases and murder, injury, robbery.

Life is precious and unpredictable. Plan your lifestyle investments and retirement planning. Wealth will be eroded if yield on investment is less than the rate of inflation. Life insurance for breadwinner spends the money within your repaying capacity if you borrow.

So, invest wisely, retire happily. Once you retire, your income fails. Nevertheless, if you have set aside a tidy sum each month while working, you will have no qualms when you retire. It will ensure you a life of dignity and independence. Invest where risk is less. Spend only on essentials, unnecessary expenditure must be curtailed to last your interest for a month. It is never too late to budget and to learn to live within ones means.

You buy expensive house, invest in dream car, go to restaurant every weekend, pay by credit card and throw party what are you doing for your last phase, is there enough wealth? Reflect all this important issues and do the adjustment in cutting down entertainment, and plan well before retirement.

With age advances, basic needs of food and clothes decreases but more money needed for health care. As cost of living is going up only 13% of aged have health covers, health insurance falls with increasing age, and most companies do not provide for health insurance after a particular age.

With the recent increase of violence against senior citizens, secure your old age with city police. Elderly feel lonely and are prone to attacks.

So sad at the end of elders life to feel despised, desolated, ditched by their own blood-children pushed, sidetracked and left all alone to live in loneliness. Even children throw them there old ones still bless them and wish good for their children. Both the situations are bad in life that is to have property or not to have property.

When they long for the company of children and there care, they are abandoned and left alone, life is like merry go round- at young age you are up and at the end, you are down. They had never imagined when they conceived the child in the womb and nourished them. That life would takes 'U' turn and darkness surrounds all around. Once something so dear and part of you leaves you for yourself to be all alone, no comfort, all turn there backs at you.

The elderly care home makes them feel at home away from their own home. Where they try to make their life purposeful and happy where they live life on their own terms. One thing you can do is turn towards God and get solace that your own do not need you; you have accomplished your task entrusted by God to you. Do not dishearten or break, there will come invisible hand to protect you. As Gods promise, I will be with you until the end of your life. Anchor on him he will accompany you.

We were taught to respect our elders, but today's youth is different. As long as they need the help of there parents to look after and cook for the family, they are wanted. No sooner they become helpless, they are unwanted. Locking phones saying the bills are too high. They must have courage to counter their condition. India, a land, here elders, parents, teachers and noble souls were respected and their feet touched for their blessings. Today the same people as unwanted and abused by their own children and others, what a downfall of this country, which once was considered the mother of civilization, human values and traditions. How can we stop this?

There are certain eternal truths, which do not lose their relevance with time. When life is full of health and glee work thou as busy as bee. In fact, in the modern era's increasing lifespan and reducing work period, it is even more necessary to ensure your *money* earned by working, now works for you; be careful with money. In country where the majority is employed in the private and unorganized sector are not entitled to any benefit from either pension or the other state welfare schemes. Put your money government backed scheme, the highest degree of capital security is assured.

Human care—Animal and birds may get sanctuaries but there is none for humans. Reality unfolds worse situation of deprived set of old aged, neglected women and unprotected children. Industrialization, westernization, urbanization and migration have considerably changed the value system and structure of families. Modernization and globalization has added to negligence. Malnutrition, disable, destitute, illiteracy, child labour, no safe drinking water, urban areas lack drainage facilities, rivers polluted we can go on describing heart breaking situations.

VALUE OF PARENTS

An 80 years old man was sitting on the sofa in his house along with his 45 year old highly educated son suddenly a crow perched on their window. The father asked the son, what is this? The son replied it is a crow. After a few minutes, the father asked the son second time what is this. At this time, some expression of irritation was felt in sons tone when he said to his father with a rebuff, it is a crow. A little after, again same son shouted at his father, why do you keep asking me the same question repeatedly, although I have told you so many times it is a crow. Are you not able to understand this? A little later, the father went to his room and came back with an old tattered diary, which he had maintained since his son was born. On opening a page, he asked his son to read the page. The son found flowing words in the diary. Today, my little son aged three was sitting with me on the sofa, when a crow was sitting on the window. My son asked me 23 times what that was. It was a crow. I hugged him lovingly each time he asked me the same question repeatedly for 23 times. I did not at all feel irritated. I rather felt affection for my innocent child. While the little child asked him 23 times what is this? The father had felt no irritation in replying to the same question all 23 times and when today the father asked his son the same question just 4 times, the son felt irritated and annoyed him. So.

If your parents attain old age, do not look at them as a burden, but speak to them a gracious word; be cool, obedient, humble and kind to them. Be considerate to your parents, from today say this aloud, I want to see my parents happy forever. They have cared for me ever since I was a little child. They have always showered their selfless love on me. They crossed all mountains and valleys without seeing the storm and heat to make me a person presentable in the society today. Be good and serve your parents-no matter how they behave.

For example, the old couple sat huddled near check in at the airport, holding onto two tickets and their meager belongings, waiting for their son, who had gone to get their seat number. Minutes passed in to hour, still no sign of the son. Prodded by his wife, the old man timidly walked up to the check in counter to seek the status of their flight. His heart almost stopped to hear the flight had taken off with their son, and they were holding cancelled tickets. Why did he do this to us? They were happy in heir small world at the chawl, where all neighbors lived like a single family, sharing each other's joys and sorrows. There only son was given the best education possible, went abroad on a job, got married and settled there with the occasional phone calls.

There were no reproaches, no demands, suddenly unexpected, the son decided to talk them along to stay with to sell off all their belongings, including there room in the chawl, deposited the money in his name and gave those two tickets. On reaching the airport after a teary farewell to their old friends, he made them sit while where he arranged everything. That was the last they saw him. Officials at the airport were more human, they tried to contact the number in the S. in vain, finally, one of their old neighbors were contacted who came and took them away. With there kindness a few days was spent at the balcony of the chawl and was moved to old age home. With the why still unanswered.

For example, the funeral prayer was moments from being lit when a movement on the bier triggered panic among the staff at a crematorium in southern India. As they rushed to exam the elderly woman under the shroud, her three sons suddenly abandoned their mourning and fled. 75-year-old widow narrowly escaped being cremated alive by their own children fed up with caring for her in her battle against cancer; the family had taken her to a hospital, expecting her to die there. Some days after she was discharged while still in a stupor rather than taking her home, her offspring drove their mother straight to the crematorium.

For example, Family throw granny on a garbage heap. An old woman was found lying on a heap of rotting garbage. She told the rescuers she had been thrown there by her daughter and grandsons who wanted to get rid of her. Died in old age home.

For example, an advocate had engaged contract killers to murder his father over a family dispute involving property.

For example, Life story- a young man was getting ready to graduate college. For many months he had admired a beautiful sports car in a dealer's showroom, and knowing his father could well afford it, he told him that was all he wanted. As graduation day approached, the young man awaited for signs is his father had purchased the care. Finally, on the morning of his graduation his father called him into his private study. His father told him how proud he was to have such a fine son and he told him how much he loved him. He handed his son a beautifully wrapped gift box, curious, but somewhat disappointed, the young man opened the box and found a lovely, leather-bound bible. Angrily, he raised his voice at his father and said with all your money, you give me a bible?

And stormed out of the house, leaving the holy bible many years passed and the young man was very successful in business. He had a beautiful home and wonderful family, but realized his father was very old and thought perhaps he should go to him. He had no seen him since that graduation day. Before he could make arrangements, he received a telegram telling his father had passed away, and willed all his possession to his son. He needed to come home immediately and take care of things.

When he arrived at his father's house, sudden sadness and regret filled his heart. He began to search his father's important papers and saw the still new bible, just as he had left it years ago. With tears, he opened the bible and began to turn the pages. As he did so, a car key dropped from an envelop taped behind the bible. It had a tag with the dealer's name, the same dealer who had the sports car he had desired. On the tag was the date of his graduation, and the words, paid in full. How many times do we miss gods blessings because they are not packaged and we expected?

In human one eats one place the other parents cannot even have a meal together. Elder abuse and harassments, we have lost our culture and ethos of love and care for the elders. Not allowing them to use phone, inadequate food given, lacks clothing's, medications, rape, indecent assault, verbal intimidation, shouting, threats of physical harm, withholding affection, removal of decision making powers, injury, hitting. Is home for senior citizens the safest place to put our parents? Or do we have to rethink our lives to accommodate the old age needs? Our parents just like our mother did, when we were young to look after us. They have added meaning to their years by doing tings they are passionate about. The zest of these golden oldies proves the later years can be as beautiful as the summer of their lives. How often we live our lives for the happiness of others, only to find the end comes nearer and nearer and we are run out of time to discover where out own happiness lies.

The realization 'death is inevitable' takes place strongly during late adulthood. How do nurse counselors help patient to cope up with such distressing thoughts? What is the major psychological concern that comes up with an increasing age above 60? Which are the various therapies used and techniques used? Family support being an essential factor, how family is integrated in this process.

World Elder's Day- October 1st. The United Nations has declared international day of older persons. A day on which to recognize the contributions made by the older persons be remembered and celebrated with joy. To remember that there is no substitute to children taking care of their own parents. Our elders deserve love and protection, may the younger get inspired and value the dignity of there parents.

NURSE UNDERSTANDS ON PATIENT OF ALZHEIMER'S DISEASE

Alzheimer's disease is a form of dementia. Dementia involves progressive decline in two or more areas of cognition, usually memory and one or more of the following:

Language, calculation, visuospatial perception, constructional praxis, judgment, abstraction and personality.

Dementia of the Alzheimer's type constituted at least half of all dementia. 10 to 15% of people develop over age of 65. 19 % of people over age of 75 and 47% of people over the age of 85 years.

It increases greatly with increasing age.

The cause not been found, although several risk factors have been identified increasing age is a risk factor. Genetic factors can influence, environmental, metabolic factors also pay a role. Nearly all persons with Down syndrome develop dementia. Head trauma lack of education and myocardial infraction have been linked, disordered immune function, viral infection are causes yet not proved.

Alois Alzheimer has first described dementia in 1907. Areas of cell loss in the brain of the person; learning and reasoning, memory storage and recall, language abilities and consciousness changes.

Clinical manifestation and diagnostic findings is characterized by a relentless impairment of decision-making and can progress for a decade of so. Memory disturbances are first feature of the disease. Family member or co-workers often notice the memory loss before the individual does. The individual may demonstrate poor judgment and problem solving skills and become careless in work habits and household chores. He does well in familiar surrounding and lack ability to adapt new challenges, can follow well-established routines. The person may become irritable, suspicious and indifferent. Agitation, apathy, dysphonic, cognitive impairments.

In second stage, the person demonstrates language disturbances, impaired word finding speech becomes empty words used in wrong context. Repeat words and phrases. Difficulty in using everyday objects such as toothbrush, comb, razor, and utensils.

It creates safety problems. He may leave a burner on in the kitchen to forget to extinguish a cigarette. Taking everything in the mouth to suck, chew or taste, sees bugs crawling on bed or throughout the house wandering at night in common.

Third stage mental abilities are lost, including speech. Voluntary movement is minimal, limbs become rigid and lost all ability of self-care, lose of normal alertness.

Diagnosis through the ECG, CT, and MRI can be done.

Lab test such as BUN, creatinine, liver function test, serum test, can be done as doctor's order.

There is no cure to enhance memory. Brain continues to atrophy and the limbic system becomes dysfunctional patient uses abusive language and becomes suspicious of others.

Impaired verbal communication- make needs known and interact meaningfully if person speaks only single words or short phrases, the nurse should do likewise. Speak slowly and simple firm volume and low pitch, tone of voice calm.

The patient may forget why he was upset. Reach him by touching, holding a hand, putting an arm around waist. Altered through processes, maintain orientation to maximum. Intervention to enhance memory, reorient by placing a calendar and clock.

Risk for injury- in home electrical devices, toxic substances, loose rugs, hot water tap, inadequate lighting, unlocked door, and dangerous objects should be kept out of reach. Cooking should be supervised. Driving skill should be evaluated at regular intervals. Boost patient's confidence and self respect, constant encouragement, urging to teach step by step approach is necessary.

Keep dry, clean clothing and bedding. Constant supervision, to live with damaged thinking is to live at risk. Neat house with fever things to trip over or knock over, hazards are more easily seen. Remove furniture with sharp corners, most accidents happen in kitchen and bathroom.

Assist family in understanding symptoms related to memory loss, nature of the illness, symptoms, and stages of diseases, progression and behaviour manifestation. Provide written materials to reinforce education and understanding. Family grieves for the loss of the person they used to know.

Alzheimer's disease- memory tips- is there a thief hiding in your home. Mother forgets to serve the Idli she cooked-normal; mother forgets she already cooked it- problem.

Alzheimer's disease is a disease of the brain. Leads to loss of memory; if the disease strikes the old person at home, he cannot be left independent. He forgets to eat. He forgets he has to go to toilet. If he goes out, he cannot remember his home address. Loving family members can thus be lost if not taken care 24 hours. Ronald Reagan, Margaret Thatcher are victims of it. But there is a hope.

Be in the Moment

You cannot remember something if you are not learned it. So focus on learning.

Pay attention to your environment so that you can encode this information into your brain.

To learn how to stay in the moment, do not focus on the past or worry about the future while you are learning.

Do not multitask, as you create a brain drain when you focus on more than one activity.

Create a learning environment.

Note the kind of environment which helps your learning and try to create it while you learn.

If you are visual learner, make sure you have tools to create visuals that will help you to retain information.

If you are an auditory learner, purchase a tape recorder so that you can use it to repeat instructions or information.

Use All your Senses

While you are learning something, involve as many senses as possible to help retain the experience.

Drawing and writing includes the use of motor skills that help you to remember information as you stimulate motor pathways.

Talk to another person about what you have learnt, as this will incorporate more senses in the process.

Use Mnemonic Devices

Visual images use to remember things, e.g. To remember a name Ajay, use image of actor Ajay Devgan.
Use positive and amusing images as brain remembers them well.
If the images are colorful and three dimensional, it is easier to remember.
Make silly and amusing sentences to remember a list of things.

Rhymes-create rhyme to remember things, like this one, in fourteen hundred ninety two, Columbus sailed the ocean blue.

Retain a Positive Attitude

If you do not want to learn something, chances are you would not learn it. If you constantly tell yourself and others that you have a bad memory, this action actually hampers the ability of your brain to remember.

Get organized—Once you have fixed locations for all medications, important phone numbers, valuable papers, useful tools and keys, wallets, and glasses you will minimize searches for a misplace item.

Research—Portable kit to detect Alzheimer's in early stage has a chance to slow the diseases advance with the development of a new device that allows an inexpensive and easy to administer test to detect the cognitive decline associated with its early stages. About 24 million people worldwide are thought to have these diseases. Families usually wait until their mom or dad does something somewhat dangerous, like forgetting to take their medicines or getting lost, when the person has already lost the significant portion of their cognitive function. With this device will help before symptoms occur and become serious.

Researchers say Arthritis drug restores speech in Alzheimer's; though still they it is early findings as still research continues.

Parkinson's diseases—Why early diagnosis and treating it right from the start matters? Parkinson's disease is a chronic neurodegenerative disease affecting over 1 million people in he US. Earlier it used to be a disease of old age, but more and more young clients in their 30s and 40s are being diagnosed PD. The lack of early markers for detection of the disease makes it difficult to identity the ones that will be at risk. When increasing number of genes being discovered, we may have to change the way we think about the disease. A combination of genetic susceptibility and environmental toxins may be responsible for causing the disease.

Since the 60s, Levodopa has been the corner stone of the therapy for clients with PD. As we learn more about the disease, we realize that it is not all about correcting the dopaminergic dysfunction since there are so many non-motor symptoms of PD, which are minimally responsive. The fight against PD continues as researchers and clinicians alike toil day and night to develop insight into pathogenesis, genetic and management of PD.

Many of us fall to recognize that there are some non-motor symptoms, associated with Parkinson's disease. These symptoms are not directly seen in the ay we move or handle things, but affect our lives in several ways. Various symptoms like depression, anxiety, hallucinations, sleep disorders, autonomic symptoms and sensory symptoms constitute the non-motor symptoms in Parkinson's disease. A global multidirectional search is on for a cure for Parkinson's diseases or at least better management of its symptoms. This includes therapeutic options, stem cell and surgical intervention. Science is doing whatever they can, to find solutions to address difficult problems whether it is Parkinson's, Alzheimer's, cancer, AIDS, the fight continues.

Nurse and Nursing Art as Science and Nurse in Clinical Field with Procedures

Introduction to Nursing

Nursing owes much to the influences of Florence Nightingale. The word nursing comes from root word, nutritious means to nourish, to cherish, to protect, to support, to sustain etc. it also means to train, to educate, to supply with essentials of growth.

The first mother was the first nurse woman protecting their children, talking care of elderly and sick members of the family. Simple procedures were adopted by her like application of cold water over the forehead to reduce fever, application of pressure on bleeding injury.

WHAT IS NURSING?

It is an art, science and vocation. According to the ICN/international council of nurseing nursing is unique function of a nurse that is to assist the individual sick/well in the performance of those activities, contributing to health or its recovery/or to a peaceful death that he would perform unaided if he had the necessary strength, will or knowledge.

WHAT IS COMPREHENSIVE NURSING?

It is a systematic process of problem diagnosis problem analysis, development of plan of care and continuous assessment of evolving plan of care. It is an individualized plan based upon scientific principles and concepts utilization of specialized skills and techniques for the care of whole patient to meeting the physical, psychological, spiritual, social, economical and intellectual needs of the patient.

WHAT ARE THE ELEMENTS OF NURSING?

Nursing is nurturing caring for and about people
   Nursing is a services to the individual the family and the community
   Nursing can be either preventive or therapeutic

Nursing is educative

Nursing is a direct service, one of direct conduct between the nurse and the patient or between nurse and the patient or between nurse and family.

Nursing is adapted to the individual needs of the patients even though the person suffer from the same kind of disease their needs are different/each individual is to be considered to be a unique person.

Core of nursing—Promotion of health, prevention of illness, restoration of health, alleviation of suffering

Essentials of nursing—The science of nursing, the art of nursing, the spirit of nursing

Scope of nursing—The individual, the family, the society

Principle Applied to Nursing Procedures

Safety—Prevention of mechanical thermal, chemical and bacteriological injuries to the patient and worker

Comfort—To provide comfort to give satisfactory to the patient and workers

Use of Resources—Right use, economy of time, energy and material

Good Workmanship—It is the art of doing

Individuality—Consider needs and problems of a particular patient

WHAT IS NURSING PROFESSION?

A profession is an occupation with ethical components that is devoted to the promotion of human and social welfare.

Professional nurse is a graduate of a recognized nursing school who has met the requirement for a registered nurse in a state in which is she ascended to practice

WHAT IS THE HISTORY OF NURSING?

Prehistoric time, life was very simple and he made few changes except when compelled to do so. He lived close to nature and soon associated spiritual values to all natural objects, believing that a thing in nature like a tree or river had a spirit or soul. Such a religion is known as Animism. They believed diseases associated with which craft, magic or by some spirit. Thus starving, beating, loud noises, magic rites etc were tried. If evil spirit was thought to live in a special part of the body holes were made to allow it to escape.

In Judeo Christian era, women provided nursing services at home as part of their ethical and humanitarian responsibility like caring children, aged and the sick members of the family. Nursing evolved as a natural response to the desire to keep healthy as well as to provide comfort to the sick. This was reflected in the caring, comforting, nourishing cleaning aspects to the patient knowledges of these simple skills which were passed down from generation to generation.

Nursing in Medieval Period

Nursing in medieval period in Europe many nursing orders developed during that time Assisi was founded. The poor Clares who cared for the sick and lepers, and during 17th century, St Vincent de Paul founded the sisters of charity who cared for the sick. This pattern continued till the industrial revolution in 1800 until the time of Nightingale of England.

WHAT IS MODERN NURSING?

Miss Florence Nightingale (1820-1910) was born in a prominent English family with the benefits of excellent education and knowledge of social conditional and reforms of the time. She believed that nursing should be a separate career and not the part of religious responsibility.

Can you Explain Nursing in India?

Nursing in India goes back to 1500 BC. It was found diseases were attributed to demons and treatment was given primarily to that medicine had passed into the hands of Brahmins who were scholars and members of priestly class. Banaras became center of medical education. Halls of healing was founded. This time Sushrata bought practice of surgery to high standard Sushrata and Charaka famous physician were the leading authorities of ancient Indian system known as ayurveda means science of life. He gave detailed instructions for ensuring absolute cleanliness in all departments of operating room, cleanliness of instruments was stressed. He was the man who described the technique of suction, plastic surgery, cranial surgery and cataract operation. Sushrata defined the relation of doctor, patient, nurse and medicine as the four feet on which cure must rest.

Ancient people believed more prevention than cure doctors also well trained not only in medicine and surgery but also in prevention of diseases.

From 500 BC to 300 AD was period of Buddhism, King Ashoka established a large number of hospitals and health centers.

WHAT IS MILITARY NURSING?

In March 25, 1888, ten fully qualified certificate nurses landed in Mumbai. The Indian nursing service was founded. The first lady superintendent was Ms. Locke. It developed very slowly until Second World War of 1939. Forty-five nurses recruited to India in 1914 and attached to Queen Alexandra. Military nursing service formed in 1927 and it had 12 matron, 18 sisters and 25 staff nurses. They were responsible for supervision and training in nursing section. It was mission hospitals, started training of Indians as nurses and Christian girls were mainly attracted towards nursing training.

Can you Explain the Present Scenario of Nursing in India?

Development of nursing in India was progressing. The trained nurses association of India was established in 1908 and Indian nursing council in 1949 as per act of parliament 1947 various efforts were made by government of India by forming a number of committee such as Shety committee, Kartar Singh committee etc.

A National Convention of Nurses was held in 1988. It had an opportunity to discuss nursing problems with the president and prime minister of India. The central council of health recommended-

1. Improve training of nurses in clinical specialties
2. Open more postgraduate courses for nurses
3. Strengthen regulatory mechanisms
4. Funds for strengthening of nursing services

Explain the Concept of Hospital

It derived from Latin word 'hospitlasis for a guest' in French' 'hospos'a host, a guest. It is an institution in which sick or injured person are treated as well as healthy persons are helped to promote and maintain an optimum level of well being and prevent diseases.

Due to advance medical technology the hospital has progressed from a custodial institution where sick people went only as a last resort to emerging modern, comprehensive medical care centers in which patient expected to be treated successfully. Now they have followed up of community link and reach the families in the home situation.

Hospital divided into four **categories** that are public, voluntary, private and corporate hospitals.

Public Hospitals are run by the central/state govt or municipal bodies on a non-commercial basis. It can be general hospitals or specialized hospitals or both general hospitals are those which provide treatment for common diseases, where as specialized hospitals provide treatment for specific diseases, specific groups of people like infectious disease, cancer, eye, cardiac diseases etc.

Voluntary/Charitable Hospitals are those which are established and incorporated in societies, registration act.

A board of trustees usually managers such hospitals

The main source of revenue is public and private donations and grants and aid from central govt/state govt. and organizations.

Private Hospitals are generally owned by individuals or groups of people and are run on a commercial basis

Corporate Hospitals are run by limited companies, formed under the companies act. They can be general, specialized or both.

EXPLAIN THE HOLISTIC APPROACH TO NURSING

Proponents to holistic health believe that the time has come to give serious consideration the spiritual dimension of the individual which reaches out and strives for meaning. When people find a balance between their life values, goals and belief systems for aids have experienced beneficial, even transforming outcomes as a result of meeting spiritual needs and purpose in life. It is intangible, something that transcends physiology and psychology. As a relatively new concept which includes integrity, principles and ethics, the purpose in life commitment to some higher being and belief in concepts that are not subject to state of the art explanation.

IMPORTANCE OF SPIRITUALITY IN NURSING CARE

Spirituality can positively influence the immune, cardiovascular, hormonal and nervous systems, improving coping skills specially with chronic illness such as arthritis, diabetic, heart disease, alleviates stressful feelings and promotes healing, encourages a sense of relaxation, can lower pressure and reduce feelings of anxiety and depression. Health is no longer viewed as a passive state of being, but as a dynamic process of achieving higher levels of wellness within each dimension of health. Beliefs affects once viewing problems, influences behaviour, moods and helps in resolving your problem and becomes supportive.

When we analyze the above, we find **elements such as—**

Nursing is caring for people, nursing is a service to the individual the family and the community. Nursing can be either preventive or therapeutic, nursing is educative, and nursing is a direct service between nurse and the patient and his family. Nursing is adapted to the individual needs of the patients. Even though a persons suffer from the same kind of disease their needs are different/each individual considered to be unique person.

WHAT ARE THE OTHER HOSPITAL DEPARTMENT?

1. **Admitting** department for the purpose of admitting patient to the types of room he desires.
2. **Cashier and crediting** department—Make the necessary financial arrangements.
3. **Pharmacy** department gives prescribed medications of the patients are obtained here.
4. **Laboratories** directed by pathologist who is trained in the method detecting changes that take place in the tissues and fluids of the body during disease.
5. **Radiologist** department; a radiologist reports X-ray radiation therapy procedures are administered under his direction.
6. **Dietary** department function is to plan, propose and serve meals for patients.
7. **Social service** department obtains aid for the patient and their families.
8. Physiological/occupational therapy department.
9. Chaplain, house keeping and maintenance, purchasing, central supply department are some of the other departments of hospital.

WHAT ARE THE RISK FACTORS FOR SICK AND HEALTHY?

1. *Age*—increases or decreases susceptibility to certain illness, e.g. risk of heart diseases increases with age, the risk of birth defects and complications of pregnancy in women bearing children after age of 35 years.

2. *Environment*—in which a person works or lives can increase the likelihood that certain illness will occur, e.g. chances of tuberculosis due to air pollution in cotton mills.
3. *Lifestyle*—many activities, habits or practices involve risk factors, e.g. poor nutrition, personal hygiene, over eating, lack of exercise.
4. *Illness* is a state in which a person's physical, emotional, intellectual, social development or spiritual functioning is diminished or impaired, compared with previous experience.
5. *Acute illness*—usually short duration and is severe, symptoms appear abruptly, subside after short period.
6. *Chronic illness* persists usually more than 6 months and can affect functioning in any dimension. It can fluctuate maximum functioning and serious health relapses that may be life threatening.

WHAT IS PERSONAL HEALTH?

Achieving and maintaining an optimum personal health level through fundamental health habits is simple routine practices developed for the purpose of giving greater freedom and more efficient use of body and mind. Even early in the using programme the student should be able to share and teach the fundamentals to patient. Learning to cope with stress is preventive care because it can give disease like bodily reaction like headache, backaches, feelings of anxiety, depression etc are signs of stress.

WHAT IS COMMUNITY HEALTH?

In broad term it is accepted as referring to organized efforts of all agencies in the community that are inducted towards promoting health including both private and government agencies. The average modern community local resources for health include the private physician, the hospital, the health department and private health agencies.

PURPOSE OF ADMISSION OF PATIENT

1. It is to receive the patient according to his condition to welcome and provide comfort and safety with immediate care;
2. To be safety for any emergency; to assist the patient in adjusting with hospital environment and to establish nurse patient relationship.

   Prior to patient's arrival the room bed can be prepared and modified by admitting office. For ambulatory patient bed should be in normal position where as if the patient has to arrive on a stretcher the bed should be in lowest position for easy access to bed. Nurse makes sure that the equipment are ready and in functions properly to use for patient on arrival.
3. *Reception* is a place where the first impression of a hospital is formed. The kind of reception provided by the clerk is of importance. They should convey then tactfully that the chief aim of all hospital personnel is to make the period of hospitalization as pleasant as possible.

4. *Admitting office* where basic information's are obtained, e.g. name, age, address, occupation, reason for admission and admitting physician. This information is entered in register and placed on admission sheet which accompanies the patient to the unit. The patient gets ID number which serves to identify his record during hospitalization.

5. In *emergency* patients are admitted in acute condition requiring immediate treatment because every moment is precious for life saving immediate treatment has to be started.

6. *Transporting* the patient from OPD to IPD patient who are allowed to walk escorted by the nurse. Wheel chair should be available to those who are week or lame to walk. Seriously ill patients should never be left alone.

7. *Ward reception* patient is welcomed by a nurse and ensured his confidence and cooperation and oriented to ward unit.

8. *Preliminary observation done;* helping the patient to occupy the bed. Patient comes on trolley then he is transferred with assistance. Vitals recorded at regular intervals and recorded in chart and specimen sent for investigation.

9. *Car of the valuables* and clothing given to the family and if he keeps anything with him it is his own risk.

HISTORICAL BACKGROUND OF MAN AND MEDICINE

The medicine, man, the priest, the herbiest and the magician brought relief to the sick- there were errors and false theories and mistaken interpretations down the ages as it was ever changing concept. The scope of medicine has broadened recent years.

1. *Medicine in Antiquity*—Dominated by magical and religious beliefs

2. *Primitive medicine*—Feeling of sympathy and kindness in time of suffering. Primitive man attributed pain, suffering, calamities to the wrath of gods. Evil spirits-influences of the stars and planets. Appeasing gods by prayers of rituals and sacrifice driving out evil spirits by witchcraft. With stone and flint instruments performed circumcisions, amputations and trephine of skulls. Primitive medicine is timeless. It still persists in many parts of the world. In India, snake bites by Mantras, leprosy as a punishment of ones past sins. Traditional healers found everywhere even to this day.

3. *Indian medicine*—Ayurveda and siddha system; The early Indians set fractures, performed amputation, excised tumor, repaired hernias, excelled in cataract and plastic surgeries. Ayurveda is the 'tridosha theory' vataa-pitta-kapha, disturbances in the equilibrium diseases occurred. When there is perfect balance and harmony said to be healthy.

4. *Chinese*—Medicine based on principle of 'yang-yin M/F. The balance of the two opposing forces meant good health. Bare foot doctors and acupuncture have attracted world wide attention in recent years.

5. *Egyptian*—Time, art and medicines was mingled with religion. Egyptian physician were co-equals of priests trained within temples. They often helped priest to care for sick brought to the temple for treatment. They believed disease was due to absorption from the intestine of harmful substances which gave rise to formation of pus and impurities.

6. *Mesopotamian* called as cradle of civilization demons caused disease. Liver was considered seat of life.

7. *Greek*—Hippocrates, Father of Medicine was born on the 460 BC island of Cos, in Aegean Sea Radical new approach to medicines, i.e. application of clinical methods in medicines. Where there is love there is healing – oath has become the keystone of medical ethics. It sets a high moral standard for the medical profession and demands absolute integrity of doctors it will always regard as masters of medical art.

8. *Roman* had a keen sense of sanitation, they made roads, pure water, drainages built sewages and established hospitals for sick, preserved health to diseases.

9. *Middle Ages*—Dark ages-rejection of body and glorification of spirit - people seldom bathed, no progress in medicines. Monasteries headed by monks, saints and abbots came up. They rendered medical and nursing care to the ill.

10. *Dawn of Scientific Medicine*—Marked by political, industrial, religious, medical revolutions – people claiming their just rights with civilization standards of living improved.
    i. Revival of medicines → Ambroise Paré (1510–1590), Father of Surgery.
    ii. Sanitary awakening →
    iii. Rise of public health →
    iv. Germ theory of disease →
    v. Birth of preventive medicines → James Lind advocated the intake of fresh fruits and vegetables, discovered vaccines, causative agent, made of transmission – development laboratory detection.

11. *Modern Medicine* : → Two major branches: curative, preventive – moved to specialization rational, scientific approach – control – other factors caused diseases – namely social economic, genetic, environmental, psychological which are equally important which are linked to man's lifestyle and behavior.
    Multilateral causation – risk factors – epidemiology
    The concept of Health Center first rooted in 1920 by Lord Dawson in island in 1931.

12. *Medical Revolution*: → Medicines moved from the organism to organ and from organ to cells to molecular properties.

13. Today highly technical – acquired new capabilities – manipulation and body and mind, i.e. genetic counselling, genetic engineering parental diagnosis of ser, in vitro fertilization, cloning, organ transplantation, the use of artificial kidney machine, the development of an artificial heart, the practice of psychosurgery etc. new revolutionary stage.

This is how medicine has evolved down the centuries. Medicine will continue to evolve so long as man's quest for better health continues.

Other factor affect health is marriage, children, noise, pollution, and mass media. TV, newspapers, violence and terrorism, crowded urban living, disrupted biologic rhythms, abortion, VD, social instability.

Diseases are a state of imbalance of one or more cell components or conditions of cell fluids. Maintenance of body balance, psychological and emotional balance, spiritual and philosophic balance with this broad view health becomes a tremendous task restoring balance of individual.

Between illnesses and wellness there is the ambiguous area neither well nor especially ill. To maintain equilibrium between health and illness.

Alarm stage is response to the alarm the body fights back. When body unable to adapt, an adaptation disease may follow from faulty adjustments to stress. Health and illness and life depend on the quality of that adaptation.

Message for nurses on the importance of being a N-U-R-S-E is nobility of demeanor and professional integrity. Understanding her patients and anticipating his every need. Quality care to the patient.

Undertaking responsibility, being accountable for her actions and showing respect for every individual as a person of dignity and worth and skillful.

Over the last century, nursing education has moved from hospital based schools to collages and universities. This trend helped in establishing nursing as a profession.

Her dual role of nurse as educator and practitioner, for that she needs better learning experience, better role models, and good quality nursing care, better coordination between nursing service, and education and personnel development. For that she also should take individual interest and get involved in all round development and keeping abreast with the advancement in knowledge and technology.

With drastic changes in lifestyle at home, at workplace, and in society at large, a re-look at changing role of nursing and nursing practice. A situation, we are set to face.

To be an educated nurse who continues attendance educational cases to improve her professional skill so that their status in the world, would be enhanced.

The caring hands and empathy of the care giver sets positive triggers, by some process not known to the scientific community, and supplemented by a congenital psychological preparation which a nurse can best provide, the patient tends to become fit.

Ethos: Be punctual set an example to others. Be courteous, it does not cost anything. Be helpful, this only generates good will. Be humble, it never hurts anybody.

The patient is a center of our hospital. Never forget that. Avoid unnecessary tests and expenses. Medicines as far as possible, the patient is already under stress. Make his stay as pleasant as possible-but short. What if you were a patient? How would you have wished to be treated? Treat your patient thus. Teamwork is fun; take your place on the team. Enthusiasm turns work into pleasure.

Share the misfortunes of the poor. Help disabled. Look after the sick. A small act will awaken a great strength within. Supply a lion like force to your heart. Do not hold it back.

Nursing Care I

Nurses who are already staffs and need to revise themselves what they have already learnt and know but have forgotten as the years passed could revise themselves with up to date knowledge by refreshing themselves in continuous education through nursing practice of the procedures.

When enough time is limited and vast comprehensive topics in short time to go through and revise becomes difficult, sometimes, this book will give information in a flash. Quick and easy look-ups handy tool to enhance your competence and what is necessary. All needed apt information of all up to date latest vital topics which are mention in content are focused in nut shell. This allows the reader to quickly identify important information and to see how nursing practiced in short time. This will give added confidence to a nurse and provide as a guide.

Hygiene is a set of practice that one conductive to the preservation of health such as cleanliness. In normal everyday life, we meet our own needs for hygiene during illness, however problems such as vomiting, diarrhea, excessive perspiration, prolong time in bed can increase needs for hygiene at the very time and decreased ability to take care of them. Meeting hygienic need includes cleansing body, perineal care, providing oral care, changing linen etc. as nurse provides for cleanliness and comfort she can also assess the persons over all condition teach appropriate hygiene, comfort and self care and assess the persons psychological needs.

There are *four levels of nursing care* that patients when come to the hospital has, such as in *first level* of care a patient needs an encouragement for eating. He does his daily care by himself such as does his own bathing, oral hygiene, hair combing, goes to bathroom all alone ect.

Second kind of patient who needs some help in eating, bathing, daily care, adjusting position and the one who feels mild debility.

The *third* kind of person is the one who cannot feed himself but is able to chew and swallow. He is unable to do self care, needs bed pan, able to partially turn and lift him but cannot turn without help. It could be acute illnesses, medical or surgical case, tracheotomy etc. and the *fourth* one patient who cannot feed self and have difficulty in swallowing, is completely dependant, critically ill, needs nursing care in eating, grooming, medications ect.

The qualities of a nurse that will enhance such patient performance of services, efficacy, appropriateness, availability, timeliness, effectiveness, correct manner care provided to archive desired outcome.

As nurses, none of us like to make mistakes, still mistakes happen. Nursing errors like technical error can be prevented from reoccurring. Judgmental error choosing the wrong strategies can be correct by seeking advice. Normative errors are serious which itself doubts the ability of a person to be a nurse. Though nurses needs to take risk with patient, but the process of safe risk talking must be learned through clinical practice.

How effective are nurses in identifying and managing ethical issues of nursing practice? How do they resolve ethical conflicts, ethical decision making in nursing practice? Nurses are human beings with human values and spiritual beliefs yet how can cultural beliefs of people be incorporated? What happens when the nursing care plan is in conflict with specific cultural practices? How should nurses respond to conflict between patent and family members in the homecare setting? What is the difference between withholding and withdrawing treatment? How does the hearing impairment affect the quality of life in older patient/? What is the good, right the morally correct things do? Who gets sick? Why? Who stays healthy? Why? These are some questions she needs to ask herself and find answers.

Therefore, nurse needs to maintain safe work environment and give the following basic care.

WHAT ARE THE PROCEDURES OF DAILY LIVING THAT A NURSE NEEDS TO KNOW AND PRACTICE?

They are as follows:

What is Hand Washing?

Handwashing: Hand washing is important in every setting, it is an infection control measure or prevent the spread of microorganism. There is a Medical Handwashing, Surgical Handwashing and Social/Community Handwashing. Infectious diseases can be transmitted through contaminated hands so handwashing is most important for a nurse before any procedure. It is an effective infection control measure, which helps to prevent spread of microorganism. A vigorous handwashing under a stream of water for at least 10 seconds using soap is must, as soap contains antibacterial agent, which has a lasting bacteria static effect.

In addition, soap reduces the surface tension and facilitates removal of microorganism. Wash palms and finger, back of the hands, wash fingers and knuckles, thumb, fingertips, interlocking of hands, wash wrists and arm by running water and use friction in cleaning.

For the purpose of removal transient and resistant bacteria from fingers, hands and forearms.

It prevents the risk of transmission of infection to patient, and reduces the risk of transmission of organism to oneself, prevent cross infection. Because many pathogenic organisms grow in the hospital, nurses must know how to wash hands with its purpose. Infection is transmitted between individual with different pathogenic organisms. Cross infection occurs in the hospital through direct or indirect contact, e.g. while disposing of excreta, urine, stool, sputum, discarded dressing.

In surgical handwashing, the hand is thoroughly cleansed for about for about 3 to 5 minutes. When washing hands, they are held above the level of the elbows. So the water runs from least contaminated areas to elbows greatest contaminated area. A sterile towel is used to wipe the hands and arms, starting from the palms to the elbows. Before assisting to the operation hands should be washed for about ten minutes. Scrubbing with brush finger nails in running water. 10 stroke along finger nails. 10 stroke along all sides of fingers. Using betadine scrub or antimicrobial antiseptic agents to inhabit microorganism. Hand washing should be done when there are known multiple resistance bacteria before invasive procedure; in special care unit such as ICU and TO.

Warm water dissolves dirt and grease easily so it is more effective warm water to cold water. Soap lowers surface tension of water therefore should be used in sufficient amount to remove dirt.

Steps of medical sepsis file the nails short; ensure nails are free of nail polish. As short nails are likely to harbors resident and transient's microorganism. Remove jewelry and wrist watch as microorganism can be inside the setting of jewelry and under rings.

WHAT IS THE IMPORTANCE OF HEAD BATH AND HAIR COMBING?

The appearance of once hair reflects the general health of a person. The cleanliness and grooming/brushing of hair frequently is related to ones sense of well being. For a woman hair is the crowning glory. It is a factor on making a good impression on another person. Hormonal change, lack of good nutrition, unsound mental health affects the hair. An unclean scalp contains dirt, dandruff; excessive sweat due to this there can grow microorganism and parasites. Oily scalp also accumulates dirt, dust. Keep scalp clean by brushing to keep pediculosis away. Daily care by brushing and combing is must. Regularly shampoo in order to maintain cleanliness and promote growth. It helps in establishing good circulation, reduces itching, and infection and hair looks neat. It prevents and removes tangles.

WHAT ARE THE IMPORTANT POINTS TO REMEMBER WHILE GIVING THE HAIR WASH?

Take two bath towels one to protect pillow and the other to dry hair. Keep the patient flat in bed and remove pillow and back rest. Move patients had and shoulder to the edge of the bed. Place the pillow under the shoulder, so that the head is slightly tilted back. Roll newspaper and mackintosh in to a horse shoe shape. Place bucket on the low stool. Message all areas of the scalp with the finger tips. Add water to lather soap/shampoo. Wash and rise to remove soap until hair is clean. Squeeze all water from the hair and dry it with towel.

WHY PERINEAL CARE?

It involves cleaning external genitals and surrounding area. Since perineum area is warm, moist and not well ventilated and there are many orifices like urinary meatus, vaginal orifice, there are more chances of organism to enter into the body. The principle is from cleanest to less clean area. The urethral orifice considered as cleanest area and anal orifice is dirtiest area. As it is lying near anal orifice there is more chances of cross contamination and entry of organism from anal orifice to urethral orifice causing urinary tract infection.

Greatest risk for acquiring an infection of patient who are bed ridden, catheterized, recovering from rectal or genital surgeries, postpartum or postnatal period, menstruation time, genitor urinary tract infection, incontinence of stool and urine, excessive virginal discharge, patient who are unable to do self care etc.

If fecal matter is present clean buttocks and anus washing from front to back cleansing dry area thoroughly, cleansing reduces transmission of organism from anus to urethra or genitals. Put patient in dorsal recumbent position with flex knees and spread legs. Wash and dry upper thighs, wash labia major and wash carefully in skin folds. Wipe the area in direction from perineum to rectum. Same way cleanse thoroughly labia minora and vaginal orifice. In male patient, wash tip of the penis at urethral meteous first using circular motion.

Asses the condition of perineal skin, any itching, irritation, ulcers, edema, drainage etc. principles of body mechanism must be utilized changing position. Maintain proper body alignment. Avoid pressure especially over bony prominence by adequately padding. Use pillow, splints, and footboards to protect and maintain position. Friction and excoriation can disturb the skin integrity, which in turn can cause infection.

WHAT IS THE IMPORTANCE OF BACK CARE IN NURSING?

Back massage consists of rhythmically rubbing, squeezing and stroking tissue of the back, buttocks, neck and upper arms. It is straight, deep, firm strokes that is light, circular friction. It increase in local circulation and prevents pressure ulcers. It provides physical and psychological comfort and relaxation. It helps to detect early signs of bedsore, to keep skin clean and dry, it refreshes the patient and relives fatigue. Back care followed by change of position and comfort devices is vital. Put patient in lateral or prone position, expose the back, and prevent unnecessary exposure of the body by covering rest of the part. Keep skin smooth for massaging and avoid friction by applying oil, glycerin.

Effleurage or stroking from base of the buttocks up to the shoulder over upper arms and back to the base of buttocks.

Give continuous rhythmic rubbing increases circulation to superficial tissues and produces blanching and oxygen and nutrient reaches cells. Kneading or Petri sage is done by using palmer pressure by picking up tissue between thumb and finger and release before pinching or twitching. Give friction by exerting pressure in small circular motion around and not over bony prominences give gentle pressure with finger.

Low Back Care

Low back care- get out of bed by rolling on to one side near the edge of the matters, push up to a straight position by pushing off the bed with your arms while keeping your spine straight and swing your legs over the sleep of firm matters. Sit erect without slouching, use your leg muscles while rinsing from chair. When you stand for a long time, bend one knee to reduce stress on your low back. Maintain a body weight, exercise and walk or swim to strengthen your back muscles, wear low heeled shoes, eat a diet high in fibers and plenty of fluids to soften the bowel movements and reduce strain. Use proper body mechanism when lifting. Get adequate help if the object is heavy. Use the muscles of your legs, not your back, by bending at your knees to get closer to the object to lift. Never turn and lift at the same time.

WHAT IS BED BATH?

Know the anatomy and physiology of the skin. Skin is one of the sensory and excretory organs. It has important function such as protection, secretion, excretion, temperature regulation and sensation. Skin has three layers such as epidermis, dermis and hypodermic/ subcutaneous layer.

Epidemic layer is an outer layer and generates new cells. It contains melanocytes, which produce melaoes and dark pigments of the skin. As seilds against water loss mechanical and chemical injury and prevent entry of pathogenic organism.

Dermis is thicker layer containing collagen and elastic fibers. It contains nerve fibers, blood vessels, sweat glands, sebaceous glands and hair follicle.

Subcutaneous tissue contains blood vessels, nerves and lymph, fatty tissue serve as a head insulator for the body. It is the largest organ covering the whole body.

Bathing a patient who is confined to bed and who cannot have the physical and mental capability of self-bathing/self care.

Such patient as unconscious, semiconscious, strict bed rest, paralysis, heart failure, plaster cast, traction, etc. who needs daily bed bath.

Important Points to Remember

Before starting the procedure all the necessary equipments should be at hand and conveniently placed and avoid leaving the place until the entire procedure has been completed.

- Conserve the energy and the patient by avoiding unnecessary exertion. Only small areas of body should be exposed and bathed at a time.
- Each stroke be smooth and long rather than short and jerky
- Support should be given to the joints in lifting the arms and legs while washing and drying these areas
- Wash hands and feet placing this in basin clean thoroughly the fingers and toenails
- Special attention given to axilla and groins
- Upper part of the body bathed before the lower parts

- We wash clothes squeezed and made a mitten then apply soap and clean the area.
- Wash, rinse and dry the back with brisk circular movements
- Give back care on points and wear upper garments before lower extremity bath
- Powders used to prevent friction and absorb moisture
- Small amount of spirit in the back care used as it evaporates causes raid and excessive cooling of the body and also causes drying of the skin
- Nurse should maintain good posture and balance the body during bed bath *Sequence* should followed- face, neck, farthest arm, near arm, chest, abdomen, back, farthest leg, near leg and pubic region
- *Body mechanism* using alignment posture in lifting, bending and moving use center of gravity Good alignment is necessary when sitting, sanding or lying down. It helps to conserve energy, gives stability of the body maintained by base support. Injury and strain on lower back can be avoided, moving an object on a level surface requires less effort.
- Bed bath *purpose* is to clean the body and refresh the patient. It also increases and stimulates circulation and provides comfort and sense of well-being.

It helps to increase elimination through the skin and relieve fatigue and induces sleep

It provides active and passive exercise and to regulates body temperature, which helps to improve muscle tone and to provide comfort. Special attention to pressure points, and skin folds as skin is a soft flexible, membranous covering that is made up of epidermis and dermis layer; sebaceous glands and sweat glands are found in the skin; which secret sebum/oil.

Therefore, bath is an important intervention to promote hygiene. Cleaning done from cleanest to the less clean area .Water temperature for sponge bath 100-115° F. Ideal time for bathing is morning before breakfast along with morning care, and it should not be given soon after a meal. You have to wait for at lest one hour after meal.

There are different types of baths:

Sitz bath decreases pain and inflammation after perineal surgeries or pain relief from hemorrhoids

Hot water bath to relives muscle spasm and muscle tension.

Cool water bath to decrease fever and to reduce muscle tension.

Complete bed bath, partial bed bath/back rub where the secretions accumulate like face, hands, axilla, back, perineum, self-help bed bath.

Bathroom bath/shower bath/tub bath etc.

Baby bath-

Hygienic care-babies are bathed daily. They are cleansed of the blood, vernix caseosa or the stool.

Babies do not perspire for the first month. The newborns temperature regulating mechanisms are underdeveloped. So measures to avoid overheating and chilling are important. The nurse should use right judgment in selecting the clothing. The clothing should be according to the environment temperature. If the environmental temperature is too hot they develop prickly heat, a pin head popular rash on the face, neck and in places where skin surfaces are rough. When selecting the soap, select mild soaps, the soaps contains less alkali.

Types of bath

Sponging-sponge baths are given to infants who are actually ill. It is given in bed itself using a soft sponge cloth.

Tub bath- this is the common method of giving bath to a baby. The baby is submerged into the water in any tub or basin. Nurse's responsibility in tube bath- checks the temperature, respiration and color of the skin. Using powder on the skin may give rise to allergic rashes. Dress cord with spirit and cord power.

Warm water 37.8°C / 100°F

Articles—A tray contains bath tub, jugs -2, buckets-2,mackintosh and towel, bath blanket, soap with soap dish, cotton balls, oil, spirit and cord power, kidney tray, baby dress, apron

Lap bath—When tub baths are not possible, members keeps their babies on their lap and gives bath

Oil bath—Premature babies and sick babies are given oil bath. Oil is applied all over the body and it is wiped off with cotton balls or rag pieces. When the baby's body is covered with vernix caseosa, an oil bath is given to remove it.

Ideal time for bath—Baby should not be bathed within an hour after feed because moving may cause vomit. Most babies go to sleep after feed. Bathed before second feed, see that baby is not too tired or hungry.

WHAT ARE THE PRINCIPLE OF SKIN CARE

Intact skin and mucus membrane serve as the first line of defense for the body against injury and diseases. Pressure on the skin can cause tissue injury. The tissue over the body structure like occipital, shoulder blade, the ribs, the spine, the coccyx, the hip bones, elbows, ankles and heels exerting pressure against the mattress pressure decreases blood flow so decreased supply of oxygen and nutrients results in ulcer.

Change of position and soft, smooth and unwrinkled bed prevents bedsores. We need to give a special attention to patient who are thin, old. Friction causes injury, careless handling of bedpans, rough handling of skin such as prolonged message without lubrication, use of rough sponge leads to bed sores.

Prolonged application of heat and cold cause tissue trauma

Excessive moisture in contact with the skin for a period can result in tissue irritation. Patient suffering from acute or prolonged fever with profuse sweating; Patient with incontinenance of urine and stool; Patient with excessive vaginal discharge, and excessive drainage from wounds need special attention to prevent pressure sores.

WHAT IS A BEDSORE?

It is an ulcer occurring on the skin of any bed-ridden patient. Particularly over bony prominences or where two skin surfaces press against one another. Due to pressure, the circulation becomes slow and finally death/necrosis of the tissues occurs. Patient susceptible to it are acutely ill, whose general condition is rapidly deteriorating. Such as elderly bed ridden who make very little movement. Obese, thin emancipated having very little subcutaneous tissue pad at bony prominence. In addition, patient like Edematous, neurological, malnourished are victims of bedsores.

Pressure sore patients important complain which develop from confining the patient to bed which can be prevented by skilled nursing. Causes observe patients body weight redness, movement difficulty, loss of skin sensation; incontinence increases the risk of pressure sores five fold, friction, impaired circulation, and edema.

The ripple bed has an alternating pressure point pad used over the patients ordinary matters under the bottom sheet to provide regular, frequent automatic redistribution of the pressure areas.

Pathogens grow well in a warm and moist environment. Greater number of organism greater number of infection. The body temperature is suitable for the growth of microorganism. Sweat provides a moist environment. If hygiene is not maintained excessive perspiration, interact with bacteria and cause offensive odor. Any injury to skin should be treated properly. Persons suffering from communicable diseases should be isolated and precautions for current and terminal disinfection should be taken care of.

The skin that is poorly nourished and dry has less ability to protect and is more vulnerable to injury. Maintain health of the skin, well balanced diet containing vitamins and protein is necessary. Dehydration leads to cracks and crust formation. So patient with fever, excessive sweating with vomiting, diarrhea, on diuretics, not able to take fluid should be more cared. Poor circulation impedes nutrition to the skin and cause skin damage.

Message around boney prominence stimulates circulation, warm bath dilates superficial tissues and provides nourishment and helps in elimination of waste products. Sensory receptors in the skin are sensitive to heat; pain, touch and pressure. The temperature of water is regulated according to the tolerance of patient. Soap acts by lowering surface tension of water that aids in the emulsification of fat. By application of soap, bacteria are dissolved and removed from the body.

Make conscious effort to prevent bedsore that is mark of good nurse. Identification of the patient who is prone for bed sores. Assess the patient daily for redness, discoloration or blister. Keep patient clean and dry. Every two hour change position. Keep the patients skin well lubricated to prevent cracking by using powder. Protect the damage skin. Attain pressure points as often as possible. Call assistance to lift the patient before and after talking bedpan. Use special mattresses such as water or air mattress. Cut short finger nails. Use adequate amount of cotton under splint and plaster casts to prevent friction. Use comfort devices to take off the pressure of the linen and to increase blood supply. Encourage the patient to move in bed. Change linen as soon as they are wet. Teach patient hygiene.

WHY MOUTH CARE?

Oral cavity bounded by the lips in front, the cheeks on sides, mandibles, maxilla at the floor, palatine and born in roof and pharynx at the back. It contains tongue, teeth, gums and opening of salivary glands. Teeth consists of three parts, the crown the neck and root. Outer white part is enamel, inner to enamel is dentine, inside is pulp cavity, which contains blood essentials, and nerves root is surrounded by gum.

Effect of neglected mouth results in gingivitis, glossitis, root abscess, stomatitis, dental carries, periodontal diseases, pyorrhea, purulent discharge and tissue atrophy, severe pain and without supporting structures the tooth becomes very loose and falls out.

Formation of sorde and brown crusts, which is formed on the teeth due to lack of oral hygiene and neglected of mouth care a sticky color less layers of mucus forms containing which if allowed to remain the teeth becomes calcified called tartar is the primary cause of gum disease or dental carries. If there is, Bleeding gums do not use hard and stiff brush for brushing and take vitamin C as deficiency of vitamin C causes scurvy. Due to bad breath and if mouth is not clean properly, there will be decomposition of food materials left behind the mouth. Therefore, clean mouth makes a person feel fresh and comfortable, society acceptance, so have frequent mouthwash to prevent the complications.

Mouth is the portal of entry for food and digestion is starts here. To feel fresh and clean, to prevent mouth infection, to stimulate salivation, to prevent infection of parotid glands, to help to increase appetite, to prevent dental carries and tooth decay. The patients who are unconscious and helpless, patient on fluid or liquid diet, paralyzed patient, seriously ill, patient having local diseases of the mouth, malnourished and dehydrated patient who will require mouth care.

Solutions used in mouthwash are potassium per magnate used as a oxidizing agent which keeps mouth fresh. Acts as antiseptic and deodorant makes mucus membranes soft. In addition, Hydrogen peroxide, Normal saline, Soda -Bi -Crab etc too is used. Glycerin borax used when lips are dry and cracked. Seriously ill patient, unconscious patient should be removed dentures to prevent dislodging and blocking air passage. Dentures are kept in water when not in use.

WHAT ARE THE COMMON PROBLEMS OF THE ORAL CAVITY?

The oral cavity is an ideal place for bacterial growth by providing warmth, moisture, and food supply from the residual foods on and in between the teeth. A neglected mouth can cause various types of infection in the oral cavity. Halitosis is offensive odour of breath. It could be due to poor oral hygiene or a health problem. Dental caries causes decalcification of the enamel resulting cavitations of the tooth. Once the decay has started there is no cure.

Dental plague is a soft thin film of food debris with it teeth appear dull and yellowish cast. Tartar plaque remains on the teeth and becomes hardened and forms calculus. It is the primary case of gum diseases and dental caries. In pyorrhea, the pus formation in the sockets of the teeth. Sordes is born crusts which are formed on the teeth and lips are called Sordes. Bleeding gum, glossitis, root abscess, stomatitis, and parotitis to prevent these complications good oral hygiene and have frequent mouth care, prevent dehydration, after brushing teeth massage the teeth and any problem consult doctor.

Dental problems- due to cavities some children lose permanent teeth in school years which changes the shape of child's face and no amount of bridgework fully helps for lost teeth. Some teeth may be defective from the start, yet tooth decay is due to sugar, sweets, soft drink, lack of balance in diet, and vitamins, modern diet contribute towards it.

A tooth needs proper brushing at least twice a day. The upper teeth should be brushed downward, and the lower teeth should be brushed from below, upward. This should be done thoroughly too both the inside and outside surfaces. Using sweeping motion, so that bristles reach the cervices between the teeth, thus helping to remove any food particles.

Gums should be carefully messaged when brushing the teeth. Soften brush should be used. When the gums are soft teeth are likely to loose and fall out.

A clean mouth contributes towards an attractive personality and a happy disposition. An unsanitary mouth usually arises from neglect. Teeth are as important to your health as they are to your appearance. Nurses should educated patient for oral hygiene and good mouth condition.

WHAT IS NAIL CARE?

The nails are the portions of horny layer of the skin. Nails grow from the epithelial cells lying under the lunula at the proximal end of each nail. The cells of the nails are translucent parts. The part under the skin is called as nail root. The portion above the nail is called as nail plate. The portion, which is cut, is called as nail blade and the portion upon which the nails are embedded is called nail bed. The average growth of nails is approximately 1 mm a week. Fingernails are transmitters of bacteria. Dirt accumulates under the fingernails where bacteria grow. To keep the nails clean in order to prevent worm infestation.

Common foot and nail problems are corns, athletes/tinea padis it is a fungal infection cracking of skin or blister between toes and soles of feet occur because of wearing tight shoes.

What is the Pediculosis and its Treatment?

The state of being infected with lice is known as pediculosis. Lice are small wingless blood sucking insect which are found in head, in body/pedicel's capites. Pediculosis corporis perineal area, eye lashes. A patient complains severe itching of scalp and scratches giving rise to abscess formation. Restlessness and insomnia, lice are blood suckers cause anemia.

Parasicidles used- DDT 5% or 10% with talcum powder to dilute it. Carbolic lotion 1:40; equal part of kerosene and coconut oil. Apply it thoroughly on the scalp and is left for over night. Next day thoroughly bath is given and linen should be changed. For eggs repeat the procedure after one week. Nurse's responsibility is to asses order to see specific precautions, asses the general condition of scalp and hair. Protect the eyes.

How is the Carbonization of Bed Done?

Carbonization is cleaning of the cot and matters with carbolic acid solution prepared in the ratio of 1:20 with water, which has disinfective action against spread of infection.

Purpose to control cross infection, prevent microorganism etc.

To clean bed thoroughly, we need to mope the bed, starting cleaning from head to foot and back of the bed from foot to head.

Importance of Giving a Bedpan Explains

Bedpan is given to a patient who cannot move to toilet. Cover bedpan with cloth. Lift the bed clothes and fold gown up high, under back, remove the waist clothing, fanfold the bed clothes, remove sanitary pad, ;T' binder and keep it in kidney tray. Ask patient to flex knees and press heels against the bed, at the same time place your hand under the patient's pelvis raise the hips and slip the bedpan under patient. Place pillow under the back if required. Leave the patient for sometimes but do not forget. When bedpan is removed, turn the patient on his side and clean the anal area with washed with rough cotton balls. Toilet paper can be used too. Discard waste in container, cover bedpan and keep on stool and give comfortable position to patient.

Empty Bedpan Immediately

Notice color of stool, consistency, and amount, presence of blood, mucous and undigested food particles or worm should be notice. When patient ask for bedpan give attention to this job priority. Helpless patient more than one nurse required. Disinfect bedpan after use. Pay attention not to injure to operation stitches. If patient wants can allow for his own cleaning; Take care that patient does not get injure to his back, bedsore with friction. Avoid unnecessary exposure and discomfort.

Which are the Comfort Devices or Mechanical Devices Used?

They are as follows:
- *Back rest* is a mechanical device, which provides support for the patient in the sitting position
- *Pillow which gives relaxation, may substitute knee rest* and thus relieves pain and abdominal muscles and tendons beneath pillow because of the fear of thrombus formation and pulmonary embolism. Change of position at frequent intervals is necessary.
- *Footrest* is a device, which is firmly placed which helps to maintain the normal position of the feet at right angels of the leg. It prevents foot drop and gives comfort. Hard pillow, sand bags or footboard may be substituted to support the lower extremity even in offices.
- *Bed cradle helps to* support and to take off the weight of the top bed clothing and prevents it coming in contact with the patients of burns or to apply heat of drying plaster casts or used to supply desired warmth.
- *Bed blocks* are made up of wood or metal and are used to raise the foot end or head end of the bed. Bed blocks are used to prevent shock, to arrest hemorrhage, to retain enema and used after giving spinal anesthesia.

- *Sand bags* are used to immobilize a part as in fractures and to relieve discomfort. It also may be used to support the body and to prevent foot drop or wrist drop.
- *Air cushions* are made up of rubber and it can be infected with air. It is used to take of the weight of the body and to relieve pressure on certain parts of the body. They should not be used directly in contact with the skin they should be covered.
- *Rubber and cotton rings* are used to relieve pressure on certain parts of the body like elbow and heel.
- *Air and water mattresses* are used for very thin and very obese patients and those who are prone to pressure sores thus pressure against body prominences or areas subject to development of pressure sores will be reduced.

WHAT ARE THE TYPES OF POSITIONS USED IN NURSING CARE?

- *Knee-chest position*: The patient lies prone on the knees and chest. The head is turned to one side with a cheek on a pillow. A small pillow may be placed under the chest. The arms are above the head or they may be flexed at the elbow and rest along the sides of the head to support the patient partially. The weight of the patient should rest on the chest, knees, the knees are flexed as in a kneeling position, and the thighs are at right angels to the legs. This position are used for examination of the rectum and vagina, for sigmoidoscopy, postpartum mothers to do there exercise, etc where as patient with arthritis or joint deformity may be unable to lie in this position.
- *Dorsal recumbent position*: Patient lies on his back with the legs separated knees flexed and soles of the feet flat on the bed to table. One pillow is placed under the head. This position is used for assessment of head, neck, anterior thorax and lungs heart, breast, extremities and checking peripheral pulses.

    Also vaginal examination, rectal examination, operative procedure of the vulvas areas, and catheterization of the urinary bladder.

    This is not used for abdominal assessment as it causes contractures of the abdominal muscles.
- *Fowler's position* is more erect, in which an effort is made to maintain the position of the patient in sitting posture as merely upright as possible. In this patients have to raised to 80-90 degree. This position can be maintained by means of a backrest and additional pillows. The arms should be supported on pillows so that patient sits with arms supported in an armchair fashion. An air cushions under the buttocks and a pillow and bolster to prevent the patient from slipping. This position improves cardiac output, promotes ventilation and eases eating, talking and watching TV, relieves breathing, difficulty/dyspnea. Relieves tension on the abdominal sutures, helps in drainage of the abdominal cavity and helps to relax the large muscles of the back and thigh. This gives him a sense of well being and enhances self-care. It is contraindicated after brain or spine surgeries. Precautions such as change of position is important to prevent circulation from getting sluggish and development of thrombosis, pulmonary embolism specially when knee pillows are used for longer period of time which gives pressure on the blood vessels.

- *Lithotomy position:* Patient lies supine with hips flexed, calves, and heels parallel to the floor. The buttocks are brought to the edge of the examining table and the heels in stirrups. One pillow is placed under the head. The legs are well separated and the thighs are well flexed on the abdomen and legs on the thigh. Used in gynecological examination and treatment.

  Surgical procedure involving genitor-urinary system and assessment of female genitalia and rectum.

  It is difficult for patient with immobilizing arthritis or joint deformity. If the position is prolonged, there is a danger of embolism. This position embarrassing and uncomfortable. Patient with arthritis, joint deformity may be unable to assume this position.

- *Prone position:* Face down patient lies flat on the abdomen with head turned to one side. The head rests on a pillow. One or both the arms rest in a comfortable way either beyond the head or at the sides of the head. Used to assess the hip joint, posterior thorax; Patient with injury, burns and the surgeries of the back.

  To give comfort, relieve pressure from pressure sore, after anesthesia to prevent aspiration of saliva, mucus and blood. Contraindicated for patient with respiratory or spinal problems and after abdominal surgeries.

- *Supine position/dorsal/horizontal recumbent*: Patient lies flat on back with legs extended and knees slightly flexed. Supine is horizontal position. Pillows may be used under the head knees and calves to raise heels off the mattress, cotton rings at the elbow and heels, air cushion under the buttocks to take off the pressure and there by prevent pressure sores. In bed-ridden patient, a footrest is used to prevent the foot drop. Used for comfort, assess vital signs, physical examination of head, neck, and anterior thorax and for checking peripheral pulses. After surgeries involving the anterior portions of the body. This position provides access to pulse sites and prevents contracture of abdominal muscles. Patient with cardiovascular and respiratory problems may be unable to life flat.

- *Lateral/side lying:* Patient lies on the side with weight on his hips and shoulder pillow support and stabilize upper most leg, arm, head and back. In this position trunk is right angel to the bed increase the base support and comfort. One or both legs are bent and both arms are extended in front of the body because body weight is borne on the shoulders and hips semi prone all same in supine position.

- *Cardiac position* patient propped in sitting position by means of a backrest and pillow place on over bed table in front with a pillow on it. On which patient can lean forward and take rest. A small pillow for patient of cardiac asthma who cannot breathe easily

Position flat with the mattress in a completely horizontal position is to prevent pressure on any one body area and prevents pooling of blood in any particular area.

Trendelenburg improves blood flow to the brain and assists with drainage of pulmonary secretions. Reverse trendelenburg helps prevent reflux of gastric juices and allows adequate lung expansion.

Fowlers position facilitates lung expansion and breathing, *Hi-low position* with the entire bed raised to its highest level, lowered to its lowest level or positioned somewhere in between, this refers to the heights of the bed and highest adjustments may be made without interfering with the mattress positions, higher levels allow the nurses to work without bending over and injuring her back. Intermediate levels can be helpful in transferring the patient to a stretcher or the device that is at a different level.

Ideal features of hospital bed: Easy, comfortable, movement of the patient into various body position including face down, vertical position and maintenance of patient in any required position without allowing the patient to slide out of position or downward in the bed. Lack of friction and shears on the side skin to prevent tissue breakdown, allow for circulatory changes, solid, firm body support when needed for nursing care, medical treatment or emergency measures, such as cardiopulmonary resuscitation, independent control by patients who have minimal mobility.

HOW WILL YOU HELP THE HELPLESS PERSON IN BED?

To maintain muscle strength, encourage patients to move themselves as much as they are able. The strongest person should be at the patient's hips as this is the heaviest part of the patient. Pulling requires less energy than pushing your arms of lift sheet help protect patients skin for effects of frictions. Cradling helps avoid trauma to the patients' cervical spine. Side rails help prevent falls. Gradually the patient will be moved up to the desired position. Lifting force will be at the area of the greatest weight.

Weight should be equally disturbed between two nurses facing the direction of movement avoids twisting the nurse's back. Keeping the feet apart provides a wide base of support for stability. For over head trapeze is used; it should be high enough toward the head of the bed that pulling on it and flexing the elbows will indeed help the patient to move upward. Assess patient's skin condition, pain or discomfort caused by move, check any tubes present to be certain they are still in place and functioning correctly and secure them as necessary.

When the hip and knees are flexed, blood pools in the hip area and increases the danger of phlebitis pressure can cause injury to a vein wall and result in thrombus formation. Wrinkles are uncomfortable and cause pressure. Good body mechanism reduces muscles strain. Check bed linen for smoothen, replace head pillow, it should be large enough to support the vertical curvature but small enough that it will not cause cervical flexion contractures, and other positioning devices as needed, cover person raise rails, lower bed, replace call signals. Assess patents feelings such as lightheadedness, fainting, sweating, and diaphoresis. Be caution patient fainting, falling to floor; maintain center of gravity.

Impaired physical immobility- a patient who is immobilized will have high risk for injury, trauma, ineffective individual coping, impaired adjustment, fatigue sleep pattern disturbances, impaired social interaction, self care deficient e.g. feeding, bathing, grooming, toileting, body image disturbances, self esteem disturbances, hopelessness, powerlessness, anxiety and fear.

Inspect the skin of all immobilized persons every 2-3 hours as pressure from bony prominence can result in tissue breakdown. Maintenance of tissue integrity requires a constant supply of oxygen, nutrients and vital chemicals.

A method of removal of metabolic waste products, an adequate blood supply.

Born is living tissue and requires a balance of catabolism and anabolism, associated trauma or infection increases metabolic needs. The stresses and strains of mobility and weight bearing stimulate formation of ectoblastic cells. Bone decalcification occurs when there is immobility. The normal anatomy and physiology of the upper extremity is best suited to performing a wide range of motion, where as that of the lower extremities is best suited to weight bearing major nerves and blood vessels crosses the axilla as they extend down the arm. Movement of voluntary muscles promotes venous return to the heart.

Pain stimuli mechanical thermal and chemical agents; receptors for pain are nerve endings found chiefly in skin, muscles, joints, tendons, duramater and arterial walls. Trauma to the musculoskeletal system stimulates pain receptors.

WHAT ARE THE DIFFERENT TYPES OF BED MAKING?

Types of beds—Simple/closed bed, open bed, cardiac bed, blanket bed, admission bed, operation bed, fracture bed, amputation bed, rheumatic bed etc.

It provides comfort, safety, rest and sleep are important in maintaining health and promoting recovery from disease. Special care should be taken to provide comfortable beds to patient during their stay in hospital. It gives unit/ward a neat appearance, provides cleanliness and prevents bedsores. It enhances to establish interpersonal relationship, to economize the time and materials and energy. We can also teach the relatives how to take care of the patient at home.

Scientific Principles

a. principle of microbiology
b. principle of safety
c. principle of mechanic
d. economy of time

In bed making, remove sheets from the bed, lift the mattress and while loosening the bed linen never pull sheets with force. Always fold bed linen from top to bottom. Turn the mattress from top bottom or with three fold when bed is unoccupied.

Always arrange bed linen in correct order with closed side away room you before making the bed it should never touch the bed. While tucking bedding under the matters the palm of the hand should face down in order to protect your nails. Keep the open end of the pillow away from the entrance of the ward. Soiled linen should not be thrown on the floor but it should be kept in dirty linen box. Discard the soiled linen and sent to the laundry. Dusters to dust the mattress and sheets One dump duster to dust the furniture A bowl with antiseptic to carbonise the furniture.

After completing the bed making see that, the locker and chair are in place and that all the beds are in line. When making an occupied bed try not to cause discomfort by shaking the bed or moving patient unnecessarily.

Have all equipment on hand and arrange conveniently to handle in order of use. Wash hands before and after procedure. Do not expose patient unnecessarily. Do not cover his face while placing the linen. Start from head to foot and from clean to unclean, maintain body mechanism.

Make the bed smooth, unwrinkled and firm. Keep reasonable distance from the face at the patient to prevent cross infection. Protect patient from draught. Do not mixes clean linen with soiled ones?

Microorganism are found everywhere on the skin, on the articles used by patient and in the environment. Nurses need to take care not to transfer organism from source to new host by direct or indirect contact and prevent multiplication of it.

Never place the woolen blanket next to the patient's body except bath blanket and do not allow patient to lie on the mackintosh without lining. Practice economy of time, energy and material.

Arrange the bedclothes in such a way that they allow freedom in the daytime but come over the shoulders at night and the top linen loose over the feet. Make adaptation according to weather climatic differences, individual needs, customs and habits of the patient.

Always get extra help to make a bed for helpless patient and prevent them from falling. The side rails may be used if extra help is not available.

Inspect the cot, matters and pillow daily for the presence of vermin's and destroy them if found on the bed. The nursing principles such as individuality, comfort, safety and good workmanship should be kept in mind during the bed making.

Nurse's responsibility in bed making is preliminary assessment. Check the doctor's order for specific precautions regarding the movement and positioning of the patient. Assess the patient ability for self-care. Check the furniture and linen available in the patient unit.

Assess Articles Needed

- *Amputation/divided bed* are prepared for a patient amputated of the leg to take off the weight of bedclothes of side of operation. It is a bed, which is divided in two parts to visualize the amputated part of the lower limbs without disturbing patient. The purpose is to keep the stump in good condition, to be able to see the stump for hemorrhage. Make frequent observation and do the procedures without disturbing patient. Take extra top linen, bed cradle, two sand bags, tourniquet and dressing tray in case of emergency. Pillow with waterproof cover, and handle the patient skillfully.
- *Rheumatism/burns bed*—Purpose to carry weight of bed cloths from painful joints. Avoid direct contact with top sheet in case of burns.
- *Cardiac bed* is used to help the patient to assume a sitting position, which can afford him greatest amount of comfort with least strain. To relive dyspnea caused by cardiac diseases. Additional pillows, backrest and cardiac tables, air cushions, knee pillow, footrest.
- *Fracture bed*—Used for the fracture of the extremities to provide firm support by use of firm mattress that rest on a fracture board. Most fracture beds fitted to pulleys and weight where the insertion of the bedpans is difficult or lifting the hips is contraindicated.
- *Closed bed/ an empty bed/unoccupied bed* to receive the patient, it is fully covered with counterpanes to protect it from dust or dirt on admission of the patient. It provides a neat and tidy appearance of the unit.
- *Blanket bed—therapeutic bed-* cradle is used to immobilize the painful joint. The patient is dressed in woolen clothes. Additional warmth may be given by using the hot water bottles or by use of electric cradle. Foot board may be used to prevent foot drop.

- *Operation bed*—Pillow should not be used. To receive the patient conveniently prepared for the patient who is recovering from the effects of anesthesia after surgery. To be prepared to meet any emergency. To receive patient safely and comfortably quick transfer from the trolley to the bed without loss of time provide care. To provide warmth, prevent shock, injury, soiling and meet emergency. Keep temperature tray, BP apparatus, IV stand, hot water bag, oxygen cylinder with tubing and catheter, suction apparatus, bed block, artery forceps, tongue depressor, airway, kidney tray, gauze pieces etc ready. Why are *posture* and *positioning* often of more important?

Why are the Gloves Used?

They are used in medical asepsis to protect the nurse from pathogens they serve as barriers when the nurse handle contaminated articles. It is also worn in case of patient with poorer resistance. Gloves used for this are clean not sterile; it should be changed between two activities. Wash hands, dry and apply power to facilitate insertion and put on clean gloves. After attending the patient remove it and discard it in container with antiseptic solution.

Disposable sterile gloves—Wash hands and open the packet of proper size on a flat surface above waist level to prevent contamination. It is not powdered apply powder lightly to hands slip on easily. Identify right and left hand. Carefully pull the gloves over the dominal hand and ensure thumb and fingers in proper spaces. Carefully pull the second gloves over the non-dominant hand. After that, interlock hands together.

How do you understand cross infection as a nurse and methods of cross infection?

Direct contact—Organism can transit infection from person to person trough kissing, sexual contact, droplet infection and infected hands

Indirect contact—Contact with secretions and excretions of the infected person.
Through fomited-like instruments, utensils etc.
Through contaminated food and water
Through insects
Through dust
Through carriers
How will you prevent cross infection?
Hospital should be well ventilated.
Maintaining general cleanliness of the hospital sweeping and mopping with antiseptic solution daily.
All articles should be kept clean and dry. Roof should be sweeped to remove cobwebs once in a week. Bed, lockers, stools etc washed and cleaned. Mattress and pillows exposed to sunlight and aired.
Safe food and water supply in kitchen and pantry are protected from flies
Safe disposal of excreta and urine, stool, sputum
The bedpans, vermeils, sputum cups ect should be cleaned and disinfected before use
Safe disposal of refuse, discarded dressings garbage etc.

Destruction of rodents and insects play a major role on the spread of diseases, so they should be destroyed.

Prevention of direct contact with the infected person/barrier nursing, isolation technique.

Respiratory isolation—In case where the pathogens spread on droplets from the respiratory tract. In this masks were generally worn by nurses/gowns are also worn particularly when handling the small infants. The nose and mouth cover with tissue paper and dispose properly. If handkerchief is used, clean and disinfect it, restrain member of visiting take precaution while collecting sputum, keep reasonable distant from the patient from the droplet infection and nurse who is having respiratory diseases should not attend the patient.

Enteric isolation is indicated when pathogens in transmitted feaces for this type of isolation there is no need to wear mask, but wear gowns and gloves while hand washing soiled articles. Hand washing emphasized both the client and nurses. The excreta may be disinfected by eldding lime before disposal. The soiled articles such as linen should be disinfected before it is sent to dhobi.

Wound and skin isolation—In this, pathogens are found in wounds and can be transmitted by the contact with wound discharges usually gloves and gowns are used of this type of isolation safe disposal of dressing and discharges from the wound and disinfection of articles are very important stick isolation techniques should be followed. While coming for client with abscesses, boils, infected burns, gas gangrenes, anthrax, rabies, tetanus, venereal diseases, scabies etc of all these articles should be kept separate.

Great care should be taken by the nurses to prevent cuts or abrasions on their hands. Frequency and through hand washing reduces the chances of infection.

Blood isolation is intended to prevent transmission of pathogen that is found in the blood. So any equipment that comes in contact with the patient's blood should be carefully disinfected before touching another object or person.

General precautions: Maintain high degree of cleanliness.

Health teachings are to be taught to patient and relatives about spread of infections and its prevention.

Emphasis on hand washing after elimination, before eating and after handling patient or his articles.

Personnel caring for the sick should have immunization against communicable diseases.

Person with lower resistance should be protected.

If possible patient should be nursed in separate rooms, otherwise there should be at least a sufficient space between the beds, and screens may be provided to separate one patient from the other.

Medical aseptic practices—Medical aseptic refers to all practices used to protect the patient and his environment from the transmission of diseases producing organisms.

An article considered to be clean when it is free from pathogenic organism. Rinse the article first with cold water. Then wash with hot water and soap. It has emulsifying action and reduces surface tension, which facilitate removal of dirt. Use bristled brush, it helps to remove the dirt from the grooves and corners. Isolation gown should be made with long sleeves, long skirt and high neck to cover the clothing of the wearer. The isolation gowns should be used only once and then discarded. Hold the gown at the neck on inside permitting to in fold open part of the gown should be turned towards the nurse. Slide the hands and arms down the sleeves. Overlap the gown at the back as much as possible. Gown is worn only in the patients unit and never outside. It protects nurse's uniforms from contamination and controls known infection spread by indirect contact.

WHAT IS THE IMPORTANCE OF TAKING TEMPERATURE?

It may be defined as the degree of heat maintained by the body. It is the balance between heats produced and heat loss from the body.

The clinical thermometer is used in measuring body temperature and is available in both Fahrenheit and centigrade scales.

The principle on which the thermometer is constructed is the expansion of mercury when subjected to heat.

The thermometer is made of glass and consists of an end bulb containing mercury and a stem in which the mercury rises. This column of mercury remains at the height to which it rises and must be shaken down before talking it.

A constriction near the bulb prevents the mercury from receding and thus provides a more reliable reading.

Bulbs vary in size and shape to fit the different orifices.

It is accurate talking temperature by under the tongue and rectum, where good blood supply takes place.

The body temperature should be evaluated in relation to the patients usual temperature emotional state, time of day, activity and method used.

Oral temperature may affect by hot, cold food, fluids, smoking, mouth breathing, gum chewing.

Rectal method more accurate reading in children, unconscious; Contraindication in diarrhea, surgery

Oral temperature should not be taken within 30 minutes stimulates above mentioned. It is wiped after removing towards the bulb with rotary motion because friction is necessary for cleanliness.

Subnormal temperature is significant as high one as it may indicate shock, hemorrhage, or decreased body functioning. Rectal temperature is most accurate because it shows inner body temperature.

Most conscious patients are aware of the fact when their temperature elevated. Thermometer should not be kept longer than is necessary.

Types —core temperature is the temperature of deep tissue of the body, e.g. cranium thorax, abdominal and pelvic cavity. It is 37°C' and remains constant.

Surface temperature is the temperature of the skin, subcutaneous tissues and fat.

Regulation of body temperature: Neural control of hypothalamus in the brain controls body temperature. When body temperature deviates from normal hypothalamus activates heat loss and heat production impulses from hypothalamus are sent to periphery, which cause vasodilatation and vasoconstrictions.

Oxidation of food metabolism of protein, carbohydrate and fats affects temperature that is one gram of carbohydrate gives 4 calories of heat. One gram of protein gives 4 calories and one gram of fat gives 9 calories.

During Muscle activity, the stored glycogen is converted into sugar causing heat and blood supply to the skin increases and individual feels hot.

Strong emotions and excitement, anxiety and nervousness, etc stimulates autonomic nervous system, which causes stimulation of different organ in the body including secreting glands. Due to this heat is produced in the body.

Hormonal effect-increased activity of thyroid gland and adrenal gland produces heat. Ovarian hormones produces rise in temperature. When these hormones are produced in the blood, it stimulates oxidation process and produces heat.

Nursing responsibilities-identify the patient. Check the diagnosis, date, type of surgery. Any special instruction of taking the temperature in particular route.

Explain the sequence of the procedure to get the cooperation of the patient. Meanwhile time record patient's vitals; Have a clear understanding of tools- how to use its limitations in patient's situation. Keep the patient in comfortable position. Prevent cross infection.

Keep the thermometer three minutes while talking pulse and counting respirations. To get accurate reading hold it against the light. Electronic equipments use as standard one. Note temperature at bedside and other special sheets.

Watch precaution handling thermometer, comfort, economy and safety. Place watch within range of vision. Rectal thermometer is lubricated to reduce friction; Thermometers are easily broken, handle with care.

Boiling point 100°C / 212°F. Freezing point 0°C /32°F.

Commonly used antiseptic names and strength-

Savlon concentrate 10 ml mixed in one liter of water that is 1:1000

Eusol solution 12.5 gram boric acid, 1.25 gram bleaching powder in 100 ml water. Always use freshly made solution

Mercurochrome 2% solution dressing wound and preparation of skin

Potassium permanganate 1:5000 to 1:10,000 used in mouthwash, Sitz bath, irrigation of bladder

Lysol 1:100 solution.

Nursing Care II

WHAT IS THE IMPORTANCE OF WOUND CARE IN NURSING ? EXPLAIN

Wound is a cut or break in the continuity of any body structure.

Open wound is caused by a sharp blow or object. Open wound allows the entry of organisms and loss of fluid. It is in which there is destruction of the skin or mucus membrane, thus exposing the underlying tissues to the open air.

Closed wound has no break in the continuity of the skin and is damaged of tissues under the skin. They are caused by direct blow, blunt instrument or crushing. Blood vessels may be damaged and bleeding takes place into the tissues.

Surgical wound is an intentional type performed during surgery incisions under aseptic care. A wound is made under sterile conditions. Its edges are usually smooth and clean, healing will be quick. At the time of incised wound is free from infection. If the patient has received a steroid therapy, he will show delayed wound healing. If the patient is diabetic he will have complicated healing process and non-healing unless diabetes is treated.

The diet rich in protein, vitamin A and vitamin C, minerals particularly zinc. Undue pressure over wound is avoided, and a free cool circulation of air should be ensured, movements of part encouraged for better circulation and quick healing. If surgical wound is infected it may start oozing pus, foul smell. Therefore dead tissues to be removed to facilitate drainage of discharge, remove sloughs.

Some surgical wounds that are severely infected do not heal may be treated by debridement to remove all necrotic tissue. The nurse's responsibility is to prevent infection, prevent injury, assist healing, prevent cross infections and restore the function of the part. She must reduce the incidence of infection. Septic wounds need special care and aseptic technique.

Traumatic wound is an unexpected caused by accidents and occurs under septic conditions.

Incised wound are caused by sharp instruments, razor, knife and sword. It is a clean cut with sharp, smooth and regular edges.

Lacerated wound is torn, a cut with rough and irregular edges and bleeds profusely.

An *abrasion wound* is scraping or sliding of the skin surface. The removal of surface tissue by friction with a hard surface

A *penetrating wound* caused by an object passing through the skin, can be perforating and can cut open whole thickness of a wall of a cavity or organ.

A *clean wound* contains no pathogenic microorganism and *microorganism will invade contaminated wound.*

The *infected wound* also called *septic wound* where organisms invaded and clinical signs on infection produced.

Infection brought under control then healing process stars. This is called *proliferative phase*.

A scab is formed over the wound, the cells multiply, the blood vessels and the circulation established.

If patient has young age, adequate blood supply, good stamina and proper nutrition, and rest, immobilization, and absence of infection he recovers fast.

Due to old age, poor health, inadequate blood supply, diabetics, presence of infection wound healing is delayed. Wound healing is influenced by the extent of the injury, types of tissues injured, the presence of pathogenic organism and the presence of certain diseases. Many new cells must be formed in the healing process. Healing is slow in malnourished, anemic person.

A wound that is healing without infection is called **clean wound**. Separation of the wound edges is called **dehiscence**, here doctor may re-suture the wound or binder over a sterile dressing and allow it to heal. The care of the wounds is for purpose of aiding their healing and preventing infections or other complications but caution is needed when new cells are formed in the healing process.

Complication due to this there will be pain, fluid collection, hemorrhage, infection, abscess formation, cellulites, necrosis or gangrene, contractures.

Protect the wound with dressing, use sterile technique, clean it thoroughly, use antiseptic in and around wound, use antibiotics, immobilize the part with slings, bandages, splints or plaster, keep it clean and dry, elevate injured part.

Wound may be irrigated, surgical debridement to remove scalpel any dead tissues or slough, incision and drainage of abscess.

Change the dressing and apply waterproof ointment. Principles microorganism are present in environment, on the articles, and on the skin and bacteria travel along with dust particles.

Anything that touches the wound is to be sterile.

Wash hand before and after, sterile articles must be covered until it is time for use. Prolonged exposure makes them contaminated.

Consider the wound area cleaner then skin around; clean the wound from center to the periphery.

Practice strict sterile technique to prevent cross infection.

All materials touching the wound should be sterilized.

Instruments used for one dressing cannot be used for other dressing until sterilized. Create sterile field around.

Spread sterile towel around the wound. Pickup a dissecting forceps and remove the dressing, ask assistant to pour cleansing solution into the bowl.

Nursing responsibility to check the diagnosis and the general condition of the patient

She has to know the Purpose for which the dressing is to be done.

Check the condition of the wound the type of wound, type of suturing applied, application of medications etc.

Wound drains is inserted into a surgical wound, where large amount of drainage is expected and when keeping wound layers closed is especially important.

Accumulation of fluid under tissue prevents closing of the wound edges.

The drains are to be pulled out or shortened from day to day until it falls out on its own or as soon as its purpose is achieved.

The amount, color and consistency of drainage must be observed daily and documented. The drain site is considered as the most contaminated.

The skin around the drain is cleaned from the drain site outward.

Note the character of drainage such as serous clear watery plasma.

Sanguineous bright red in color and indicates fresh bleeding.

Sero sanguineous pale, watery drainage

Purulent thick yellow, green or brown drainage

Types of drains *gauze wick* used to keep the sinus open, so that healing can take place from the base of the wound.

Intercath or paediatric feeding tubes are used after mastectomy or thyroidectomy where a continuous transudate is expected.

These drains are installed with a continuous suction. *'T' tubes* used in cast of cholecystectomy.

Rubber tubes are used after chest surgery.

A water seal drainage system is attached to this type of drainage.

Corrugated drains used after incision and drainage of an abscess.

Delayed wound healing- Diabetes, malnutrition, poor tissue perfusion, steroid dependency, smoking; it can be prevented by using appropriate safety devices such as knee and elbow pads in sports. Use caution when using sharp objects, stop smoking, increase intake of protein and calories, control bleedings during surgery, and provide vitamin A to reverse the effect of long term steroids. Use antibiotics, use wound drains to limit dead space.

Wound assessment- what is the size of the wound?

Where is the wound located anatomically?

What is the colour of the wound?

Is the granulation tissue/epithelial tissue formed?

Are there signs of infection in the wound/is there any drainage?

What is the condition of surrounding skin?

Is it intact, red, indurate or macerated?

Is the wound painful?

Is it shallow open wound, moist wound, wet-to dry, debridement wound?

Are there blisters, abrasions, ulcers, deep wound with eschar?

Is it clean wound with profuse drainage? (Hydro gels have cooling effect, maintains moist environment, relives pain, and permits autotypic detriment, easily removed unless they dry out. Calcium alginates retain moisture, absorbent, left intact for several days. Normal saline speeds healing because solution is iso-osmolar and it keep wound bed moist. Hydrogen peroxide, beta din, acetic acid retards wound healing.

WHAT ARE THE TYPES OF SUTURES?

Interrupted suture is tied and knotted separately.

In continuous sutures, one thread runs in a series of stitches and is tied only at the beginning and at the end of the run. A suture is either surgical catgut or non absorbable materials.

Surgical guts absorbed readily.

It is easily handled.

Available in multitude of size

It can be used to suture beneath the skin.

When the wound is deep, a curved needle is used.

Cutting needles are three edged triangular needles.

These needles may cut into the tissues to allow easier passage of the suture.

Traumatic needles or eye needle

Traumatic needles with no eye

WHAT IS THE RESPONSIBILITY OF A NURSE IN FLUID BALANCE?

Like a fish torn from the sea, a human being deprived of water cannot live for long. Water is necessary to life and health. It is required in all body issues. The body fluids, such as blood, CSF fluid and lager percentage of water is needed in metabolism. In an infant 80% and in adult about 60% body weight is water. It is known as intracellular and extra cellular fluid. It also includes blood, saliva, digestive juices and other secretions. As part of the blood, it carries nutrients to the cells and waste substances away from the cells. Without fluid, the skin dries and cracks.

Water is vital to life and health. It is needed in digestion and other internal activities of the body; it carries nutrients to the cells and waste substances away from the cells. There is continuous loss of fluids in the form of urine, sweat, Faeces, and in air exhaled etc. it must be replaced to keep the correct balance of fluid for good body functioning. Hot weather activity perspiration and respiration, rate of metabolism, fever, stress, surgery, certain diseases and drugs affect fluid imbalance. The amount eliminated should be equal fluid intake.

Water lost also through vomiting, diarrhea, drainage from wounds, oozing from burns area, hemorrhage. It can cause shock, decrease urine out put, dehydration, thirst, weight loss of skin elasticity, salt holds water unless fluids are not restored and replaced may result in death. Nurses play important role in maintain fluid balance, by encouraging oral fluids, input out put chart, observation of signs of fluid imbalance etc.

Both fluid and electrolytes are important to maintain good health. The average adult having moderate activity and at moderate temperature requires about 2000 ml of fluid daily. Dehydration exists when the fluid intake is inadequate. The fluids are lost in body through vaporization from lungs through breathing, perfused sweating in fever, increased urine output, diarrhea, vomiting. Whenever body loses fluid, it needs to be replenished. The amount of fluid lost is affected by the weather, activity, rate of metabolism, fever, stress, surgery, certain diseases and drugs. Normally 900-1000 ml of fluid is lost daily.

To restore the fluid volume intravenous infusions are given if (1000 ml is to be given in 8 hours then 480 minutes patient 20 drops/ml therefore 41 drops/minute. *Complications* of iv fluids- circular overload, infiltration, hematoma, thrombophebitis, pyrogenic reactions, air embolism, infection at the needle site, allergic reaction, nerve damage) transmission of diseases. Nursing activities play an important role in maintaining fluid balance. Accurate measuring and recording of all fluid intake and output, careful observation for signs of fluid imbalance is nursing responsibilities. A carefully kept record of all fluid taken and excreted is of invaluable help to a doctor in treating a patient

The need for food, water and oxygen is common to all living organisms. What ever be the specific cause promote adequate nutrition to all body tissues.

For survival of cells, respiration, ingestion, digestion, absorption, circulation, synthesis of new materials, breakdown of materials for energy, response to the environment, exertion, and reproduction.

All cells require a continuous supply of oxygen, water, and nutrients for maintaining their functions.

The behavior of an individual is affected by nutritional state. Established food habits are difficult to alter eating, habits usually change during illness.

Administration of oxygen inhalations to relieve anoxemia or hypoxemia that is deficiency of oxygen in blood.

Also *indicated* in cyanosis, breathlessness, bronchial asthma, pneumonia and pulmonary edema, cardiac insufficiency, peripheral insufficiency, chest injury, anemia, poisoning, shock and circulatory failure, hemorrhage, under anesthesia, critically ill, asphyxia that is drowning, electrical shock, strangulation, inhalation of poisonous gases, during operation, obstruction in air-passage like foreign body, enlarge thyroid.

Oxygen is given by means of a mask, oxygen tent, trough the nasal tube or catheter.

Since oxygen acts as a drug, it must be prescribed and administered in specific doses in order to avoid oxygen toxicity that is tracheal irritation and cough, dryness irritation.

The dosage of oxygen is stated in terms of concentration and rate of flow.

Administer oxygen without introducing infection into the respiratory passage.

Lubricate catheter, test oxygen flow, and wipe the secretions.

Measure the length of the nasal catheter to be introduced into the nostrils.

Measure from the tip of the nose to the ear lobe

Mark the length with ink. Stay with patient till he is at ease.

Keep him warm and comfortable. Evaluate his progress by observing vitals.

Record the time, check apparatus, change the nasal catheter at every 8 hours, and change the nostril.

Oxygen to be stopped gradually, reduces the volume first, and then gives it intermittently.

Watch the patient for any deteriorating symptoms after the removal of it.

Irrigation is the washing or flushing of an area, using a large volume of fluid in order to cleans.

An *instillation* is a process by which a liquid introduced into a cavity drop by drop.

Painting of throat medications are applied to the throat by way of spraying and painting. Gastric lavage means to wash out stomach with solution.

Used in emergency treatment in gastric dilatation and poisoning

Tidal irrigation used in spinal cord injuries that may interfere with the normal functions of the urinary bladder.

Endo-tracheal intubations- in order to save the life of a patient

It is a passing of a tube into the trachea through the nose or mouth to administer oxygen, to remove secretion, to ventilate lungs, to establish and maintain airway, to administer anesthetic in operation room.

Suction through this is less effective and it is more traumatic because it can cause extensive and permanent damage to the larynx and the vocal cord.

In cases of severe burns and laryngeal edema, it is less practical.

A wide variety of tubes are in use for oro-tracheal or Naso tracheal incubation.

Very often patient have obstruction in their airway by a flaccid tongue falling back and obstructing the airway, inflammation and swelling of the mouth and pharynx following fracture or surgery of mouth.

In such situation, insertion of an oral/nasopharyngeal airway helps to keep the airway clear to some extent.

It is a fearful experience if the patient is conscious.

Suction and Drainage

Water seal drainage system—Called as closed drainage, which allows air and fluid to escape from the pleural space with each exhalation and to prevent their return flow with each inhalation.

Water seal acts as a one-way valve, permitting the unidirectional flow of air and fluid out of the pleural space, but permitting none to enter from the drainage system.

A water seal means the water in the bottle seals off the atmospheric air, preventing atmospheric pressure from entering the chest drainage tube and thus from entering the pleural space.

It is indicated after thoracic and thoraco- abdominal surgeries after chest injuries involving the pleura and the spontaneous pneumothorax.

In a thoracic surgery, the parietal pleura are incised and the pleural space is opened.

Atmospheric air rushes into the pleural space and the lungs collapse.

Additional air may continue to leak into the pleural space through the openings in the pulmonary pleural incision. the body's ability to reabsorb air and fluids from the pleural cavity is limited.

So the closed drainage system is used postoperatively to remove air and sero-sanguineous fluid from the pleural cavity.

It re-establishes normal negative pressure in the pleural space.

Promotes re-expansion of the lungs and restores the normal pulmonary ventilation.

It prevents return flow of air and fluid back into the pleural space from the drainage apparatus.

Prevents shifting of the mediastinum and collapse of the lung tissue by equalizing pressure on both sides

Proper placement of the catheter- Usually two catheters are placed in the chest

One of them is placed anteriorly through the second intercostals space to permit the escape of air rising in the pleural space.

The lower catheter is placed posterioly through the 8th and 9th intercostals space in the midaxillary line to drain off fluid accumulating in the lower portion of the pleural space.

The lower tube has a larger diameter than the upper one to enhance free drainage of the fluid.

These catheters are connected to separate water seal drainage from each tube and then to remove the non-drainage tube without disturbing the rest of the system.

When there is only one chest tube, it is placed in the lower portion of the pleural space. It must be located lower then the patient's chest.

This helps drainage by gravity. Moreover, prevents the back flow of air and fluid into the pleural space.

When shifting the patient from one place to another, the drainage apparatus may be placed over the bed to trolley after clamping at to places.

The length of tube not too short, it should give patient enough freedom for movement in bed, as short tube may pull off and the connection may get separated.

Maintain the patency of drainage tube. Observe the drainage amount, milking the tube helps to dislodge clots formed in it.

Fowlers position the patient helps to localize the fluid in the lower portion of the pleural space.

Continuous and gentle suction can be used when patient coughs and respirations are too weak to force air and fluid out of the pleural space through the chest catheter.

Postural drainage -is the drainage of secretions by gravity from various lung segments by the application of specific positions.

Supportive technique to postural drainage bronchodilator medicine, hot stem inhalation, cupping percussion forcefully striking the chest wall with cupped hands.

It is contraindicated when cyanosis and exhaustion are increased by its use.

Patient with increased intracranial pressure and head injury.

Patient with unstable vital signs, who cannot maintain particular position even with assistance.

Gastrointestinal decompression is the removal of fluid, flatus and other contents from the stomach and intestine through a tube passed into the stomach or intestines.

Purpose to drain fluid or gas that accumulates above the mechanical obstruction in the stomach or intestines

To prevent or treat post-operative vomiting and distension caused by the lessening of peristalsis following surgery, obstruction in the gut.

To deflate the stomach or intestine in case of dilatation and bring them back to there normal functioning

To aid in the healing wound in case of surgery, to prevent or check hemorrhage in case of esophageal varices

Types of tubes used- short tube called Nasogastric Levine, long tubes 6-10 feet long abbot miller, Harris, canter tube are in common use. Insertion through the nostril.

IMMOBILIZATION AND AMBULATION

Restraints are protective devices employed to prevent a patient from harming himself or others, to immobilize a part, to restrict the activity and to promote a feeling of security in a patient who needs control. They are useful in preventing injury to patients. It gives safety or protection and prevents a patient from falling from the bed or chair. They are released every two hours.

It is applied smoothly without obstructing circulation to maintain normal anatomical position. If numbness, loss of sensation, cyanosis it is removed at once. They are released every two hours to relieve pressure and improve circulation and provide comfort to patient.

They are made up of linen, canvas, leather, plastic, metal or wood.

Common types *Anklets and wristlets* used to restrict the activity of limbs in a patient who is potentially harmful to himself or others.

Also to prevent the patient from removing any appliances used in the treatment.

Simple one can be made by padding the wrist/ankle with this layer of cotton/gauze and a bandage is tied over this using a clove hitch and tied to bed.

Elbow and knee restrains—to prevent flexion made by making pockets or slots on a piece of cloth into which tongue blade will fit into

Then restrains wrapped around elbow/knee joints.

Mitt restrains used for children or confused patients in order to prevent patient removing tubes, dressing, prevent injury, scratching.

Prepared one available e.g. a sleeve of a shirt to stockinett

Body jackets—chest restrains, patient sitting on wheel chair to maintain his position and prevent him from falling.

Mummy restrains used to restrict the movements of the limbs in a small child during the procedure.

Safety belts are made up of electrically non-conductive materials.

These are used on stretches and operation tables in order to prevent the patient from falling.

The belt, which goes around the patient's waist, is attached to longer belt, which is then tired to the bed frame under the mattress.

Splints, plaster casts, sand bags, bandages, binders, slings etc. are used to restrict the movements of different parts of the body.

Side rails are attached to both sides of the bed to prevent patient from getting out or falling out of the bed.

It must be kept raised if patients who have altered levels of consciousness, the elderly, the debilitated patients and children.

Hazards such as tissue damage under the restrains due to constant friction.

Damage to the other parts of the body, development of pressure sores development of hypostatic pneumonia due to immobility.

Ischemia or nerve damage due to constrictive restraints.

Foot drop and wrist drop, asphyxia and aspiration pneumonia in-patient who is in supine position and has altered levels of consciousness and vomits. Psychic injury, where patient feels that he is punished.

Splints are used temporarily to support/immobilize injured part of the muscular-skeletal systems.

They are applied in management of fractures, sprains, strains, dislocations, lacerations, degenerative disorders or in a patient who is unable to sustain a part in functional position.

Types of splints are straight, Thomas, Braun, internal splinting, cervical collars, plaster of Paris slabs.

Plaster casts—Made from plaster of Paris are devices that incase an injured part in order to protect, to support and to immobilize it during healing process and are used to prevent or correct a deformity.

It is soft and malleable when moistened with water, but hard and durable when dry.

It becomes firm rapidly but takes time to dry.

During this setting period, there should be no movement, which may produce a crack in the cast and make a cast a weak.

Eventually this water evaporates leaving a dried mature cast which is light in weight.

Stockintte is a soft knit material which is an tubular form, resembles a footless stocking it without seams and is available in rolls of various widths from 5 to 40 cm to cover any part of the body.

It protects the skin under the plaster cast and forms a lining for the cast. It is also helpful to protect the edges of the plaster casts.

Padding with cotton is necessary to protect the skin and bony prominences under the plaster cast.

It is applied directly over the skin or over the covering of stockinette, it should be smooth and without wrinkles.

Special orthopedic tables are used for the application of the cast. It has devices to support the uncasted area leaving the area on which the cast applied is lift free.

Types of plaster casts wrist, above elbow, below knee, above knee plaster. Spica cast may be applied to the hip, shoulder and thumb joints.

Body cast-body jacket and *Bivalve casts* splitting it along both sides to treat surgical wound, to prevent uncomfortable abdominal distension, to allow space for tissues swelling it along both sides, prevent deformities.

Complication of plaster casts-impaired blood flow, nerve damage, tissue narcosis and infection, cast syndrome, wound infection and complication due to immobility

Removal of *plaster cut off*, apply an elastic bandage for few days, no forceful attempt should be made to remove the dead skin. Scrubbing the skin with strong cleansing agents should be avoided.

Traction is one method of reducing a fractured born.

Closed reduction/manipulation is performed by manually applying the traction to lock the ends of the fragments together and thus restore the normal bone alignment. X-ray films are taken and a plaster is applied.

Open reduction done under surgical asepsis. Metallic screws and plates, pins, wires, nails or rods placed through the bone fragments or fixed to the side of the born or inserted directly into the medullary cavity. *Hazards* of it may be introduction of infection into bones, accidental injury to the major nerves and blood vessels during surgery. Additional damage to the born caused by friction of devices, impaired circulation. *Reduction traction* means the restoration of a displaced bony part to its normal alignment, position and length. It is used to bring the displaced fragments of the broken bone into close approximation to one another and to maintain proper alignment until the healing take place completely.

It is mechanical pull to a part of the body for the purpose of extending and holding that part in a desired position. Traction is applied in the direction and *counter traction* is applied on opposite direction.

Purpose of traction is to restore and maintain the proper alignment of the broken bones, in a fracture site, relieve pain caused by spasm, prevent deformity, correct deformity, treat dislocations and spinal cord compression due to prolapsed intervertebral disc, to immobilize the part.

Skin traction wide bands of adhesives directly to the skin and applying weights to these bands.

Buck's extension and *Bryant's* traction and *Russell* are common.

Skeletal traction is applied directly to the bone.

Under strict antiseptic precautions a rustless pi or wire is inserted through the bone fragment distal to the fracture and out through the skin on he opposite side of the limb.

A metal U-shaped spreader is then attached to the wire or pin and the weights are attached to the spreader. Used in fracture of the femur, tibia, humerus and cervical spine

Specific tractions are pelvic, head halter.

VAGINAL IRRIGATION/VAGINAL DOUCHE

'Douche' is applied to a stream of fluid directed to a body cavity to flush that cavity. A vaginal irrigation is the washing of the vagina by a liquid at low pressure. It is similar to the irrigation of external auditory canal, in which the fluid immediately returns after being installed in. it is the flow without force of plain or medical water into the vaginal cavity and out again.

Purposes

- To cleanse the vaginal canal, removing an offensive or irritating discharge.
- To relieve inflammation and congestion of the genital tract – to arrest hemorrhage
- To stimulate the circulation of pelvic organs and promote absorption of exudates
- To stop hemorrhage
- To clean vagina in preparation for surgery

Solutions Used

- Sterile water 1500 cc, normal saline
- Sodium bicarbonate 2%
- Vinegar (acetic acid) 1%
- Salvon 1 in 1000 Potassium permanganate 1 in 4000
- Dettol 2% 11 in 60
- Bichloride of mercury 1 in 4000

The temperature of the solution is adjusted according to the purpose of the douche. Prepare the solution at 105°F/40.5°C and allow it to cool. To apply warmth the douche can be given as hot as the patient can tolerate, that is with 110°F (43.3°C).

Instructions

- Douches are given only on doctor's order. Not given during menstruation period, pregnancy.
- Thorough hand washing done, use gloves to prevent cross infection
- Remove pads, clean perineum, and use solution in correct strength.

The height of the irrigation can 24 inches from the level of patient's hips (pressure ½ pounds) should not exceed one pound.

The douche nozzle kept wet and lubricated regulate tap 105°F/40.5°C. It should take 20-30 minutes to give 2 pints – if glass nozzle is used examine for cracks – apply medications after douche if ordered – do procedure in adequate light.

Articles

Irrigating can with tubing and a clamp can fill with the irrigating solution.
Douche nozzle
Cloves 1 pair
Jug with extra fluid for irrigation
Bedpan or douche pan
IV pole
Apron

Sponge holding forceps and wet cotton swab and dry cotton swab – in csontainer
Cotton applicators
Medication if ordered
Macintosh and towel
Kidney tray/paper bag
Extra sheets and garments
Check name, diagnosis-doctors order, vitals, and perineum lesions if any
Explain the procedure
Maintain –privacy and screen-close door
  – remove backrest and extra pillow
  – bring the patient edge of bed
  – place mackintosh/towel
Cover patient with both blanket-fanfold expose only perineum-
Bottom garment raise above waist level-
Dorsal recumbent position-
Place pillow under the back for comfort

Eye, Ear, Nose and Throat Disorders

Administering prescribed treatments safely
  What is the physiologic effect of a warm irrigation on the eye?
  How spread of eye infection be prevented? Types of drugs used with purpose – eye disorders
  Important technique of administering eye drops, eye ointment, eye compresses, eye irrigations
  Why eye drops be directed towards the outer cantus?
  Purpose of ear irrigations
  Of what significance nasopharynx is continues with that of Eustachian tube.
  How would you make a normal saline solution for throat irrigation?
  Comfort → therapeutic effect → economy → safety.

Surgical Intervention →

Surgical operation is always a stressful for patient and family. Uncertainty of the outcome of operation fear of changed body image, dread of associated pain, fear of anesthetic, altered personal plans.
  Metabolic changes after surgical trauma listless, weak, no appetite, little interest in people and surroundings.
  Fear, will it be success? Will I wake up? Will I be paralyzed by the anesthetic? How will the operation affect my future life?
  What are chief causes of anxiety? Importance of position – post-operation pain and other type of pain.
  Describe surgical shock, internal hemorrhage thrombophlebitis of lower extremity, pulmonary embolism, infection of surgical incision, inability to void.

Postoperative abdominal distention

Measure employs to maintain an open airway

Skin preparation – areas covered from equipment and solutions needed – points of shaving process

Moving unconscious/semiconscious patient to safety from the bed to a stretcher and then to the bed

Following general anesthesia, what fluid and foods anticipated that the patient is able to tolerate.

Observe the isolation technique– identify scientific principles

Describe in detail an effective method of hand washing for use in carrying out isolation technique.

Kinds of protection required for various forms of isolation.

Room private – door closed

Gown worn by all entering room

Mask worn by all entering room

Hand washing on entering and leaving

Gloves worn by all entering room

Article discarded or wrapped – sterilization gown should lap well in the back to afford complete protection for the uniform.

Placing contaminated linen into bag within the unit avoid cross-infection

Therapeutic agents – support Respiration:

Respiration is a vital function of life. Oxygen exchange depends on the partial pressure of gases in the air and in the bloodstream. Relieve anoxia oxygen used.

Check order – oxygen flowing at the proper rate and pressure. No smoking. Is mask or canula positioned properly? oxygen turned off when disconnected from patient, maintain proper concentration. Is patient relieved of distress after oxygen started – is oxygen discontinued gradually? Is the patient observed frequently? How do oxygen get into the bloodstream?

Explain how an oxygen analyzer works. Fear of patient and relatives who receives oxygen your explanation.

Hood device for administering oxygen to pediatric patients so that oxygen concentrations may be easily controlled.

Administration of Injection

Articles

Tray with cover

Syringes and needles of various size

Transfer forceps in a jar containing antiseptic solution

Sterile cotton swabs, gauze in sterile container

Methylated spirit in container

Bowl with a water

Kidney tray and paper bag

Distilled water

Drug ordered

File to cut open the ampules.

Identify patient correctly

Explain the procedures

Provide privacy

Avoid mealtime

Have a friendly conversation

Make patient relax and comfortable position suitable for the type of injection

If giving Injection on hand gives, lying down position with patients hand flexed at the elbow

If giving on the buttocks, place the patient in a prone position or a lateral position with the knees flexed

Select the site suitable for the route

Dorsal gluteal site, draw an imaginary line of two bony landmarks that is greater troches of the femur and the posteriors superior iliac spine or divide the buttocks into four regions by imaginary line.

Superior iliac crest 'V' shape ventro gluteal site

Select appropriate syringe and need, obtain spirit swab

Recheck orders, label and expiry date

Calculate dose, premix solution be drawn for injection take solvent in syringe introduced into vial or ampoule, clean top, open as directed, mix powder, rotate vial in palm of the hand. Use strong needle to pierce rubber stopper. Mix well, change needle, cover it, select site, clean with spirit, pull back piston with left hand, if blood appears quickly withdraw needle.

Numerous blood vessels and nerves are lying below the skin. Careful selection of site can avoid injury to these areas.

A *drug* made up in a capsule in such a way that there is slow release of its contents. Medications are manufactured in a variety of forms or preparation to make them more useful or easy to administer. Drugs are classified according to their chemical composition, clinical action, and therapeutic effect on body systems, her purpose and uses by the symptoms relieved by the drug etc. the safe and accurate administration of medium is one of the most important responsibilities of a nurse. She should know name of the drug, classification, route and time and action, dosage, standards, type, source, order, prescription, weight and measured used, storing ad symbol and abbreviation, legal aspects etc.

Explain nurse's relationship with co-workers

Factors contributing to ward teaching

Responsibility of the staff nurse in student education

Importance of public relations in a health care set up

Relationship of staff nurse with the head nurse

The types of in service education

Various ways of fostering public relationship

Points needed to establish good inter personal relationship

Purpose and methods of clinical teaching

Principle to be kept in mind while giving health education

Objective of ward management

Objectives of forming time schedule in using services

The characteristics of good hospital policy

A criterion is on which the quality of nursing care can be evaluated important principle of administration.

State the Scientific Reasons and Answer the Questions (Assignment)

Why do we need to lubricate Nasogastric tube while passing it?

Why do we need always-fresh specimen for laboratory examination?

Why does urinary bladder need to be emptied just before doing a paracentesis?

Why Lumbar puncture is done between second and third; third and fourth lumbar vertebrae?

Why is it plaster of Paris stored in airtight containers?

Why are all the metallic articles removed from the body, while preparing patient for an X-ray?

Why oxygen passed through water before administering to the patient?

AB group blood is known as universal recipient and O group as universal donor- reason

Why do we need midstream specimen of urine collection for culture?

Why do we have to maintain strict antiseptic technique in doing dressing of the wound

Why stool for ova and cysts are to be sent fresh to the laboratory?

Why is oil base solutions avoided in nasal instillation?

Why tracheotomy tube sections done only five to ten seconds at one time

Skeletal traction provides a better traction than skin traction reason

Endoscope should not be kept moist and it is not autoclave reasons

Why only upright position slightly leaning on the cardiac table with arms and shoulders raised is used in Thoracentesis/

A: C" shaped position with full flexion of the spine is given in doing lumbar puncture why?

Patient after lumbar puncture instructed to lie flat in bed for 12 to 24 hours and foot end raised why?

Injection vitamin "K" is given to a patient several days prior to liver biopsy reason explain

A test dose is given to the patient before full administration of a day for X-ray explain laxative is given following barium swallow or barium meal explain.

What is the contraindication of colon irrigation?

Which are the principles to be observed during bandaging?

Which are the devices used to limit movement?

Classify wound according to its severity or injury that are the ways wound healing takes place.

What are the common types of drains used?
Mention the types of sutures and needles
What are the indications of intravenous infusion?
Which are the complications of intravenous infusion?
What precaution to be taken while blood transfusion?
What are the methods of steam inhalation and the drug that is used mention?
Which are the methods of oxygen administration?
Indication of oxygen therapy and the hazards of oxygen inhalation
Which are the solutions used for gastric lavage and vaginal douche?
What are the hazards of bladder irrigation?
Types of urinary catheters used
Types of colostomy and nursing problem that can occur while caring for the patient
Causes, sign, and symptoms of cardiac arrest
Mention the sequence of CPR
Indication, complications of tracheotomy
What are the parts of tracheotomy tubes, points to be kept in mind while suctioning
Parts of water seal drainage apparatus
Factors affecting the chest drainage
Indications for postural drainage, position and contra indication of postural drainage
Types and hazards of restrains
Types of plaster and its complications
Methods of performing biopsy
Indication and complications of different scope
The common used contrast agents in X-ray
Allergic symptoms that develop following angiography
Define the term wound, gangrene, contractures, suture, dialysis, hematoma, embolism, topical medications, gastric lavage, CPR, tracheotomy, postural drainage, biopsy, traction, vaginal douche.

CHAPTER 23

Nursing Care III

THERAPEUTIC AGENTS–SUPPORT RESPIRATION

Respiration is a vital function of life. Oxygen exchange depends on the partial pressure of gases in the air and in the bloodstream. To relieve anoxia, oxygen is used.

Oxygen is a drug. It has beneficial as well as undesirable effects. Oxygen administration can depress respiration drive in person with chronic obstructed pulmonary disease (COPD). Oxygen is a dry gas, it supports combustion, oxygen cannot be stored in the body, while oxygen is flowing, continue to evaluate the effects of oxygen therapy.

Check the flow rate on the flow meter periodically. Provide oxygen during all activities. Change the delivery device, humidifier and water reservoir daily, discard disposable equipment as necessary. Continue to observe the effects of the therapy. Recheck liter flow and device. Record positive effects of therapies to note if respiratory rate decreased to normal, heart rate returned to normal, breathing pattern improved and distress relieved. Also record negative effects, e.g. increased confusion, lethargy or other signs of carbon dioxide retention.

Report results of all blood gas measurements to physician. Never remove the oxygen source sudden it may cause a severe drop in the patient's oxygen. Respiratory changes can herald various problems in ventilation and gas exchange. Decrease breath sounds on the affected side indicate atelectasis. A rapid pulse is one of the first signs of a lack of oxygen. If the person seems irritable, confused, restless or disoriented, there problems may be hypoxia. Help with positioning may be needed to prevent pooling of lung secretions.

Oxygen administered in different ways → *Nasal canula* or inhaler, by *facemask*, or by shielding device. Different concentration of mask 28%, 40% tents are seldom used now, hoods are used.

Central oxygen banks- from which *oxygen is piped* throughout the hospital.

This method eliminates the necessity for bringing cylinders to the bedside. Some hospitals have installed hyperbaric chambers for giving oxygen under pressure. When piped oxygen not available oxygen is supplied for therapeutic purposes in cylinders that contain 244 cubic feet of oxygen under 2,200 pounds of pressure per square inch and pressure reducing regulator must be attached to the cylinder valve outlet. A regulator has two gauges.

One indicates pressure in pound per square inch the amount of oxygen in cylinder and other registers flow to the patient in liters per minutes.

ADMINISTRATION OF MEDICATION THERAPEUTIC AGENT

Nurse needs to look into- List all the medications ordered to your patient.

For what purpose is, each medicine ordered.

By what route is each being given?

What is the safe dosage range for each?

Precautionary measures and adverse symptoms

Which needle has the larger lumer, the 25 gauge or the 18 gauge?

For each of the four recommended intramuscular sites, identify the particular structures to be avoided during injection of needle. Anatomic boundaries – sites

Subcutaneous/Intramuscular – why to aspirate before injecting

Is the equipment sterile, skin properly prepared – needle sharp – air expelled – positioned patient – identification of site injection proper angel, is pressure exerted after the needle withdrawn – is ordered amount of drug given – is insertion, is withdrawal quick – arm/leg in a relaxed position – equipment clean and disposed.

Read Label 3 times: calculation accurate label clear – carry ID card – identify patient at bedside - drug give in time.

List medication errors – common abbreviations related to dosage, application, time, hour and route.

The nurse should be able to identify the container and medical gas cylinders by its colors. Respiration is the process whereby the tissues are provided with oz and coz is eliminated. The central mechanism in the brain which controls respiratory effects much be working and the nervous pathways from this to the muscles it controls must be intact.

Air contains about 20% of oz, this is adequate to saturate the hemoglobin of the blood in a patient who's respiratory and circulatory systems are normal. In many surgical conditions the respiratory and cardiovascular systems have suffered from severe interference. The result is that the circulatory hemoglobin is reduced in amount or is inadequately saturated with oz. for this reason the % of oz in the inspired air has to be increased. The distress of respiratory failure is often due to coz retention, not to lack of oz.

How the Medicine Trolley Prepared?

Tray with cover

A bowl of clean water

Ounce glass, Minim glass, teaspoon, dropper

Drinking water in a glass or feeding cup.

Mortar and pestle to crush and powder tablets

Medicine slab and spatula

Duster or towel

Kidney tray and paper bag

Plastic measuring cups

Medicine cards

Give position may aspirate fluids swallowing raise head end and extra pillows.

Give a mouth wash.

Ill tasting (lemon juice)

Read physician's orders and copy correctly

Compare the label – expiry date – measure

Calculate dose – shake tablet / cap into lid in medicine cups – do not touch with hands.

Pour liquids from side of bottle – hold measuring cup at the eye level and thumb nail correct measurement – do not pour excess wipe the mouth of bottle and close bottle tightly. Return to shelf. Do not mix medicines

Identify patient with medicine card, read name on bed – call by name, ask patient to repeat name, verify identification – give water/fluid to moister mouth – give medicine one at a time – stay with patient until he/she has taken – check patient's mouth

Verify swallowing.

Provide water after medication.

Remove towel – wipe the face

Record

Wash hands

Replace card

How will you Prepare the Administration of Injection?

Tray with cover

Syringe and needles of various sizes

Transfer forceps in a jar containing antiseptic solution

Sterile cotton swabs, gauze in sterile container

Methylated spirit in container

Bowl with water

Kidney tray and paper bag

Distill Water

Drug ordered

File to cut open the ampoules

Identity patient correctly – explain – provide privacy avoid meal time, friendly conversation, relaxed comfortable position – suitable for the type of injection.

On hand, give lying down position with the hands flexed at the elbow.

On buttocks, place the patient in a prone position or a lateral position with the knees flexed.

Select a site suitable for the route

Dorsal gluteal site, draw an imaginary line of two bony landmarks i.e. greater trochanot of the femur and the posteriors superior iliac spine or divide the buttocks into four regions by imaginary line.

Superior iliac crest 'U' shape ventrogluteal site. Select appropriate syringe and needle, obtain spirit swab.

Recheck order – label – expiry date – calculate dose – premix – solution be drawn for injection take solvent in syringe introduce into vial or ampoule – clean top – open as directed mix powder – rotate vial in palm of hand use strong needle to pierce rubber stopper mix well – change needle – cover needle with cover – keep in sterile tray and cover it – select site clean with spirit – pull back piston with left hand – if blood appear quickly withdraw needle.

UNDERSTANDING OF GASTROINTESTINAL DISORDERS

Scientific Principle

Very little absorption occurs in the stomach

Peristalsis is stimulated by a bolus of food

Glands of the mucous membrane when irritated secret increased amount of mucous

Gastric mucosa acts as a protective lining HCL responsible for the low PH of gastric juices production of acids in the gastric juices are derived from chlorides of the blood. Gastric antacids counteract HCL.

Siphon action depends on difference in atmospheric pressure. The negative pressure / vacuum liquid flowing from a higher level to lower

Liquid exert pressure because of their weight.

How is it Inserting a Rectal Tube Done?

Relaxation of the sphincters guarding the anus facilitates passing the tube and is promoted by encouraging the patient to take deep breaths during the process of insertion; very gentle, slow insertion of tube is done.

A well-lubricated tube may be inserted smoothly past anal sphincters if there is (pillow) no obstruction.

Combined length of the anal canal and the rectum is about 6" to 7" in length, 3" or 4" inserting may be sufficient. If inserted further curve of the sigmoid flexes may cause injury to mucosa.

Patient lie on left side—descending colon of left side if patient sphincter control not sufficient then give bedpan while administering the solution – gloved during procedure. The head of the bed should not be elevated more than few degree, when drugs are given by rectum, they must be well dissolved to aid absorption, sodium chloride solution 0.9%, is isotonic non irritant – prepared ordinary salt with water.

Solution commonly used → soap, sodium chloride, magnesium sulfate, glycerin, sodium biphosphate, mineral oil 150 Ml 4 to 6 ounce Barium sulfate colon X-ray drug aspirin, and suppository form.

Fluid Flow maintains pressure – about 12" above the rectum is the usual height.

The solution is prepared at 105°F (40.5°C) comfortably warm to the mucus membrane.

Assess bowel sound before and after treatment record amount of fluid returned, the colon, consistency and amount of faeces, blood, mucus, or other unusual material.

Teach → sound nutrition, exercise, activity adequate fluids, and self-care.

Cleansing, retention, return flow, enema.

What is Gastric Lavage or Stomach Wash?

Gastric lavage means a washing out/irrigation of the stomach; to cleanse the stomach operation of stomach, to obtain bacteria that is swallowed with lung secretions cells for cytological study. Aspiration of gastric contents – fluids food or gas. To wash out or irrigate the stomach with a solution frequently as an emergency treatment in gastric dilatation with poisoning.

For the purpose to remove the ingested poisons irrigate matter from the stomach. Relieve nausea and vomiting cleanses stomach as a preparation for surgery.

Siphon device used for drawing a liquid from a higher level to a lower level. It has short and long arm. The short arm is placed in the liquid to be emptied and a long arm is carried down to the lower level. The air must be first removed. Fluid flows because of the difficult pressure in the two arms. Fluid will flow from the shorter arm to the longer arm until the air enters system and produces equilibrium once again.

In gastric lavage, the gastric tube acts as the siphon tube. The part of the tube that goes into the stomach acts as the short arm and the part of the tube that lies outside the body acts as the long arm of the siphon. The end of the tube that goes into the stomach lies under the level of the fluid in the stomach and the other end of the tube goes below the level of the stomach. When the air is expelled from the tube, the contents of the stomach will drain out.

Plain water is particularly useful when the poison is unidentified. Normal saline types of poison – antidotes given, 500 Ml fluid is introduced.

In Funnel Method the tube is introduced either orally or through the nose. Making sure tube is in the stomach; aspirate the contents first and save it for lab in case of poisoning. Attach a funnel to the tube and fill it with the irrigating fluid. Expel air and allow fluid to run – to discontinue pinch the tube and pull it quickly, give a mouth wash and dry the face.

What is Gastric Intubations?

It is an introduction of a tube into the stomach for therapeutic or diagnostic purposes

The tube is passed via nose or throat (inserted through a surgical opening, i.e. Gastrostomy) purpose of gavage, levage or gastric aspiration artificial feeding.

For stomach, the Levin tube used which is narrow and can easily be passed through the nasal passages.

A duodenal tube often used is the Miller Abbot tube, which has a metal tip and a balloon on one end. The balloon is inflated after the tip has reached the duodenum. There is a partition inside the tube one passage for introducing air, water, or mercury to inflate the balloon.

The inflated tubes stimulate peristalsis and the other for drainage to flow out

Other tubes used are the cantor tube.

Harris tube and the ships tubes

Each time the patient swallows, the tube is advanced through the esophagus toward the stomach. It is passed smoothly along the posterior wall of the pharynx and into the esophagus; otherwise, it may accidentally slip into the trachea and obstruct the patient's airway.

A positive test for determining that the tip of the tube is in the stomach is aspiration of stomach contents.

If the tube has slipped into the trachea the patient will experience difficulty in breathing and it may become cyanotic.

The conscious patient will cough vigorously nurse must listen with stethoscope over the stomach as air is injected through the tube with a syringe. Clear bubbling sounds could be heard.

After a poison is taken, immediate action should be initiated to remove it from the stomach before it enters the duodenum to save patient's life. If the tube is to be passed into the duodenum, it is carried down from the stomach by peristalsis after several hours.

A disposable tube is economical and can be discarded after use.

Drainage bottle used in gastric suction to be washed well to prevent odors as well as transfer of pathogenic organism.

Litmus paper may be used to test the aspirated material; stomach fluid has acid reaction intestinal will give alkaline reaction. There is losing of sodium chloride it is replaced by infusion of salt solution chemical antidotes – acid – alkali vice-versa. The gastric tube acts as a siphon, siphon suction requires a bent arm. Gravity suction using this bottle method. Electric action pump

The pressure in the stomach is at atmospheric pressure, the stomach contents will flow into the area of less pressure or into the upper bottle.

Before the tube is withdrawn, a clamp is applied to cut off air pressure on any fluid that remains in the tube and to prevent its dropping out as it passes the trachea.

Nursing responsibilities → aid elimination, relieve intestinal flatus, administer medication.

How will you Set-up Enemas Tray?

Tray containing
    Enema can, tubing, glass connection, screw clamps.
    Rectal tube adults or rectal catheter placed in a kidney tray
    Mackintosh and towel
    Jelly/Vaseline
    Rag pieces in a container
    Hot/cold water in jugs
    Soap jelly in a bottle
    Ounce glass
    Paper bag
    Specimen bottles SOS (in case of need)
    Bedpan
    Fluid
    Provide privacy – cover patient with sheet/bath blanket
    Remove the back rest and pillows
    Place mackintosh towel under buttocks close to the edge of the bed
    Remove bottom garments or raise waist level.

Drape patient – expose only anus.

Wash hands.

Attach the tubing to the enema can and clamp.

Prepare solution 30 Ml soap jelly – 600 Ml water.

Remove froth – hang can on stand and adjust the height at 45 cm from anus.

Attach rectal tube to the tubing – loosen the screw clamp allow small amount fluid run into kidney tray, regulate flow – pinch tube, lubricate tip, 2 to 4 inches – lubricate rag piece, insert the tip 8 to 10 cm while patient exhale deep breath – 500 to 1000 ml stop if patient develops discomfort. Remove gently, hold with rag firmly against anus.

Place tube in kidney tray

Observe patient.

Question Assignment

How is aspiration of gastric contents done?

Three kinds of tubes that may be put in stomach principle of gastric lavage.

How far rectal tube inserted?

Why it is this distance – equipment used – explains difference in amount of solution given for a retention enema and for cleansing enema.

Mouth wash after tube is removed, lubrication tube clamped, solutions used, temperature correct, strength correct etc.

Suctioning an Endotracheal/Tracheotomy Tube

Patient on mechanical ventilation do not suction routinely.

Explain procedure

Collect necessary equipment → sterile suction catheter, sterile gloves, sterile water, sterile cup or basin, sterile tousle, goggles.

Wash hands

Use sterile technique to open sterile package fill cup with water, put on sterile gloves and connect catheter to suction source. Designate one hand as contaminated for disconnecting, bagging and operating the suction control.

Lubricate catheter tip with water and gently insert catheter until obstruction is met. Do not apply suction during insertion. Apply suction intermittently while withdrawing catheter in a rotating manner. If suction volume is large – continuously

Limit suction time to 10 seconds.

If secretions are tenacious, instill SNL normal saline solution into the airway.

Dispose of catheter by wrapping it around fingers of gloves and pulling gloves over catheter discard all equipment in proper waste container.

Some tracheotomy has two cannula – an outer which remains in place and inner which can be removed for cleansing – mucus that accumulates on the inside tube – it is not sutured – several precautions are required – tapes should not be changed 24 hrs after the insertion procedure, 7 days tubes not changed – if tube disloged replaced it at once – unlock inner cannula – drain water from cannula – immerse cannula in sterile water, shake and dry – give – semi-Fowler's position.

Management of Artificial Airways: Tracheotomy: Explain

Tracheotomy is an artificial opening made in the trachea into which a tube is inserted:

To establish and maintain a patent airway

In emergency, it is done to relive the respiratory distress.

In prophylactic, the need is anticipated and a tracheotomy is done.

According to duration, it can be temporary and permanent.

In a high tracheotomy, the incision is above the so-called isthmus of the thyroid.

In a low tracheotomy, the incision is made below the isthmus of the thyroid at the level of third and fourth ring of the trachea.

Indication- observation in the air passage in the upper part of the trachea due to tumors, stenos is edema of the larynx and trachea and intrusion of foreign bodies.

Unconscious patients with respiratory depression

Patients undergoing major surgeries of the mouth and neck such as hemiglossectomy, mandibulectomy, laryngectomy, radical neck surgeries etc. ; laryngeal and tracheal trauma and paralysis.

Patient with head, neck, chest injuries

Infection of mouth, diphtheria, tetanus, poliomyelitis, accumulated secretions, and neurological disorders, severe burns, poisoning, etc.

A variety of tubes is available which are made up of plastic, stainless steel, sterling silver. Care to be takes not lose any part of it or else completely set becomes useless.

Complications- excessive secretions, foreign bodies, swelling of the mucus lining can cause obstruction.

Accidental expulsion during coughing, suctioning, while changing the linen, untying gown.

Infection of the wound, erosion chocking.

No time should be lost to act, delay causes worsening of the situation.

Follow strict aseptic technique to prevent introduction of infection, select proper size, and length tube, patient should not be left lone.

Assess sign symptoms of respiratory distress such as chest wall retractions, stridor, restlessness, apprehension, confusion, exhaustion.

The patient is positioned on the back with pillow under the shoulder.

Hyperextend the head and neck, so that the trachea becomes prominent

Supervise the patients self care, teach him what to do if the tube becomes dislodged, how to prevent accidental aspiration of fluid, hair, cotton, while taking bath.

Swimming is prohibited; use a face mirror in front of them when they wash their face to prevent entry of soap and water into the stoma.

Care taken when using after shave lotions, neck power, spray directed towards face, neck and chest.

Teach the patient how to talk, take a deep breath and then close the tube with a finger and then speak one or two words.

Again, take the breath and do the same.

- *Placement of endotracheal tube/tracheotomy* both tubes have inflated cuffs. Fenestrated tracheotomy tube with cuff deflated, inner cannula removed and tracheotomy tube capped to allow air to pass over the vocal cords.
- *Speaking tubing cuff inflated* – the second tubing is connected to a source of compressed air/oxygen. When the ports on the second tubing is occluded, air flows up over the vocal cords allowing speech with an inflated cuff.
- *Types of tubes* → (a) Disposal oral/nasal with cuff stopcock and pilot balloon (b) Shile and portex tube with cuff – inner cannula – decannulation plug – pilot balloon (c) Bivona tube one cuff is dilated on tracheotomy tube.
- Inflate cuff to minimal occluding volume. Place stethoscope over the neck and auscultate listen for air leak while slowly injecting air into cuff. Continue until no leak is heard. If the patient does not require mechanical ventilation auscultate while ventilating minimal leak technique to inflate using this technique, first determine minimal occluding volume. Then withdraw 0.1 ML of air, allowing a small leak.

Attach a pressure recording manometer to the pilot balloon port with a stopcock and attached syringe – pressurized the tubing leading to the manometer by injecting a small amount of air into the tubing. Close stopcock to the syringe.

Measure cuff pressure after a deep inspiration or after a breath, using a manual resuscitation bag.

Cuff pressure should be <20, 25 cm H_2O to prevent tracheal necrosis. If the cuff will not hold air, the tube must be replaced.

Explain Catheterization

Urinary catheterization is the introduction of catheter through the urethra into the bladder for the purpose of removing urine.

Drainage of urinary bladder by means of a rubber tube inserted through the urethra for the purpose of empting the bladder. Various factors cause difficulty in voiding. When patient is unable to void or to provide for continued emptying of the bladder to obtain sterile specimen of urine and used in paralyzed muscle damage patient to release distention and help in voiding.

To measurement of residual urine, (bladder may not be completely emptied at each voiding often associated with a partial obstruction of the bladder outlet e.g. enlarge prostate. which leads to bladder infection and calculus formation). Retention of urine (patient experiences difficulty in voiding in strong emotions, fear, embarrassment, surgery, injury to spinal cord, urethral strictures, hypertrophy of the prostrate gland, child birth) Complete emptying of a bladder prior to surgery or delivery. After surgery when a patient unable to void e.g. radium implant into vagina.

The urinary meatus is never sterile, due to vaginal orifice and anus, organism are introduced by catheter. To get clean specimen external meatus cleansed by soap and water or mild antiseptic solution; 50-100 ml voids is discarded and 100-200 ml void is taken in sterile specimen bottle.

Types of catheter used are rubber, metal, glass and Foley's that is self retaining catheter. Bacteria are present in air; therefore catheter is kept covered until ready to use. Plastic catheters on time used and discarded. Catheter size-French scale; small number 8 to 10 for children; number 14-16 for adult female; number 20-22 adult for male are used. Disposable catheterization set with all materials use sterile rubber gloves.

For adequate visualization of perineal area dorsal recumbent position given

Support helpless patients thighs with pillows will aid her in proper position. Protecting the fingers with sterile cotton balls/gauze will help to keep them from slipping while exposing the meatus. Press upward and backward labia majora with thumb and finger-locate above vaginal orifice. Drape patient in modified dorsal recumbent position with draw sheet or bath blanket, after fan folding bedding.

Three swabs- each swab used only one cleaning stork. Labia majora then minora- lubricate tip of catheter hold it three inches from the lubricated tip with gloved finger of a free hand. Inserted 2 to 3 inches the urine appears. Hold it steady resting hand on pubis as flow decreases; it is gradually withdrawn about half inch at a time.

Foley's catheter is typical indwelling which is constructed with a double lumen. The main channel is for drainage of urine and the other for inflation of balloon through the sidepiece, using saline or water. Foley's catheter after it has gone to bladder 5-30 cc water in injected, and when balloon is distended which inflates a balloon like bulb below the tip of catheter inside the bladder. This bulb then does not allow slipping out of catheter through internal urethral orifice. Tie the tube to prevent leakage of water; when removal of catheter remove injected water through its thinner end. When water is withdrawn, and then gently removes catheters. Female catheter taped to the inner thigh and, male it is taped on the abdomen. Connecting tube must be long for patient to move above freely in the bed.

In *male drape* patient by applying bath blanket to upper chest, fold upper bedding down to mid-thigh, make mackintosh piece across thighs under the penis if necessary. The foreskin of the penis is retracted, to expose meatus.

Then Cleansed with Dettol solution, wiping with backward motion from meatus

Catheter is lubricated about 18 cm and inserted until 18 cm/60 degrees until urine comes, no force is used.

Types of catheterization are urethral, cardiac, arterial, ureteric, and *supra-pubic catheterization*. In supra-pubic catheterization catheter is introduced into urinary bladder through an incision made above symphysis pubis to relieve acute retention of urine when urethral cauterization with rubber catheter fails.

Indwelling/self retaining catheter is introduced through urethral meatus to bladder in certain cases where continuous evacuation of bladder content is required. The catheter can be put temporarily or permanently for long time. Foley's catheter is used in this. It is indicated in for collapse of bladder, neuorgenic bladder, after prostrate operation, for incontinence of urine, for continued drainage of urine, for recurrent retention of urine.

Articles

A sterile tray
Sterile catheter (Foley's)
Small bowl with 2% Dettol
Cotton swabs
Gauze piece
A pair of gloves
Sponge holding forceps
Kidney tray
Specimen bottles
Bowl with liquid paraffin
Dressing towel and slit
Syringe with Distilled Water
Drainage tubing and collection bag
Unsterile tray with mackintosh and towel
Kidney tray and paper bag
Spot light
Clean linen as needed
Pint measure
Move patient to the edge of the bed
Give dorsal recumbent position
Cover patient with a sheet/bath blanket
Place mackintosh and towel
Arrange articles
Focus light
Drape patient
Both legs are completely covered with sheet.
Open the sterile tray – aseptic techniques.
Place sterile kidney tray on sterile towel
Lubricate catheter – clean perineum with cotton balls dipped in the antiseptic lotion using the forceps.
Clean labia major on both sides – step by step
Discard the swabs and forceps in kidney tray catheter introduced – pick up catheter with gloved hand – maintain position balloon on indwelling catheter is inflated. Attach the drainage tubing when bladder is empty remove catheter slowly.

Nurses help in maintenance of proper position. Sound of urination may induce urination, give hot water bottle over suprapubic area, give plenty of water or fluid orally, pour alternately warm cold water, to relieve spasm.

Explain Physiologic Process of Dying

There is a series of changes that make the nearness of death known. The process of dying is a progressive failure of the vital functions. Organs absolutely essential to the maintenance of life are known as vital organs. The three vital systems are the CNS, circulatory system and respiratory system.

When patient is told that he has a fatal or terminal illness is a shocking experience, allow the patient to pull together. In spite of the fact that each of us expects to die and expects all others to die, an element of uncertainty and helplessness is almost always present when death does occur. Few are wholly prepared for death. The patient's perception of death physiologic needs, personal, moral religious, legal and economic issues associated with death will invariably influence the patient who encounters it, whether it comes gradually or suddenly without warning.

Should the patient be told the truth? Silence deprives the patient of the empathetic communication with physician, nurse, friends and family at a time when it is most needed. Religion perception death will affect moral and religion attitude towards it. he may be prepared to die and look forward to it as a deserved rest, relief from pain or spiritual renewal. Patient may want to talk, cry, silent, wish to be alone are reactions keep patient physically comfortable and offer realistic hope that the patient's life has been well spent.

The shock may be so great as to cause patient to panic and restore impulsive, uncontrolled and unrealistic behaviour. Fright and terror may bring about patient to seek escape way out (magic – faith healing). If the feeling kept inward patient life ends in depressive state, patient becomes resigned to this state.

When patient accepts death as sense of fulfillment, he welcomes death as an end of suffering. Finds peace wishes to be alone.

During periods of stress and uncertainty, spiritual needs tend to increase in intensity. Death is a family matter, and to separate the family from patient at this time would be unkind. Relatives of dying patient pass through emotional stages similar to those of the patient. The younger the patient, the more involved will the family be, if it is an adolescent or young child. An expressive handshake a mere presence of a familiar face seems to be more helpful.

Patient view death from individual and cultural value system to be respected as a key importance.

Provide added strength and help the patient feel safe and better able to face dying with courage and dignity.

What are the Physical Signs of Death?

How is the dying patient made physical comfortable – control pain, visit close family when patient desires, encourage family members to express their feelings of grief by accepting their behaviour. Allow the time to answer questions asked by family and time to just listen to them.

Identify various emotional stages through patient passes.

What Coping Mechanism Used?

What methods are most appropriate in caring for the terminally ill patient and his family?

Long-term Illness

Chronic illness—An illness of 3 or more months duration illness/disability, i.e. permanent or recurrent and that requires a long period of care, e.g. disease of the heart and circulation, respiratory disease, arthritis, rheumatism, cancer.

The long-term illness like diabetic who will need special diet and medication for the rest of his life.

Nursing Care IV

BLOOD PRESSURE

On admission any change in health e.g. patient complains of chest pain or giddiness. Before and after surgical procedures. Before and after an invasive diagnostic procedure. Before and after administration of drugs or nursing intervention that affects vital organs. As a routine procedure to assess health status of patient blood pressure assessment is indicated.

Blood pressure refers to the force excreted by the blood against the vessel walls as it flows through them; maximum blood pressure is exerted on the walls of arteries as systolic pressure. The lowest pressure exerted on arterial wall during ventricular relaxation is known as diastolic pressure. The difference between systolic and diastolic pressure is known as pulse pressure. The normal blood pressure in an adult is 120/80 mm Hg. Blood pressure reaching above 150/90 mm Hg is known as hypertension and reading below 90/60 mm Hg is known as hypotension.

Regulation of blood pressure—Hemodynamic factor like cardiac output, blood volume, peripheral vascular resistance and blood viscosity the factors that increase the blood pressure are- raised in cardiac output, raised in peripheral vascular resistance, raised in blood pressure/and raised in blood viscosity. Or decreased blood pressure are decreased cardiac out put, decreased peripheral vascular resistance, decreased blood volume and decreased blood viscosity.

Age—The blood pressure is lowest at birth, rising at adolescence and slightly lower with aging. But due to increased peripheral resistance the blood pressure rises in elderly average person according to age.

High blood pressure is a condition where the pressure is constantly higher than normal. HBP reading is 140/90 on three consecutive measurements at least six hours apart. It various for pregnant women as 140/90 on two consecutive measurements six hours apart consistently pressure high causes the heart to work harder than it should and can damage the coronary arteries which leads to hart attack. Brain leads to stroke, kidneys leads to renal failure and the eyes leads to blindness.

Factors like smoking, a diet rich in fat and cholesterol and stress are some of the few causes, moreover 95% cases is unknown. No one has been able to determine a direct link between the factors and high blood pressure. Limit salt at the table, check food labels for sodium content, choose unprocessed foods, limits meats and cheeses, limit pickles, salty snakes, soy sauce etc. fruits and vegetables are excellent source of potassium. Exercise is the cornerstone therapy for it. do yoga and surya namaskar asana which is a beneficial, brisk walking, bicycling, rowing, swimming, rope jumping, gardening, dancing, golf, fishing etc.

- New born BP is 40 mm Hg systolic
- One month it is 85/52 mm Hg
- One year it is 95/65 mm Hg
- 6 years it is 105/65 mm Hg
- 10 to 14 years it is 110/65 mm Hg
- 14 years ad above it is 120/80 mm Hg.

Time of the day—BP is low in the morning and rises as much as 5-10 mm Hg by late afternoon and decreases during sleep.

Sex—Women have lower blood pressure than men of the same age that after menopause there pressure increases over men.

Relationship to food intake it increases after food.

Exercise and muscular activities it raises

Body built it is higher in obese in comparison to thin persons

Emotions, anger, fear, excitement, and pain it raises

Posture tends to be low in supine position in comparison to sitting and standing position

Diseases condition affecting circulatory system kidney, cranial tumorous and increased intracranial pressure cause alteration in it.

Certain drugs like narcotic, analgesic increase pressure and amyl nitrite nitroglycerin muscle relaxants decreases pressure.

Assessment of blood pressure- it can be monitored directly or indirectly, the direct method regulates insertion of thin intravenous catheter into artery tubing connects catheter with an electronic sensor it is only in operating room.

The indirect method requires use of sphygmomanometer. The nurse may use auscultation palpation or both. It is the most common technique. Sphygmomanometer consists of a cuff with tubing rubber pump a manometer. Cuff contains an airtight flat, rubber bladder covered with cloth. It has hooks to fasten the long tube attached to the rubber bladder one is connected to manometer and the other is attached to a bulb. It is used to in flute the bladder. Manometer has a mercury filled cylinder to tube calibrated in millimeter, when the mercury rises in the tube top surface of mercury forms a convex curve called meniscus. Another type of monometer is called aneroid manometer. It has a cuff which is attached to a round calibrated dial with a needle which indicates pressure.

Stethoscope—The bell of its amplifier emits low frequency sounds such as those commonly made by heart and blood within the vessels it is often used when pressure assessed.

Techniques of talking blood pressure- the nurse assess true blood pressure by listening to korot koff sound/series of sound listened while measuring pressure. The brachial artery and poplited artery are the most commonly used.

The Korotkoff sounds are the first sound is heart which is onset of phase represents systolic pressure of blood pressure is 120/80 mm Hg. 120 mm Hg is systolic pressure. The sound number represents the diastolic pressure which is noted at which either a charge in or cessation of loud and distinct sound take place tapping the faint clear sounds that graduals becomes louder the first tapping sound may be followed by an absence of sound/auscultation gap and indicates systolic pressure reading.

Murmuring slow swishing sounds that increases with cough of deflation.

Knocking crisp clean sounds, indicates first diastolic pressure reading.

No sound indicates sound diastolic pressure reading.

Alternate techniques of measuring systolic pressure- palpating the pressure- it is also known as sensory detection method. It requires only the use of sphymanometer for the return of the pulse by this method only systolic pressure is recorded.

Listing Doppler ultrasound-it only measures systolic pressure.

Electronic indirect pressure meters- helpful for people who wish to obtain their own pressure. The reading is displayed in digital numbers.

Transducers device that converts non electronic parameters like T.P.R and Bp to electronic parameters.

General instruction for talking pressure- provides comfortable position that is sitting or lying down. Select appropriate size cuff according to the age of the patient and site of talking pressure 12-14 cm for arm and 18-24 cm for the thigh for an adult.

Cuff size according to age is given below:
- Under one year 6 cm and 2.5 to 3 size length
- 1 to 4 years 15 cm and 5 to 6 cm
- 4 to 8 years 15 to 24 cm and 8 to 9
- 8 years and above 24-38 cm and 12 to 18 cm cuff with length.

Deflate cuff slowly, there should be no noise in environment view the meniscus from above the eyelevel in mercury sphygmomanometer. Inflate the cuff 20-30 mm/Hg above the disappear of the pulse. Ensure the tubing is not crocked or rented. Place the bell on the direct area of the artery. Before measuring pressure consider the factors which cause variation in normal condition. Do not take pressure more than three times in succession at the same site. Do not take pressure on arm on which IV infusion, injury, shunt or fistulas for dialysis, female with radical mastectomy. Mark the instrument error.

Assessing pressure of lower extremity the cuff may be wrapped around the thigh or above the ankle thigh pressure measurement requires larger cuff place the patient in flat prone or supine position with cuff centered mid thigh over the popliteal artery. Auscultate or palpate blood flow at the popliteal fossa. A systolic pressure measured at the thigh is generally 20-30 mm Hg higher than that or measured in the arm.

To measure in the ankle place the patient in flat supine position and place a stand and arm cuff first above dorsal is pedis artery as the cuff is deflated.

Cuff size—The width of the cuff of the bladder should be 40× of the circumference of midpoint of the limb. The length should be 80× of the limb circumference or about twice the bladder width.

Increasing pulse rates indicates a shorter diastolic phase of the cardiac cycle, with reduced coronary blood flow. This signal on increased cardiac load; decreased diastolic pressure may indicate reduced coronary blood flow, which could signal an increased cardiac load. Edema indicates decreased venous return and increased cardiac workload. A sudden drop in blood pressure and increase in pulse upon moving from a horizontal to a vertical position indicates orthostatic hypotension. After 10 minutes in a standing position, a difference of 30-35 mm Hg is mean arterial pressure and an elevated pulse indicate orthostatic hypotension. A rapid pulse is one of the first signs of a lack of oxygen.

Procedure

Explain the procedure to the patient to promote co-operation, relaxation and reduce anxiety. Wash hand to reduce cross infection. Use spirit swab to clean ear pieces and diaphragm to reduce the cross infection. Select the arm by removing constrictive clotting ensure proper cuff application palpate brachial artery and position cuff 2.5 cm above brachial pulsation above antecubital fossa. The two tubes turn towards the palm. Sphygmomanometer should be placed at eye level. If aneroid type of it is used dial should be facing up ward inflating bladder directly over brachial artery ensures that proper pressure is applied.

Wrap cuff evenly and snugly around the upper arm loose fitting cause false reading palpate radial artery with finger tips of one hand and inflate the cuff with other hand 30 mm Hg above the point of pulse disappearance and close the valve identity approximate systolic pressure. Place the stethoscope ear pieces in ear and diaphragm on the brachial artery proper placement or stethoscope ensures optimal sound reception of accurate reading. slowly release the valve and allow the mercury to fall at the rate of 2-3 mm Hg per second rapid or slow decline in mercury level cause inaccurate reading.

Note the point in monometer when the first clear sound in heart and antinue to deflate gradually noting the point at which the sound disappear or changes the first sound indicates diastolic pressure.

Deflate cuff rapidly and completely and remove the cuff continues cuff inflation can cause arterial occlusion resulting in numbness of arm. Record the reading accurately, make patient comfortable.

HOT AND COLD APPLICATION—EXPLAIN

Local Hot Application

Hot water bottles, chemical heating bottles, Infra-red-rays, ultra-violet rays, electric cradles, heating lamps/pads, short wave diathermy given known as *dry heat method. General* dry heat taken by sun bath, electric cradle, and blanket bed Heat therapy is applied specified length of time. Hot water bag temperature not more than 52 Celsius or 125 Fahrenheit in adult, child/elderly 46 Celsius/155 Fahrenheit Hot water bottle filled only two third, air is expelled, close tightly and check it for leaks. Put cloth cover to protect skin. Electrical heating pad has safety problem, moisture danger the causing an electrical shock. Heat lamp of 25 watts placed 45 cm/13 inch from the area to be treated. Disposable heat pack chemicals are activated to produce heat at a controlled temperature. Are safe and convenient to use, discarded after use. There are many ways of applying heat to bring improvement and healing.

Nurse's Responsibility

Nurse's responsibility checks the diagnosis and the physicians order. Assess the type of application to be used when specific orders are not given. Inspect the body part that is to receive the treatment for any lessons. Determine the duration and frequency of the treatment. Presence of any disorders that contraindicate the use of heat applications Condition of heat appliances check for their working conditions Check the articles available in the clients unit. Temperature of water should be checked. Record the procedure and observe the patient for its therapeutic effectiveness.

Warm soaks (local baths) hot fermentations (compresses) poultices stupes, paraffin baths, Sitz bath known as *Moist Heat method.* Steam baths, hot packs, whirlpool bath i.e. full immersion baths known general Moist Heat. Application of moist heat is use of an agent warmer than the skin which is applied in moist form to produce local effect.

Effects: Vasodilatation, Increased capillary permeability, increased local metabolism increased oxygen consumption, decreased blood viscosity, increased blood flow, lymph flow, decreased muscle tone. The maximal increase in the circulation and tissue temp occurs after 20-40 minutes of exposure. Increases nutrients, carry the waste materials and excess fluid away faster reducing edema, given relaxation of muscle tissue relieves pain, congestion, speeds up pus formation which allows earlier removal of pus permitting healing.

Purpose

Heat decreases pain decreases muscle tone promotes healing, stimulates circulation relives deep congestion, removes crust formation (softens) provides warmth, stimulates peristalsis, supply warmth and comfort relieve retention of urine, relives muscles spasm.

Contraindications: Causation in all unconscious patient, or loss of sensation, heat is not used in malignancies, patient with impaired kidney, heart and lung functions, acutely inflamed areas, e.g. acute appendicitis, tooth abscess because heat may cause them rupture, thus spreading infection weak, debilitated, paralysis will get burn and not able to respond to hot application open wounds, bleeding, edema, headache, metabolic disorders, e.g. diabetics, arteriosclerosis young and old people and patient with high temperature.

Principles

→ Water is a good conductor of heat. The flow of heat is from the hotter area to the less hot area.

→ Take hot water, wipe the outside of bag insulate the hot water bag from heat loss Vaseline/oil to apply on the skin if reddened check temperature of water.

→ Preparation of *articles*/patient unit/*steps procedure*, tray – Hot water bag with cover, jug, duster, Vaseline, lotion thermometer if available to check temperature of water.

Cold Application

→ Dry cold – Hypothermic moist cold – cold sponging, cold bath, cold packs, ice bag, ice collar, cold compress, Vasoconstriction decreases muscle tone, lymph flow, oxygen consumption, metabolism etc.

→ Relive pain, prevents gangrene, prevents edema and inflammation, controls hemorrhage, checks the growth of bacteria, reduces the body temperature cold anesthetize an area to treat epitaxis, moist cold to the eye.

→ *Contraindication:* Patient with shock and collapse – diabetes patient, muscle spasm present, patient having a sensation of numbness infection wound, low temperature, shivering.

→ *Infrared and Ultraviolet lamps*: Transmit red rays, intense heat, effect are pigmentation of the skin, production of vit D and bactericidal effects, 20-30 Months duration, wear goggles to shut out reflected harmful rays. It is used to provide heat to a localized area of the body. Infrared radiation penetrates 3 minutes of tissue at the most, thus provides surface heat.

The advantage is its dosage can be regulated easily. The application has no weight; patient can be made comfortable and left undisturbed through out the treatment. It is frequently used in the treatment of decubitus ulcers, obstetrical and gynecological causes to promote the healing of a suture area on the perineum. Precautions are check the patients skin is dry, ask the patient to wear cotton clothes. The lamp should be placed 18-24 inches above the skin area. The rays should strike the skin in right angel. Terminate the treatment at the first sign of readness or pain.

→ *Electric Heat Cradle* is a bed cradle, inside of it is fitted a light source and a thermometer installed . It is used when a large body parts is to be treated e.g. to dry large plaster body casts in burns, sheet is used over the cradle to prevent draughts. Blankets can be added over the cradle to maintain the heat levels. It is also used when the patients condition does not allow covering the skin with gown or sheets.

→ *Electric Heating Pads* are composed of an electric coil inside of a water proof rubber covering and is provided with a heat control switch to maintain the desired temperature levels. It should be covered with a flannel cloth to absorb the perspiration and to insulate the pad.

No wet dressing should be applied when EP used, - do not apply EP with pressure – increases chances of burns.

Do not lie or lean against heating pad.

- *Ultraviolet lamps* treatment is the exposure of the body to the ultraviolet portion of the light spectrum. Mercury vapors lamp or a cold quartz lamp is used for producing ultraviolet rays. The effects of the exposures are pigmentation of the skin, production of vitamin D and bactericidal effects. It is mostly used for a number of skin conditions. The lamp is placed 30-36 inches away from the skin and the duration is 20-30 minutes. Precautions are the patient and the therapist must wear protective goggles as it may cause conjunctivitis.

- *Shortwave* or microwave *diathermy* – converts electrical/vibrational energy into thermal deep in the tissues. See that all forms of metals are removed from patient's body.

Nursing Principles: Good workmanship – therapeutic effectiveness, safety, comfort, economy of material.

Sponge Bath: 110 to 115°F or 43.3 to 46.1°C

Tub Bath: 90 to 100°F or 32.2 to 37.8°C

The entire *sponge* should take about 15 minutes. Neck and right arm 5 minutes and left arm 3 minutes, chest and abdomen 3 minutes, right thigh and leg 3 minutes, left thigh and leg 3 minutes, back 3 minutes.

Diathermy → Is a heat producing high frequency current furnished by a diathermy apparatus. It is good for penetrating deep tissues like pelvic organs and bones.

Moist Heat → Compress are small light moist applications of folded gauze. Fermentation are prolonged applications of warm moist flannel stupes are short intense application of heat over the abdomen in the form of hot moist flamed, e.g. turpentine used.

Medical Fermentation → Compresses are directly to the part where there is no wound. Simple boiled water dipped, drug such as boric or magnesium sulphate or potassium permanganate solution used. It is used to relieve congestions in adjoining parts or internal organs, purpose is to withdraw a large volume of blood to the surface, the area is converted is large to relieve congestion in kidneys, axilla to hips, joint inflammation wrap completely around joint, relieve pain in stomach, never cover the nipple while applying to the breast area, avoid burning.

Surgical Fermentation/compress: → Application of moist heat using sterile gauze of other material to an open wound or an abscess purpose to produce hyperemia, aid the process of suppuration, to promote drainage, relieve pain and muscle spasm, reduce swelling and congestion.

EXPLAIN CARE OF THE PERINEUM

Clean the perineum from the cleanest to the less clean area. The urethral orifice is considered as the cleanest and anal dirtiest cross contamination.

During the perineal care, clean the area around the urinary meatus before cleaning the area around the anus.

Male perineal care begins washing at the tip of the penis. Move down penis shaft towards body, wash the scrotum last, and then proceed to cleanse the anal area. The perineal area has hair that tends to harbor organism.

Articles

A tray containing mackintosh, a jug with warm H_2O or antiseptic solution, wet cotton balls in bowl. Gauze in container, long artery forceps in a kidney tray, paper bag, clean linen, pads, dressings, soap, soap dish, towel, bed pan – place a mackintosh under the buttocks over the draw sheet – offer bed pan – ask patient to flex the knees and lift her buttocks by pressing the foot against the mattress, place bed pan – untie the pads.

Steps

Wash hands
Pour water over perineum
Clean the perineum using wet swabs
Hold the swabs with forceps and clean from above downwards towards the anal canal,
Use one swab for one swabbing
Clean the perineum – vulva – labia minora both sides – inside of labia majora both the out side labia majora both sides. - clean the perineal region and anus well. Turn the patient to one side and dry buttocks. – apply pad – remove mackintosh – change linen – arrange bed – make patient comfortable replace articles – boil forceps – remove screen – wash hands – record procedure.

Types if gastric gavage: It is an artificial tube feeding through nose mouth, esophagus to the stomach. Nasogastric, orogastric, Gstrostomy from stomach wall tube put.

Rye's Tube Feeding:
Tray containing:
Feeding cup with water
Mackintosh and towel
Cotton tipped applicators
Saline or sodadicarb solution
Ryles tube in a bowl of ice
Lubricant jelly, glycerin, paraffin
Adhesive plaster and scissors
Rag pieces in a container
Paper bag
Clean syringe/a funnel in a tray
A glass of feed in a bowl of warm H_2O
Ounces glass
A bowl with H_2O
Clamp
Suction apparatus
Nasogastric → a tube passed through the nose esophagus into stomach.
Orogastric → passed through mouth into stomach.
Patient sits on chair or put him Fowler's position or raise the head with extra pillow.
Place the mackintosh and face towel across the chest and under the chin to protect bed linen.

Keep kidney tray

Remove the dentures – put in bowl H_2O

Give mouth wash – clean teeth.

Clean the nostrils – dip swab stick

Contraindicated → gastric surgery, tracheoesophageal fistula, paralytic illus, acute abdomen.

When the patient unable to ingest, chew, swallow food but able to digest and absorb nutrients, e.g. unconscious patient infection, severe burns, malnutrition, prematurely unable to retain food, e.g. vomiting, anorexia nervosa surgery of mouth, throat, esophagus, paralysis of face, jaw, repair of palate, hair lips terminal malignancy, patient who refuse food due to depression.

EXPLAIN COLOSTOMY IRRIGATION

Check the diagnosis and the purpose of irrigation. Check the type of colostomy done; make sure of the proximal and distal loop of the colon.

Check orders – specific precautions.

Colostomy is an operation in which an artificial opening is made into the colon on the anterior abdominal wall to permit the escape of feces and flatus.

Types: → *temporary* done to relieve an obstruction which can be corrected by resection of the bowel after healing patient readmitted for closure.

Permanent conjunction with an abdominal – perineal resection after the sigmoid colon is resected; the proximal end is brought out through the abdominal wall and sutured to it to form a permanent opening for the elimination of the feces.

Patient to be prepared to accept a colostomy follow regulated dietary pattern, to establish regularity of evacuation.

Wash Hands

Fill the irrigating can with the solution and hang it at a required height. Expel the air from the tubing and clamp it. Remove the froth if any, from the solution. Untie the colostomy bag and remove the dressings, not of incision – discard kidney tray. Clean the skin around the stoma with clean cotton swabs or rag pieces or wash the area with soap and water.

Introduce the catheter is through the teat and the tip of the catheter is lubricated with water soluble jelly.

Pour some solution over the stoma.

Without force introduce catheter into the stoma about 4 inches.

Allow the solution to run in slowly, involving about 20 minutes.

Clamp the tube before the entry of entire fluid.

Remove the catheter from stoma. Disconnect it from the tubing and place it in the kidney tray.

Wait for the return flow. Complete remove the mackintosh, clean the skin around the colostomy opening and dry the skin thoroughly.

Apply a clean dressing or a clean bag over the stoma to receive any drainage that may leak out.

Patient thoroughly clean, wear clean dresses

Help the patient to get into his bed.

Take all articles to the utility room.

Clean all equipment

Rinse first with cold water and then with warm soapy water.

Chart procedure.

Nurses need to ask the following question to self and get through with its perfect answers to prove that she has basic knowledge of her profession: Assignment

In each diseases condition what nursing care will you give, e.g. hepatitis, all communicable diseases?

List the diagnostic investigation to be carried out in such patients/

What health teaching will you give to him and his family?

What health education will you give to him during treatment and the time of discharge?

Write the signs and symptoms of such patients.

Roles and responsibilities of nurse in recovery of patient.

Name different drugs used in such care.

Mention various complications and preventions.

Write down the general management of such case.

Name various treatment modalities.

What dieting advice you will give to such patient?

What health advice will you him while in hospital and on discharge?

Write the optional treatment.

Describe nursing care of patient while in the ward.

Mention side effects of drugs received.

What precautions will you take to present this condition in other family members?

What would be medical management and various methods of treatment?

Write clinical findings in detail.

What purpose does nurse serve?

What activities does nursing include?

What are the types of organization exist in hospital?

What factors determine patient care?

What are the sources of obtaining data about patient?

What is the value in keeping clinical records?

How are the records protected?

How are the qualities of nurse cultivated?

What is he future of nursing in our country?

Why do we need to follow code of ethic in nursing?

How does social change affect nursing?

What are the career options in nursing?

How is the nurse legally responsible to the patient?

What is the role of the nurse in a disaster or an emergency situation?

Nursing Care V

EXPLAIN OBSTRUCTIVE PULMONARY DISEASES

COPD

Chronic obstructive pulmonary disease obstructs airways. Chronic irritation of lungs cigarette smoking, infection and inhaled irritants also linked with emphysema, chronic bronchitis and lung cancer when cigarettes are smoked, thousands of chemical and gases are inhaled into the lungs. Smoking produces abnormal dilatation of the distal air space, with destruction of the distal air space, with destruction of alveolar walls oxygen carrying capacity is reduced, inhaling a lower percentage of oxygen than normal. The heart must pump more rapidly to supply blood.

No viral or bacterial agent has been identified as the sole cause. COPD are more prone to respiratory infection. The incidence higher in urban than in rural areas due to air pollution and occupational irritations explosion; Occupational gases and dusts can cause lung fibrosis.

With aging there is dilatation of the air space decrease elasticity of lung tissue and increased rigidity of the chest wall.

Diagnostic

History and physical examination, chest X-ray, pulmonary function tests, sputum for gram stain and culture, ABG monitoring, ECG, Exercise testing with oximetry or AGM Echocardiogram or cardiac nuclear scans.

Therapeutic

Treatment of respiratory infections Bronchodilator therapy, β-adrenergic agonists, anticholinergic agents, Long-acting theophylline preparations, corticosteroids, chest physiotherapy and postural drainage, breathing exercise, hydration of 3L/day, cessation of cigarette smoking, appropriate rest periods and exercise client and family education, influenza immunization yearly.

Effective coughing facilitates removal of secretions, clear airway, conserve energy, and reduce fatigue.

After each drainage position change and to give client time to cough and deep breathe. Chest physiotherapy consists of percussion, vibration and postural drainage – uses the principle of gravity helps loosening and mobilize secretions. Bronchodilator/hydration therapy frequently administered before postural drainage. It depends on the location of retained secretions and client tolerance to dependent positions. Procedure planed 1 hour before meals and 3 hours after meals.

A side lying position could be used for those persons who cannot tolerate a head-down position. Trendelenburg should not be performed on client with chest trauma, hemoptysis, heart disease, or head injury and other situations where patient's condition is not stable.

Percussion cupped-hand position hand should be cupped as though scooping up water.

In hospital wall oxygen or compressed air is used. At home an air-powered compressor.

Nebulization rapid acting medicines—Patients placed in position that allows for efficient breathing upright position breath slowly and deeply through the mouth and hold inspiration for 2–3 seconds. After treatment patient is instructed to cough effectively.

Home cleansing method is to wash the nebulizer daily in soap and water, rinse it with water and soak it for 20 – 30 minutes. In 1:1 white vinegar – water solution followed by a water rinse and air drying.

Nutritional considerations: To decrease dyspnea and conserve energy patient rest at least 30 minutes before eating, exercise and treatment avoided one hour before and after eating. Chewing avoided – soft food better.

PFT—Pulmonary Function Tests

Asthma

PFT, patient has reduction in forced expiratory volume FEV 25-75% with the degree of obstruction values obtained.

PFTs measure lung volumes and airflow.

Uses → To diagnose pulmonary disease, monitor disease progression, evaluate the extent of disability and evaluate response to bronchodilators. PFTs are performed with the use of a Spirometer, an instrument that measures and diagrams airflow across time. Ask patient to inhale and exhale while various measurements are taken. Patient age, sex, height and weight first obtain – information entered into a computer.

For test, patient is asked to insert the mouthpiece to take as deep a breath as possible and to blow as hard as fast and as long as possible, verbal encouragement is given to ensure patient continues blowing out until exhalation is complete. The computer determines the actual value, the normal value is *greater that 80% the test is normal – Exercise testing* involves walking on a treadmill to determine the amount of activity that can be tolerated.

PARAMETER

Total volume of air inhale and exhale with each breath 0.5 L. Expiratory reserve volume 1.5 L, residual volume amount of air remaining in lungs after forced expiration 1.5 L. Total lung capacities maximum volume of air that lungs can contain 6.0 L. Functional residual capacity volume of air remaining in lungs at the end of normal exhalation, vital capacity, inspiration capacity 3.5 L.

60% - 70% mild airflow obstruction

40% - 59% moderate airflow obstruction

Less than 40% severe airflow obstruction client with severe airflow obstruction commonly have COPD.

LUNG BIOPSY, THORACOCENTESIS

Diagnostic Studies of Respiratory System

Lung Biopsy

Purpose : → Specimens may be obtained by trans-bronchial, percutaneous, or open-lung biopsy. This test is used to obtain specimens for laboratory.

Nursing Responsibility: → If procedure done with bronchoscope, same as Thoracentesis – this test is used to obtain specimen of pleural fluid for diagnosis, to remove pleural fluid, or to instill medication. The physician insert a large-bore needle through the chest wall into pleural space chest X-ray film is always obtained after procedure to check for Pneumo-thorax and other changes.

Nurse : → Explain procedure – sign – position patient upright – instruction not to talk / cough – assist physician – apply dressing – observe – large volume fluid is removed, monitor for decrease in shortness of breath – specimen label – laboratory.

Lung Scan: → Test used to identify areas of the lung not receiving airflow or blood flow. Same as chest X-ray study. Also check for dye allergy.

Pulmonary Angiography: → Used to visualize pulmonary embolus; dye injection may cause flushing, warm sensation and cough. Apply pressure dress,

Bronchoscopy: → Keep patient NPO until gag reflex returns and monitor for laryngeal edema – if biopsy taken.

HOW IS LIVER BIOPSY DONE?

Patient placed in the desired position. LA given

Patient asked to inhale and exhale several times, hold breath at the end of expiration. This helps breath immobilize the chest wall and diaphragm. Penetration of the diaphragm therapy is avoided and the risk of lacerating the liver is minimized. Physician promptly introduces the biopsy needle via intercostals or sub costal route and penetrates the liver tissues aspirated needle withdrawn – procedure completed within 5 – 10 seconds. Patient can resume breathing. The cylindrical specimens that are trapped in the needle are collected and sent for histopathological examinations.

Patient's cooperation is essential, watch for complications hemorrhage, shock and collapse, perforation of the abdominal viscera, pneumothorax, injury to the diaphragm bile peritonitis, watch for the pallor, sweating, restlessness, dyspnea, rising pulse rate.

Abdominal Pain and Vomiting

Keep ready two of cross matched blood before sending patient for biopsy,

Patient with liver diseases are prone to bleed CBC,

Procedure causes anxiety.

Patient should be given injection, Vitamin K for several days prior to biopsy to prevent hemorrhage.

Shave and clean the area.

Patient keeps fasting 6–8 hrs before biopsy.

A laparotomy anticipated in any complication.

Give sedation SOS.

Any charge in the vital – report doctor.

Tray set-up:

Sterile covered tray containing.

Sponge holding forceps.

Syringe 5 ml with needle for LA.

Liver biopsy needle with stilettos.

Specimen bottles with cork.

Bowls to take cleansing lotion.

Aspiration syringe.

Dissecting forceps.

Dressing towels or slit.

Cotton balls, gauze pieces, cotton pads.

Gown, gloves, masks.

Unsterile tray.

Mackintosh and towel.

Kidney tray and paper bag.

Spirit, iodine, tr. Benzoine.

Lignocain 2%.

Apron for doctor.

Adhesive plaster and scissors.

Formalin 10% to preserve biopsy.

EXPLAIN NEEDLE BIOPSY

A common and important diagnostic measure in recent years is the needle biopsy. A variety of sites may be biopsied the liver, kidney, and lymph nodes are most common. Preparation, technique involved is much like that for born marrow puncture or paracentesis. A special biopsy needle is used to remove a small wedge of the organ being biopsied. The specimen must be handled like any biopsy specimen – placed in preservative solution and marked carefully. This procedure done in OT also done bedside sign consent – discomfort felt during procedure observe signs of bleeding, shock or other complications depending on the biopsy site.

EXPLAIN CERVICAL BIOPSY

It is the removal of a small piece of tissue from the cervix for the histopathological examination. It can be a punch biopsy/cervical conization, small piece removed with biopsy forceps, procedure done on OPD basis. The biopsy taken one week after the end of menses when cervix is least vascular; As it does not touch nerve ending patient feels no pain. For procedure perineum shaved and cleaned. The cervix visualized in good source of light. The bleeding from sight controlled by cauterization, few days patient may have foul discharge, patient discharged.

Report bleeding, use clean pads.

Articles for Procedure

Sterile tray:
Sponge holding forceps for cleansing
Valsellum forceps to hold the cervix
Biopsy forceps
Sims vaginal speculum
Small bowls for cleaning lotion
Gloves, gowns and masks
Legging and dressing towels
Specimen bottles
Cotton balls, gauze pieces and cotton pads
Unsterile tray:
Mackintosh and towel
Kidneys try and paper bag
Cleaning lotion
Apron
Formalin 10%
Cautery with its tips sterilized
Good source of light.

EXPLAIN RENAL BIOPSY

Open/close method
Procedure done as cystoscopy
A ureteric catheter to confirm fluoroscopy
A biopsy brush is then passed through the catheter and the lesion is brushed over several times. The brush is removed and any tissue adhering to the bristles is sent to the laboratory.

If no tissue is found on the brush, 24 to 48 hours urine specimens may be collected to catch any cell that may have been dislodged by the bristles. Postoperatively the patient may have to be given IV fluids at a rapid rate to reduce the possibility of clot formation at the biopsy site.

Percutaneous Renal Biopsy

Done under LA patient placed in prone-position with a firm pillow under the abdominal, patient instructed for deep breathe and hold it, the probe needle inserted through the skin and positioned inside the renal capsule. Biopsy tissues obtained needle removed and firm pressure is applied.

Contraindication → infection, malignant tumors, hydro-nephrosis, severe high blood pressure, coagulation disorders, renal failure, uncooperative patient.

Before biopsy through investigations such as IVP, urine culture, Hematocrit, blood urea, bleeding time, clotting time.

Bed rest; take plenty of fluids to prevent clot formation in the kidney.

Ambu – airway maintenance and breathing unit.

Methyl/Ethyl alcohol liquid in suture pack.

WHAT IS PERITONEAL DIALYSIS?

Catheter Placement: → Peritoneal abscess is obtained by inserting a catheter through the anterior abdominal wall. Catheter 25 cm long and has one or two Dacron cuffs at the subcutaneous and peritoneal ends of the within few weeks, fibrous tissue grow into the cuff and anchors the catheter in place, and prevents bacterial penetration into the perineal cavity. The tip of the catheter rests in the peritoneal cavity and has many perforations spaced throughout the tubing to allow fluid to flow in and out of the catheter.

Empty bladder, weigh patient, and obtain sign.

2 cm below umbilicus LA given – abdomen is distended with dialysis solutions. A trocar, with the catheter threaded through or over it. It is inserted into the peritoneal cavity. When patient feels pressure in the rectal area and has the urge to defecate. The trocar is withdrawn and the catheter is in the place. Midline incision umbilical – catheter insertion can cause ill effect perforation of bladder, bowel, and blood vessels infection. The catheter is connected to sterile tubing and anchored to the abdomen with tape. The catheter is irrigated heparin – to prevent catheter from clogging and help flow. 7–14 days to wait for tissue to in growth in to cuffs implantation, when catheter site heal patient can shower – it should last 18 months, keep clean, dry, apply antiseptic solution, dressing and observe sign of infection.

Solutions of Dialysis available commercially in 1-2 liters, plastic bags – the electrolyte composition is similar to that of plasma – potassium is in low concentration – solution warmed to body temperature to increase peritoneum clearance.

The three phase's cycles are inflow, dwell time and drain time. During inflow 2 liters of solution is infused over about 10 minutes, the flow rate decreases if patient becomes uncomfortable. After solution, the inflow clamp is closed before air enters the tubing. Dwell time allows for diffusion and osmosis between the patient's blood and the peritoneal cavity. Drain time takes 10 to 20 minutes gently massage the abdominal or change the position. The cycle starts again of another 2 liters of solution. For manual P dialysis, a period of 20 – 30 minutes to complete an exchange.

Three types of P. dialysis:

IPD   :   Intermittent PD.

CAPD :   Continuous Ambulatory PD.

CCPD :   Continuous Cyclic PD.

IPD   :   3-5 times a week usually over night for about 8 hours per treatment. Alarms and monitors are build into the system. Between dialysis abdominal is empty. It is easy to teach family PD at home machine.

CAPD :   Carried out manually by exchanging 1.5 – 3 L, 4 – 5 times daily dwell time 4 – 8 hours. After instillation close tubing with a clamp and bag is folded and concealed in the patient's clothing.

Complications: Infection, peritonitis, abdominal pain, outflow problems, hernias, lower back problem, bleeding, pulmonary complications, protein loss.

Hemodialysis

Silicone rubber cannula that could be inserted into the radial artery and into an adjacent forearm vein. The cannula is implanted subcutaneous and connected by silicone rubber tubing that exists from the skin. The two ends are connected by a U-shaped shunt.

The shunt can be disconnected for dialysis to allow arterial blood to flow through the artificial kidney and return to the venous side. Another external cannula implanted in the thigh using the femoral artery and vein.

How is AV Fistulas done?

Procedure: After the venipuncture the needle closest to the fistula delivers arterial blood to the dialyzer. Usually primed with saline solution; Heparin is added to the blood as it flows into the dialyzer. Once the blood enters the extracorporeal circuit, it is propelled through the dialyzer by a pump at a flow rate of 100-300 ml/minute warmed to body temperature circulates in the opposite direction at a rate of 300-900 ml/minute. Anticoagulation therapy is required to prevent clotting of blood in the dialyzer and blood illness.

Most units use routine hyalinization, which consist of a loading does given at the initiation of dialyzer and smaller doses given through out the treatment. The last dose is usually given in the last hour before the end of dialysis treatment to prevent excessive site bleeding. Bloods is returned from the dialyzer via venous lines to the patient. The system has an alarm to warm of blood or air leaks, alterations in temperature, concentration, or pressure and extremes in blood pressure readings.

Dialysis terminated by turning off the blood flow pump, clamping the arterial inflow line and flushing the saline solution to return all blood to the patient. The needles are then removed from the patient and firm pressure is applied to the venipuncture sites. Most people sleep read, talk or watch TV during dialysis hemodialysis usually lasts 2-4 hours three times a week.

Setting OPD/IPD

Complications—Disequilibrium syndrome, manifestation include nausea, vomiting, confusion restlessness, headache, twitching, jerking and occasionally seizures, muscle cramps contribute high blood pressure.

Hypotension—Precipitates lightheadedness, coronary ischemia.

Muscle cramps associate discomfort and pain

Loss of blood may result from residual blood in the dialyzer from accidental separation of cannula tubing or dialysis membrane rupture.

In a patient who had received too much heparin causes bleeding.

Hepatitis-related to blood transfusion

Sepsis

Intractable ascitis repeated fluid overload poor nutrition

Dialysis encephalopathy characterized by speech disturbances, dementia, lack of muscle coordination, myoclonic seizures

Acquired cystic kidney disease hemorrhage and bleeding into cystic kidney cause hematuria

Increase incidence of cancer

Transplantation is a solution.

What is Lumbar Puncture—LP?

A lumbar puncture is the insertion of a needle into the lumbar region of the spine, the needle enters the lumbar arachnoids space of the spinal canal below the level of the spinal cord so that CSF can be withdrawn or a substance can be therapeutically or diagnostically injected.

The CSF is formed through the choroids villi in each of the four ventricles of the brain and it circulates freely through the ventricles of the brain. The dural and arachnoids sacs extend up to the level of the second sacral vertebra and this cavity contains the CSF. Thus the region between the second lumbar vertebra and the second sacral vertebra is suitable for the withdrawal of CSF, as there is no danger of injury to the spinal cord.

Purpose

Spinal anesthesia, medication in meningitis, reduce intracranial pressure, laboratory exam diagnose disease, locate tumors or brain disorders.

Articles

Lumbar puncture needles into two sizes with stiletto, sponge holder, 5 ml syringe with needle, bowl, specimen bottle, cotton balls, gauze pieces, cotton pads, gloves, gown and masks, dressing towels or slit, 3 way adaptor, manometer and tubing to measure the pressure of CSF.

Procedure

Patient is positioned correctly and skin is prepared. Then 4th lumbar spine or L2-L3 interspaced the stiletto is removed and 3 way adaptor the manometer filled with normal saline is attached, get a stabilized pressure. Normally it is 6-13 mm Hg or 80-180 mm of water. About 2-3 ml of CSF is allowed to drip into each of 3 sterile test tubes and then the needle is withdrawn. The puncture wound is sealed.

CSF normally is crystal clear, turbulence indicates infection e.g. meningitis. Blood indicates hemorrhage, sugar content normal level 40-60 mg/100 ml.

Complications—Injury to spinal nerves gives radiating pain, infection can be introduced which may give rise to meningitis, leakage of CSF, may cause headaches, damage intervertebral disc, local pain, edema, hematoma at puncture site, temperature elevation respiratory failure and sudden death.

Explain Abdominal Paracentesis

It is the removal of fluid from the peritoneal cavity.

Acidosis is a condition that occurs with increase in blood carbonic acid or with decrease in blood bicarbonate, blood pH below 7.35.

Anuria is the failure of the kidney to produce urine.

Atrophy is the decrease in the size of a tissue or organ caused by a decrease in the size of the individual cells.

Barium is a metallic element commonly used in solution as a contrast medium for X-ray filming of the gastrointestinal tract.

Biopsy is the removal and examination of tissue from the living body.

Bradycardia is abnormally slow pulse rate, less than 60/minute.

Help the patient to sit up in bed, or allow him to sit on the side of the bed with additional support for his back and arms with this position gravity helps fluid to accumulate in the lower abdominal cavity.

Articles

Sponge holding forceps to clean the skin, 5 ml syringe with needle for LA. 20 ml syringe for aspiration of fluid. Three away adaptor and tubing, trocar and cannula or aspiration needles, BP handle with blades to make a small skin incision for the introduction of trocar and cannula. Suturing needle if incision is made, small bowls, dressing forceps toothed and non-toothed, specimen bottles, sterile dressing towels/slits, cotton alls, gauze pieces, cotton pads, gloves, mask, gowns, mackintosh and towels, kidney tray/paper bag, spirit, iodine, tincture benzoic, lignocaine 2%, apron. Dressing receptacle to collect the fluid, Pint measures to measure the fluid. Low stool to raise the drainage receptacle and adjust the height.

Stick aseptic-done for diagnostic purpose the fluids withdrawn by syringe may be sufficient. LA small skin incision-select site-occasionally soft catheter passed-fluid is removed and opening is sealed. Place a many tailed bandage apply over abdomen during the procedure to maintain the intra-abdominal pressure. Prevents shock and collapse. The vital signs check half hourly for two hours, 4 hours for 24 hours. Examine any leakage, clean articles, wash with cold water rinse in warm soapy water, dry and sent for autoclaving.

Expert nurse embraces a holistic philosophy and caring that enables them to offer a level of comfort and support that is often intuitive. It is an on going process. Nurses play key role in prevention of early intervention in all the areas as they can meet health promotion in all settings. She must be familiar with procedures as well as the equipments initiating to provide effective therapy and prevent complications.

Medical field is changing but suffering continues the same. The nurse can do much to allay and alleviate the inevitable anxieties through technical competence and anatomical knowledge and compassionate understanding. Recognizing the health needs, understanding them and meeting them. Preventing the diseases occurring and developing; and, promoting good health.

For this she requires knowledge and practice based on scientific principles. It should be reviewed and evaluated regularly. She should have clinical judgment in assessing patient's condition in determining patient's needs and planning his care. Research finding to improve her nursing practice; to improve nursing technique and increase learning. Finding new approaches and methods which will benefit patients She can get trained in highly skilled technical nursing; with understanding and high degree of skill in dealing. She should possess basic knowledge of biological, medical and social and behavioral sciences.

She should know how to bring about change through her leadership ability. Flexibility is essential specially to meet emergencies or changing situation. It should be balanced and integrated. To give the highest possible quality of nursing care that is holistic. Dealing with personnel and professional problem Nursing care that covers all activities.

What is Autopsy?

Autopsy or examination of the body after death, is invaluable for providing knowledge to clarify the cause of death. Autopsy can also serve as a monitor of clinical care and the quality of society's health. Autopsy can assist with recognition and identification of new diseases. The purpose of autopsy goes beyond providing data on the effectiveness of medical therapy. The family of the diseased may be reassured that everything necessary and possible was done for the patient. In addition, contagious illness and genetic illness can be identified and made known to the family.

Autopsy also helps clarify the circumstances of violent and unexplained death. Each country has its own laws on the need for permission for autopsy. Even though specific laws differ, there is some general similarity. Autopsy for the purpose of resolving medicolegal issues or ordered by an appropriate authority, such as medical examiner. Death that is unexpected, occurring while in surgery, in a patient who is under a physicians care, falls into this category. When there is no medicolegal reason for ordering an autopsy, permission can give only by the next of kin.

Usually a patient cannot order his own autopsy before death. Once death has occurred, the body become the property of the next to the kin, or if there is no next to kin, of a legal entity such as the coroner or sheriff. Autopsy is performed in privately and in a professional manner. An incision is made from the axilla to groin to expose internal organs. Organs are examined and weighed. In addition, microscopic study and chemical toxicology and microbiologic analyses are performed. The ideal time to perform an autopsy is within 24 hours of death. Autopsy can be performed after embalming. The family may be concerned about the final appearance of the patient at burial. Autopsy is customarily performed with great care so as not to disfigure the body. The family may meet with the pathologist and receive a copy of the findings. The cost of autopsy is usually done in hospital costs, therefore charges of it do not appear on bill.

Nurse and Her Psychological, Emotional Aspect with Client and School Health Education— Adolescence and Counseling

Diverse Roles and Responsibilities of Nurse

What does it mean to be a nurse in 21st century/ Nursing profession/nursing career/ nurse as a leader/ importance of in service education/advanced nursing field/ community nurse/ comprehensive nursing?

Health is man's most precious possession. It influences all his activities. It shapes his destines. Without health there can be no solid foundation for mans happiness. Better health induces positive attitude, conductive to economic growth and modernization. The individual becomes better citizens.

The people with good health are generally enthusiastic and try to achieve higher and higher goals in life, enrich quality of life, increasing the average length of human life for the health and happiness of humanity. It is beautifully expressed in Vedic benediction- that is May all human be happy; May all be without disease, May all witness auspicious sight, May none have to undergo suffering. Breath is the bridge which connects life to consciousness, which unites your body to your thought. Only through this breath we know that we exist. Only difference between life and death is this "Breath".

Remind yourself that this very moment is the only one you know you have for sure. Not every disease known to man but those which constitute the large bulk of medical practice. All too often we do not understand why these diseases arise. What is known from what is unknown and what is half known. All this makes nurse to think of her challenging task ahead. With this sentiments keeping in mind a nurse should work that all have peace of mind body and spirit as much as possible and she too contributes in it much by her life and profession.

Nurse means to foster, handle carefully comfort, care and assurance to the sick. The entry of woman into nursing can be traced to 300 A.D approximately. Nursing is a helping profession, it deals with human being, and it provides comfort and support in times of anxiety, loneliness and helplessness. It is sharing responsibility for the health and welfare of all people in the community.

She assists the individual and contributing to recovery. Her profession exists in response to a need of society, it is guided by its code of ethics, is rooted in caring and contributing recovery or to dignified death.

NURSING PROFESSION

Nursing profession is an occupation based on specialized intellectual study and training, for the purpose of skilled service. They are not merely academic and theoretical but are practical in their aims. Are directed by public interest, to human belief and is guided by ethical standards and educational discipline. Which requires judgment in applying knowledge to the solution of problem and accepts responsibilities for the results? It is based on socially accepted scientific principle. Develops scientific technique which is the result of tested experience. The services provided are vital to humanity and the welfare of the society. The service needs intellectual activities, individual responsibility and accountability and should continually enlarge through research and higher learning. There is a code of ethics to guide the decisions and conduct of practitioners which encourages and supports high standards of practice. Constantly enlarges knowledge improves technique by use of scientific method which are vital to human and social welfare.

Nursing is an art and science dominated with principles of skillful care which embraces the person's body as a whole, his mind and soul, his physical, mental and spiritual well being. Caring for sick and injured, helping individual, family and community to relief of illness by talking positive action. Strengthening values and guided by strong moral character, willing to share knowledge gained to help people than merely to satisfy her own intellectual curiosity, interested in progress in her profession, friendly, cheerful and pleasant showing appropriate concern with patient's emotional needs. In emergencies, make quick decisions and judgments. She should have respect for the individual dignity of every human being. Know nursing so thoroughly that every person will receive excellent care. Nursing is such an important part of the health care delivery system she needs to understand system to deliver quality care with it.

The issues facing nursing today are extremely complex with managing multiple program or agendas which requires multifaceted role, managing change resolving conflicts and making organizational goals. Now there is a need for every nurse to have a sound management base from which to operate. Management is a key to success in the professional nursing job which ultimately results in a change in primary role from clinical nurse to manager. Nurses, at all level, focus on how to deal with people, how to manage resources, and how to manage job.

In service education increases efficiency of nursing services; Nurses today must retain that special vision of what they can do and the difference they can make, and be an effective part of the answer to the aches and pains of the community. It is important to know why to educate, whom to educate, who is to educate, where is to educate, what is to educate and how is to educate needs comprehensive planning with vast subjects and specialties.

In service education develops inner power to the maximum possible extent. It makes nurse as a person of good character and useful to the society here she realizes self which enables her mind to find ultimate truth giving inner light, which lasts a life time with her profession. It helps her to earn her own livelihood; gives mastery over her field of work. In service education aims at developing the ability for efficient working and the capacity for continuous learning, so that one may adapt to the changes and judgment and produce profitable services which become an important tool and professional growth vehicle. It improves her performance, increases proficiency and knowledge expands and their professional horizons and keeps them abreast of development.

NURSING CAREER

Nursing has developed different dimensions which meet the health needs of entire community. Due to greater specialization in nursing activities her services have become comprehensive and more highly specialized than ever before. Advanced courses for higher studies are available for additional qualifications. It will help to improve the standards of graduate nurses for higher post and leading position. Medical profession is fast changing and the era of specialization and super-specialization in nursing, biomedical sciences have far advanced resulting in newer diagnostic equipments such as scanners, new drugs, need monitoring system, newer modern health care facilities, ICCU, kidney dialysis, organ transplantation, newer surgical techniques and new interventions are introduced in the curative side.

The expansions in health care have altered the role and function of a nurse which demands advanced specialized preparation of nurse. Today the number is fast growing of a persons talking up nursing profession. Due to era of fast scientific change affecting their living and working conditions. This is the space and nuclear age. Nurses therefore needs to increase her knowledge wider. There is a wide range of opportunities today. She is willing to serve any part of the country as well as abroad.

NURSE AS A LEADER

Nurse as a leader will be the most competent individual in planning and organizing the work and where she develops certain physical, intellectual or personality characteristics. A forceful personality who has ability to persuade people to a course of action efficiently has ability to get along with people; thus becomes sensitive to the feelings of a group. Listens attentively and makes sure everyone understands what is needed and the reason why. She shares responsibilities and opportunities; by helping the group to be aware of their attitudes and values.

Nurse leader has initiative qualities, technical qualities like mastery over subject, expert knowledge and expertise to work. She also should possess teaching and administrative abilities, quality of building human relations to become effective nurse leader. Needs to develop and maintain team spirit, good in planning, organizing, directing and analysis progress accurately reports and records patient's condition, treatment and responses to care. Accurate information ensures continuity and quality of care and helps in smooth running of administration. Her role is a visionary in identifying or forecasting unit needs.

Nurse needs to master the use of wealth of knowledge to improve the skill level, establish courses for super specialty. Technology will continue to advance at a dizzying pace and use of nursing data, will change nursing practice dramatically. Computerized health information networks will allow immediate access to patient data, which will reinforce the need for patient confidentially. Advances in telecommunications will improve access to medical services for rural and elderly. It will become routine for those who live in remote areas or are homebound.

Advances in technology will bring new ethical dilemmas. There will be no end to the available opportunities. International educational opportunities will increase as the global village concept takes hold. Remember God choose us to this caring profession with a definite purpose.

Nursing is a noble *profession* involving the care for and support to those who are ill and ailing. They are an integral part of any health care system. No medical team is complete without nurses. A good medical facility is highly dependent on the quality in nursing care. Surgery and medication alone does not suffice until it is accompanied by good nursing care, which is utmost important. They ensure that doctor's instructions are carried out thoroughly in respect of the patient. She serves as an organic conduit between a doctor and a patient. It requires gentleness, compassion and sensitivity.

This is innate qualities of a woman and for this reason, she dominates her profession. India, in 1947 only two nursing colleges, today there are about 930 institutions in the country imparting graduate and post graduate courses in using as well as about 1900 institutions for diploma courses in nursing. With various new technologies and advanced medical equipment coming up, to provide prompt and more efficient care. There are sociality hospitals being established in our country where a growing number from overseas also coming for treatment. In family health programme, the nursing community is critical particularly in the remote and far-flung areas, where the role of a nurse can be more diverse.

A nurse can provide counseling on healthcare matters to the local population; and can educate them about the importance of the good health of the mother for ensuring the survival of the child, which needs the contribution of the entire medical fraternity. Nurses are getting recognition all over the world and there is acute shortage. There are about 3.7 lakh active nurses in India while the requirement is for about 10.5 lakh nurses by 2012. Serious consideration needs to be given as to how to close this gap. They need recognition and encouragement. They deserve to be treated with deep respect in society. She takes care and saves the lives or cure there illness. Therefore, issues relating to their working conditions and other welfare measures needs to receive sympathetic consideration. While taking care of the health of others with a human touch; they need to pay attention to their own health.

NURSE AND FAMILY

Nurse is the pillars of the family care. Family is very much in vogue and nothing has been able to take the sheen away from this centuries old institution. Family still rules boost globally, it has been observed the test of time. Building bonds of love. Family is important as you need oxygen for breathing and family is oxygen on which we live. Family is our first priority, what we have all we owe to our family; parents are a constant guiding force in life.

They are at the core of our life, everything else comes second, their presence booster our confidence. In terms of moral support, it makes a huge support. To sustain a human relationship in sharing innermost deepest feelings, expressing feelings, talk and discuss day, your work, have a sense of humor, make each other laugh. Therefore, when patient comes to hospital comes with his unique family background and the family has special attachment to the ill member so nurse needs to take this in account that every person is unique and dear to the family.

Share the misfortune of the poor, help disabled, a small act will awaken a great strength within supply a lion like force to your heart. Do not hold it back. Remember the need has knocked at your door and has given you an opportunity to serve. Keep your character clean; remember you are an invaluable asset to the society. No one has to request the sun to shine. It is the nature of the sun to spread light and dispel darkness.

NURSE AND COMMUNITY

Improved technology and advanced science the health of the people becoming a great concern; as there are wide spread health issues. Nurse needs to understand these vast health problems of the given community. She is a mediator, an instrument to reach the center services to the homes of the family. She has to adapt people so to suit the community. She needs skills and information to up date herself to involve and plunge fully into community integration where she can get full support of the community to highlight to piece of her work.

Nurse needs strong will power, motivation, determination to do her task in the community. Where she has to go on ward in spite of lacks and difficulties. She act as a change agent for people ; for that hard work and self sacrifice and attitude of let go, never give up, is must if she strive to achieve the goal and target entrusted to her care. She has to face many difficulties and that is key to successfully community building. She is able to maintain, protect and improve the health of the public. Where she will be able to change the behavior pattern to achieve maximum health. Nurse emphasizes self-reliant health car that is significant and relevant for today's scenario where community assumes important responsibility that is modern keeping in mind the various factors that affect the health. Thus, community is empowered.

She has to know prevention and control methods. To improve habits she needs to develop awareness, she accepts respects and makes herself available, willing, emphasizes change healthy attitudes towards community. Balance diet, good water supply, safe disposal of waste, good housing, nutrition and hygiene small family, good education, occupation and health services for health and security, shelter, comfort, will promote and protect community as health is inter dependent on above factors- absence of one may lead to ill health. She needs to focus on total health stressing on all aspects.

The health services should be realistic in terms of available personnel and facilities; facilities for further training should be provided by the organization. She should be paid well to live standard living which will provide security and contentment. She needs social commitment.

What is the perfect solution for illiteracy? *'You' teach India is* a social initiative from, it aids at providing a platform for individuals to teach less fortunate children who are in need of an education. Teach India has established a strong network of partner NGOs that offers hundreds of teaching centers across country that are ready to absorb individuals into relevant teaching programs. Sixty leading colleges and schools on boards to offer volunteers, united national volunteers/UNV has joined into provide expertise in the volunteer management for teach India invite volunteers like you to join them and discover how two hours a week can help change the future of a child forever. Teaching basic one to one or a small group to make difference to the future of child and the nation. The campaign has 90% of volunteers supporting a case for the first time, creating a while new constituency adding new dimension.

The word *guru* means dispeller of darkness. Guru removes ignorance and gives us the light of knowledge. Knowledge of who we are, how we to relate with the world and achieve true success. Most importantly, how to transcend to world and reach the abide of infinite bliss. The combination of the teacher's wisdom and the energy of the student go towards making a vibrant, progressive society, importance of guru in evening walks of life, a sports person's natural gift acquires direction under the expertise of the coach, a musicians talents is honed by the dedication of the mentor.

In the spiritual path, it is the enlightenment of the guru that removes the ignorance in the seekers mind. The seeker must question, probe and analyze the truths taught so as to understand, absorb and transform his personality to the higher realms. An attitude of service/seva is the hallmark of an understanding student. The student learnt the value of humility that makes him receptive to the guru's wisdom.

Doctors will have to compulsory serve a year's internship in rural hospitals. Law making internship mandatory and discontinue the current practice of paying one lakh in bond amount in lieu of the rural stint. The minister said the bill would make it compulsory for all medical students before the degree is awarded. The govt. has proposed an increase in the bond amount from 5 lakhs to 15 lakhs for graduate and post graduate, the issue has been discussed.

NURSE'S ROLE IN COMMUNITY PSYCHIATRY

Volunteerism is a trend, which is fast catching up. How can I make my role in society leading to the empowerment of others? Beyond self-, understand poor from heart. Those who believe in living for a cause and have the passion to work towards making a better tomorrow, in the psychosocial sector make your career.

Stress is a life event that causes imbalance in a person's life. An unhealthy response to stress occurs when the demands of the stressor exceed the persons coping ability. Young students, low socioeconomic income group, students residing in semi urban area have more stress and less coping. We manage our families, our money, our property, our business; we manage whatever is valuable to us. Why would not anybody manage stress? Stress is not a part of life. Stress is your inability to manage; it is your own creation, it is your own making.

Focus on prevention and control of alcohol related problems, addictions, juvenile delinquency, acute adjustment problem like suicidal attempts. Make psychotropic drugs available, educate public involve communities, families, human resource link with other sector, monitor community, support more research in Alcohol dependence, intoxication, a withdrawal syndrome, anxiety disorder, eating disorder, confusion, denial, depressive disorder, mental retardation, hysteria, schizophrenia, mood disorder; obsessive compulsive behavior, delusion and hallucination.

Know and be aware of the psychiatric emergencies that are for example suicide is common cause of death in psychiatric patient. Self-harm self-inflicted which ends with a fatal outcome in self-injury; suicide is among top 10 causes of death in India. A crisis causes intense suffering and feeling of hopelessness and helplessness. There is a conflict between survival and unbearable stress, wish to escape, changes perception, wish to punishes self, feel guilty. In India, the highest suicide rate is in the age group of 15-29 years.

The work stress affects the body's endocrine system. The pressure builds and they are likely to suffer a breakdown.

Depression life stressors, family and marital disputes, failure in goal achievement, occupational and financial difficulties, alcoholism and drug dependence, schizophrenia, suicide happen without warning; they are psychotic/ mentally ill. Severe, disabling, painful or unbearable physical illness, resent serious loss or major stressful life event, social isolation, psychosocial factors are very important causes of suicide. E.g. failure in exam, failure in love, failure to give dowry. Lose of loved objects by deaths.

Common mode of committing suicide is by hanging, burns, drowning and jumping in front of train or vehicle. Section 309 of IPC punishable and liable to fine.

Talk all the suicidal threats, gestures attempts seriously and notify a psychiatrist and quantify the seriousness of the situation and take remedial precautionary measures, such as by removing sharp objects, ropes, drugs, deal with ongoing life stresses, teach coping skills and interpersonal skills.

Management

Women attempt 3 times as frequently as men do. Common characteristics of person attempting suicide are unbearable psychological pain. Frustrated psychological need is the common stressor, the common action is escape, and consistency is difficulty with lifelong coping.

Predisposing factors for it is psychiatric disorder (affective disorder, substance abuse, schizophrenia), personality traits (hostility, impulsivity, depression) and disorder, psychosocial (humiliating life events, separation, divorce, unemployment, multiple life stresses, chronic medical illness) family history (family stress, alcoholism, history of suicide, genetic factors) environmental factors, genetic and familial variables, biochemical factors.

Preparatory action of the self-destructive clients is to write a suicide note, giving away prized possession, use of violent method, precaution taken against discovery.

Develop contact with client, provide close one to one observation, remove all potentially dangerous objects; provide prescribed medications, identify clues triggers that precede self-mutilation behaviour, suggest alternative behaviour, identity positive consequences of adaptive behaviour. Provide basic psychological needs, monitor medications, encourage participating activities he likes, reward healthy coping. Encourage ventilation of feelings, communicate concern, calm control, and reinforce adaptive behavior. Clarify faulty beliefs and encourage formulating a new goal, using role modeling. Confirm the patient's identity; provide supportive measures to decrease panic, set limits on inappropriate behavior. Help in identifying self-strengths, weaknesses.

Reassurance, sedation, restrain when needed and uncontrollable. Disturbance in thinking behavior, interference with meaningful communication, difficulty in establishing rapport, lack insight into his illness and have poor judgment.

Some of the reasons for community psychosocial imbalance are: Family history, home circumstances, low income, low socioeconomic status, cultural and religious values, social support, early childhood history such as stammering, tics, night terrors, thumb sucking, nail biting, head banging, phobias, temper tantrum, etc.

Relationship with peer and teacher, school phobia, learning difficulties, masturbation, anxiety related to changes in puberty, number of children. Job held, ambitions, relationship with authority, present income, and reason for change in job. Family background, any gender identity disorder, duration of marriage, divorces, separation, sexual dissatisfaction, and contraceptives used, temperament.

Self-criticism, self-conscious, self-centered, abilities, achievements and failures, decision making.

To find out such psychosocial problems nurse needs to advice for detailed physical examination. Self care, hygiene.

Abnormal way of sitting, standing, walking, lying, restlessness, societal withdrawal.

Variation in mood, time mood lasts. Sad, irritable, angry, indifferent, thought block, pre occupations, ego, irrational fears, jealousy, hopelessness, haplessness, worthlessness, complete denial of illness, abstract thinking, insight.

Pre-existing brain damage, history of head injury, Alzheimer's, Parkinson's, encephalopathy, dialysis dementia, Wilson's disease, thyroid, adrenal dysfunction, endocrine causes, toxic, metabolic causes, infection HIV / Aids, dementia, poor stress management skills, low self esteem, poor impulse control, sensation seeking, childhood trauma, lack of interest, withdrawal effect, craving, peer pressure.

Human behavior cannot be understood completely. Many things affect individual consciously or unconsciously- appropriate adaptive behavior can change maladjustment. There are various stresses, which affect individual's physical, emotional behavior.

Each individual has his own private world. He has constructive and destructive behavior. Stressors occur throughout life. Acceptance depends on how nurse develops interpersonal relationship with the people in the community that is therapeutic and social, is able to help family socially emotionally.

Her ability to develop with positive self concept attitude of acceptance and tolerance respecting the status of family with mutual understanding putting oneself in other persons is going through and feeling for them promote mental health and help them to find meaning in life experience.

Thus helps to cope, understand, find out new alternative, new patterns of behavior and face problems realistically, community nurse explores family fears and anxiety, establishes contacts, talks that they are unique human being, over coming barriers, encouraging independent decision making and abilities, educates progress listening and interpreting accurately to be effective therapeutic communicator, e.g. going through financial problem, upset because husband beats help to change attitude and provide insight.

The idea of social consciousness needs to be introduced at the level of primary school or children to grow with that concept. In addition, gradually inculcated in families at home. The problem of poverty can be solving by mass education so to inculcate this spirit of social consciousness in human beings.

India has the second largest *population* in the world. The higher fertility in India is attributed to the universality of marriage, low level of literacy, limited use of contraceptives and traditional way of life. People should adopt the small family norm to stabilize the country's population at the level of some 1533 millions by the year 2050. Mothers are not having adequate knowledge; the nurse educator needs to motivate them.

The world *population* day is an event celebrated around the world on July 11 every year. The day helps to draw the world's attention to recognize population as an international concern. This day this year focuses on a global concern- the urgent need for quality family planning information and services and draws the people's attention to the effect of population on the multifarious aspects of human life.

The theme for world population day 2008 is family planning: it is a right, let us make it real. India has only 2.4% of the worlds land surface but supports 17% of its population. Stabilizing the population is essential to promote substantial development. The over all population will continue to grow as 58% of the population is in the reproductive age group and 26 million are born every year. At current levels, it may take several decades more to stabilize India's population. The national rural health mission seeks population stabilization, gender and demographic balance and mission would expect to achieve the goal of reducing total fertility rates to 2.1 by 2012. Community too has to contribute towards pooling the knowledge, and mobilizing the resources to meet the challenge.

SELFLESS SERVICE FOR AILING HUMANITY

Rescue operation during calamities, to work tirelessly and diligently with the ministry of health, leadership and management and administration programmes, contributed in close association with govt. spreading awareness of Aids and palliative care, improvement in standard of teaching and quality assurance, motivate field health workers and awareness campaign against female infanticide .

Urban family members live in a 200 sq foot and manage fine; there is always room for more. Four different families live parents, brother and wife. Work as a cook in the near by housing society. When it comes to family, there is always space for more. In fact when relatives visit from the village are welcomed them make space for them by sleeping outside the house or the veranda. There is no choice so why make difficult. Children learn to adjust like the elders. One wants to study and the other wants to watch TV.

Even today's *research* shows that there are about 67 million kids dogged by ill health. From there about 53% of these have no access to even basic medical facilities, alarming rise in rape of minors. Key areas of welfare and social development do not seem to be on the priority and development funds progressively shrinking over past 5 years.

Indian villages are the cradles of exploitation. Attitudes cannot be changed in hurry. Money continues to be a huge worry, every one is ambitious and wants to move the ladder of success.

October 2/10/2008, law passed- clearing the air for our children. On guard against the ill effects of passive smoking can have on our kids. It has negative impact on the Childs health. Every child has right to smoke free environment. Children and youth are influenced when they see celebrities smoke. They should stop smoking in public.

Public health, considered one of the fundamental functions of the state, seems to be in a state of neglect. City hospitals to be forced to become more charitable, this will bring some relief for people who fall below the poverty line. It is a positive action of govt. to give treatment at subsidizes rates. It is a duty of students who get subsidized education who serve the society. A rule is made for them to serve poorer section of society.

PHC, BMCs stocks up on drug to battle monsoon ailments, every year following the rainfall, leptospirosis and gastroenteritis claim many lives, situation under control several measures to be under taken to counter a possible outbreak. Drugs, investigation kits and awareness spread on the precautionary measures to incur outbreak. For effective results need to Sensitizing and training NGOs and private doctors for coordinating with them. Throwing rubbish out of a window and total disregard for the cleanliness of public areas.

He who has health has hope and he who has hope has everything. Value health, health is second blessing that we mortals are capable of, a blessing that money cannot buy.

Transcultural nursing is a demand of time as whole world is shrinking into a global village. It is a fact that all human beings are born, live, work and die within a cultural context and viewpoint. Health is to do with the ability to adapt to constantly changing demands, expectations and stimuli. Health is affected with genetic factor, biological, lifestyle, employment, health beliefs, politics, housing and available health services. Helping the people to change. Some developing countries now treat nurses as an export commodity that can earn vital overseas currency.

Nursing safe handling of biomedical waste continues to be a matter of serious concern for health authorities in India. Thousands of tones of biomedical waste originating from hospitals, nursing homes and clinics in the form of cotton swabs and bandages infected with blood, IV fluid bags, needles, catheters, human tissues and body parts, etc. continue to be dumped in open garbage bins on the roads in most parts of the country. Dangerous of such waste is only expected to increase for the days to come.

According to the Gazette of India, biomedical waste means any waste, which is generated during diagnosis, treatment or immunization of human beings, or animals or in research activities. This has assumed great importance the world over because of the serious hazards it poses to the environment. Authorities are still not familiar with proper waste classification; segregation, handling and disposal of the waste generated in the hospitals.

Nurse's role and responsibilities in BMW—Disinfect the waste so that it is no longer the source of pathogenic organisms. Cutting up syringes and damaging the needles. Disposable items like gloves, syringes, should be mutilated after use to prevent illegal packing and reuse. Three types of container should be available at each point namely for general waste, infected non-sharp waste and infected sharp waste. Color-coding of bags should do as per rules.

Needles, syringes other sharp instruments and objects, should be placed in a puncture resistant plastic/metal container at the workstation. Changing chemical solutions, always handling with gloves and masks. Apron and boots to be used if splashing is expected. Clear air, clean bedding and hygienic method of dust removal by wet mopping of vacuum cleaning must be recognized{< IGF important function, knowledge of infection process and the critical thinking skills involved in aseptic technique and barrier protection are necessary.

Adopting scientific approach helps to bring ethical values and high standards presented by modern technologies to uphold. If nurse is keen and enthusiastic, she is capable of overcoming difficulties. She can develop her qualities with skills in handling sick person with least discomfort. As the recovery of patient depends on technique cared used by nurses that is physical and mental comfort, proper rest, sleep, nourishment and healthy environment.

It is she who observes, records, reports investigations and treatment prescribed by physician and surgeon. Foresee possible danger or complications, is able to handle the situation with utmost skill and presence of mind. She does not waste time and does care with maximum accuracy. She contributes in welfare and well being patient. With alert reflexes each patient is treated as an individual human being. She should be vigilant enough to a professional and competent manner. She has to get acquainted with the nature of illness and various precautions to relieve pain and worry.

Nurses responsibility in giving scientific reasoning such as the use of urinometer, mask, doppler, methods of cleaning and disinfecting articles used, do and don'ts, etc.

Air should be expelled before filling a hot water bag. Air is inflated after use in hot water bag, ice bag and air cushion.

Dry dusting is avoided in sick room and dusting is done after sweeping.

Diuretics like Lasix are never given in the evening.

Pulse rate should be checked before administering digoxin.

Never expose the chest of patient while giving bed bath. Nurse should bend at their knee instead of bending the back, while doing any procedure. While tucking the bed sheet, the palm is held downward.

Never hold the thermometer touching the bulb. Mercury is used in it. A constriction is present in a clinical thermometer. It should not be taken immediately after hot drink. It is contraindicated for measuring oral temperature in small children. Rectal temperature is most accurate. Thermometer is never sterilized or boiled.

Respirations are counted without the knowledge of the patient.

Oxygen is passed through water before administering to the patient.

TPR is called cardinal sign.

Salt is added to ice while filling ice bag.

Water should not be given immediately after giving cough syrup. Water should be given through the Ryle's tube before and after Ryle's tube feeding.

While applying cold compress, it should not be covered.

Air is poor conductor of heat and water is good conductor of heat. The flow of heat is from the hotter area to the less hot area.

Small and frequent feeds are given to patient with dyspnea. Smoking is not allowed near a patient who is having oxygen administration.

Systematic ways of doing saves time, energy and materials.

Micro-organism enter in the body through food and drink.

Excessive moisture in contact with the skin for a period of time can result in the tissue irritation.

Poor circulation impedes nutrient to the skin and causes skin damage. Sensory receptors in the skin are sensitive to heat, pin, touch and pressure.

The movement of the body takes place by means of muscles and bones functioning on the principles of mechanical leverage and gravitational pull.

Blood chemistry is not uniform throughout the day. It varies with the food intake.

Entering hospital is a threat to ones personal identity. People have diversity of habits and mode of behaviour. Illness brings stress on his physical and mental health.

Each sterile supply should be clearly labeled as to its contents, time and date of sterilization.

Lift the cover of the container such a way that the inside of the lid is pointing down. Do not return the used sterile objects to the container, once they have been taken out.

Oil acts as insulator and delays the transmission of heat. Woolen materials absorb moisture slowly, but hold moisture longer and cool off less quickly than the cotton materials. Friction produces heat and lubrication reduces friction.

NURSE AND CONFLICTING CONFLICTS IN WORKING AREAS

Conflicts are an inevitable part of work life. They arise due to poor communication of management, decision/policies, insufficient resources, roles/job clashes. It hinders productivity and affects confidence levels of the people involved. But if handled effectively, they can aid in raising and addressing problems help sort out issues and motivate employees to recognize and benefit from their differences.

Conflicts can be of various types, intra-individual, interpersonal, group or even inter-organizational. Therefore, conflict resolution skills are essential since choosing the appropriate technique to solve prevent disagreements is half the battle own.

Conflict management can be resolved by discussing the causes, learning the facts and settling them by applying rules, regulations and policies. Managers can play a key role in minimizing dissonance at work by regularly reviewing job descriptions, building a rapport with subordinates, effective planning and ensuring that employees are trained appropriately. To resolve conflict there is no one best way to deal with frictions. Competing, collaborating, compromising, avoiding, accommodating is the only answer.

Enjoy the present by shedding ego. An average person always thinks he is above average. Dropping the ego is easy when we realize that we are less than a dot in this vast cosmos. When we operate from ego your relationship will be affected. Happiness and well-being become more important than the survival of ones point of view. Identity is created by what others have said about us. If others say you are a great speaker, you feel you are a great speaker. So your identity depends on others. Your image is in the hands of others.

There are two world views- material and spiritual; through which we strive to achieve the goal of lasting happiness. However, for most of us, efforts through these routes only produce fatigue and dejection. At the center of materialism is accumulation of wealth. Still we are not feeling happy even if we accumulate wealth enough for our lifetime.

That life is an illusion- if we want to find out why we don't get happiness and what else is required to be satisfied. We need to look within, in human consciousness, which not only helps in finding these answers but also brings a life of fulfillment. All the needs of the body are limited. But the need of the self is unlimited.

Due to our conditioning we fail to recognize the distinction between self and body; satisfying bodily requirements does not satisfy the self. The dissatisfaction pushes one to strive for more and more tangible items, in the false hope that possession in greater quantity will quench the thirst of self. Lack of this knowledge of self is the cause of non-fulfillment. Self in the human being draws attention to what is within us innate and intact. It brings about a dialogue between what we are and what we seek. When one evaluates all states and finds answer- moves towards fulfillment.

Wherever you turn there is uncertainty, only death is sure, but even death of your day is uncertain. Life is an unanswered question, but let us still believe in the dignity and the importance of question.

Nurse should pray daily for strength. Daily have your appointment with God. Prayer is keeping our friendship with God in constant repair. Prayer brings to an inner peace and calm an indescribable sense of well being. It removes all mental and physical conflict creating a healthy body and a healthy mind. Prayer instills positive thoughts in us about ourselves and our world and other fellow beings. It removes jealousy, greed, anger, envy and anxiety which are often the cause of our aliments and sickness. It arouses and sharpens our conscious that inner voice within each of us. That there is an unseen eye, invisibly watching you. What you do not know, you are not held accountable, but once you know what is nursing practice, you are accountable for it. Live nursing qualities, anyone looking at you will also pick up, respond and do not react, patients will remember you. So till the end of your profession maintain your dignity and self-respect. Every profession has its categories and hallmark. Live to the demands of your profession. Do not limit your abilities. Nursing education will change your attitude and behavior.

Importance of School Health

Education is one of the fundamental rights of a person. The purpose of education is to 'socialize' children so that they may imbibe the social values and norms of society and to prepare them as useful citizens. Education in India is primarily a responsibility of state. The constitution provides for free and compulsory education up to the age of 14 years. The national policy of education aims at achieving this as a goal. Education is fundamental to health. The Government concerned with the determination of educational standards, scientific and technical education and research.

Children form a sizable portion of the population and during this part of their lives; they are subjected to rapid physical, mental and emotional changes. How can one safeguard against sudden and unforeseen changes that can only adversely affect life?

The child who is physically weak will be mentally weak and will not be able to give his best in the school. The mental health affects his physical health and the learning process. They need health supervision and guidance at this changing phase of their life; so that children develop into mature, responsible and well-adjusted adults.

School is an excellent ground and field, which can provide an opportunity for the early detection of diseases, which often the child carries, infections to his home from the school. The teacher is the key person and she should be well versed in health education techniques and sincerely interested in the welfare of the pupils. Children take back to there parents the health instruction they received in the schools and when they become adults, they apply this knowledge to their own families.

Site for school building should be away from dust, smoke fumes, heavy traffic, and noisy places. School premises should be properly fenced and kept free from all hazards. Classrooms ventilated with proper light, blackboard, and visual aids to avoid strain of the eyes. Play ground facilities, cleanliness of toilets, safety, electrical wiring, and food sanitation and food vendors to be discouraged. All this will guarantee health protection of children and promote positive health.

School is the best forum for imparting such health education and for moldings the attitudes and practices of children. This can be done by promoting growth and development of healthy school living. The schoolteachers also should possess knowledge of child psychology and help bridge the gap between what the child learns at school and practices at home.

The socioeconomic environmental background from which he comes; and vocational counselling and guidance into career for which they are suited.

Teachers can organize and co-ordinate parent teachers meetings. Teacher is a counselor and educator who provide guidance to parents in this matter. She can identify and observe in the classroom sings such as- unusually flushed face, any rashes or sports, cold, coughing, sneezing, sore throat, vomiting, headache, chills and fever, listlessness or sleepiness, diarrhea, scabies, ringworm, head lice in the students.

School should be modal of good sanitation. There should be adequate safe drinking water facilities; fully equipped First Aid Box at hand in emergency such as accidents, injuries, abdominal pain, fainting, epileptic fits. Education and inspection on personal hygiene such as skin, hair, teeth and clothing, importance of exercise, sleep, nutrition, and good habit is important.

Health records of each student to be maintained where identification data and past, present health history to provide information and serves as link between parents and school.

Habits—Spitting anywhere, coughing, sneezing, while eating make funny sounds, bit nails, scratch wounds in public, scratch hair, rubbing and dragging legs, shout and scream loudly, roam around in shabby cloths. Develop good substantial manners and courtesy. When one looks at you will come to know that you are well-behaved person or they will conclude that you are ill mannered and spoilt boy. What you are within is what you are outside shown in your words, action, and behaviour. Everything counts, if you want to be a gentle man. Give respect to get respect. It takes years to build a name and a second to lose it, the choice is up to you.

Avoid health related risk behaviour and ensure physical fitness, focus on activities and sports, staff health promotion policy, provide nutritional snacks in the school. Ensure access to primary health care services; integrated family and community activities. The manual looks at holistic growth.

Education is overall development of students and health should be integrated part of the curriculum.

Daily morning inspection where the teacher is in a unique position to carry out this inspection as she is familiar with children and can detect changes in the child appearance. Teacher's observation of schoolchildren is of particular importance in India because of the limited number of trained personnel for school health work.

Young children fall an easy prey to infection and bound to have important long-term consequences. Children and young adolescents are particularly vulnerable to falls, burns, poisoning, drowning. Behavioral disturbances are another child health problem. Child has right to develop in an atmosphere of affection and security. Childs health problem vary from place to place. Awakening health consciousness in children from school itself is vital.

Periodic health check-ups such as:

Dental health, to make preliminary inspection of the teeth and do prophylactic cleansing, prevent gum troubles and in improving personal appearance, teach dental hygiene.

Eye health needs attention too; attention to remedial defects like errors of refraction, treatment of squint, detection of eye infection, give vitamin A' and basic eye health services to be provided in school.

Screening them for height, weight, hearing, vision, and healthy living habits.

Assist the handicapped child and family to reach his maximum potential to lead as normal a life as possible, to become as dependent as possible and to become a productive and self-supporting member of the society.

Thus, changes are brought about in knowledge skills and behavior for a healthy living and well-being of children. The child can act as a change agent, as child has a greater capacity to observe, learn, and transfer knowledge to others. The training of teachers on school health and essential part of the school curriculum- by using flow chart, story telling and school museum an extra hour can be devoted in imparting health education. Nurses and social workers play an important role in reducing burden from the teacher by helping.

This will help to remove misconception and correct effective communication making them to change their attitudes. Printing school health records; so that any abnormality found doctor-school-parents could do the follow up of the diagnosis made.

Mental health too affects child's learning process; school shapes child's behaviour so that they become mature responsible and well-adjusted youth. School has to plan relaxation and forms of creativity. Today juvenile delinquency, maladjustment and drug addiction being problems found in school children.

School is the place where a child is adequately prepared, where the need as a growing person are regarded and if successful, the school experience will have positive influence on children's personality development. School age children get new ideas from adults outside the family.

Healthy children are full of energy and are active. Nutritional inadequacy can lead failure to put on weight, children look small for the age, and they appear thin. Respiratory infections, gastrointestinal infections, lack of concentration, exhaustion, disturbed sleep, wasting of muscles takes place. Additional calories and protein to make up for the deficiency needed. Illness in children may differ from that of adults due to lack of reserve force.

Children need assistance in learning social interactions during the language deep, the hearing of proper words and functioning of organs. Speech is important; the impairment of central nervous system may cause speech defects in child. Functional speech disorders are due to emotional stress. The common speech defect is stuttering that is difficulty in pronouncing the starting words. During the pre-school age, children learn to listen, pronounce and express themselves in words. Give the child enough time to express itself and do not put undue emphasis. Children are not to be criticized for their speech or fluency.

Child parents relations should be explore and they need to be interviewed separately. Relationship with playmates, teacher and sibling is also important. Parent's attitude may be modified. They should provide security and support to the children. The broken families may neglect the Childs basic needs, lack of love, affection and lack of security from the parents can divert the child away from home into bad company.

Early detection and children's maladjustment at home, in school and with friends should be done. Children should be explained about the discipline. Show control as well as security to the child.

Child guidance is a teamwork job, the team comprising of a psychiatrist, clinical psychologist, educational psychologist, psychiatrist social worker, public health nurses, pediatrician, speech therapist and neurologist. The psychologist is the central figure and is helped by the others in arriving to a correct diagnosis and formulating the line of treatment. Psychotherapist restores positive feelings of security in the child. To achieve this, many methods are employed e.g. Play therapy, counselling, change in the physical environment, easing of parental tensions, reconstruction of parental attitudes etc. If sound foundations of mental health laid in childhood and adolescence, the same will continue into adulthood.

In teachers, hands lie the foundation of character formation and personality building up. The teacher inculcates in the students various kinds of skills. It is a pain taking efforts in correcting, discipline, advising, guiding and inspiring students. They are the second parents that they build up structures that last. Day in and day out they instruct students, nourish with wisdom and knowledge through their rich experience and build minds, body and hearts. They shape and form the destinies of many.

The health of the schoolchild is the responsibilities of the parents, teachers, and health administrators. Effective coordination and participation between agencies will make school health reality. The children's Act 1960. The constitution of India provides that the state shall in particular direct its policy towards securing that childhood and youth are protected against moral and material abandonment. Child welfare agencies, integrated child development services, social welfare programme, juvenile justice Act 1986 can be contacted as per need of a child.

A private school in UK recently introduced a happiness course into their curriculum. Challenge your cognitive distractions, which are negative thought process that often results in depression. Mind reading (she thinks that I am a failure) catastrophic (when I fail, I will be devastated) dichotomous thinking (I get rejected by everyone) personalizing (you take on most of the blame for any negative event) get active, look within.

The school comes next to home; therefore, there should be a healthy teacher-pupil relationship. The schoolteacher can play an important role by detecting early sings of maladjustment by parent counselling, child guidance, etc.

Therefore, school health inculcates healthy practices and positive health to envelop the knowledge and attitude for better health. Recognize students as change agents in health promotion. So that it can promote appropriate social and emotional behaviour and develop school home community cooperation in health promotion. Through which changes are brought about in knowledge skills and behaviour for a healthy living.

Study as if you were going to live forever, live as if you were going to die. Attitude is little thing that makes difference. Putting extra bit is important mantra for success.

Therefore, during school years the child is able to write his on success story, discover his identity, and become the master of his destiny.

CHAPTER 28

Adolescent Health/Sex Education-I

Due to modern living and high Tec world in which the youth lives things in and around have changed dramatically fast. Sexual experimentation is common among adolescent, due to peer pressure, physiological and emotional changes and social expectations contribute to early heterosexual relations. Adolescent pregnancy continues to be a major social challenge for our nation. It occurs across socioeconomic classes, in public and private schools, among all ethnic and religious backgrounds and in all parts of the country. They need special attention to nutrition, as well as health supervision and psychological support. Nurses/ teachers play a key role in counselling teenagers on ways to avoid pregnancies. After pregnancy has occurred, the nurse/elders can assist them in obtaining medical care and developing skills that will enhance their infant's development.

Today there is need for extensive educational efforts to prevent the spread of HIV/AIDS, and STDs. HIV infection is increasing rapidly in India. Though it is known that HIV is transmitted through three major routes, namely sexual, parental and from HIV infected mother to child, the major indirect contribution is transmission is of ignorance about HIV infection.

Increasing proportions of adolescents are being infected and the infection does not have cure and is fatal. It is easily preventable by adopting safer practices and lifestyles. They are more vulnerable due to the peculiar psychological stage of development during puberty. They are more curious about human sexuality and are likely to experiment, which needs to be prevented. They at the formative years need authentic scientific information and not searching from peer and pornographic literature. Parents and teachers needs to discuss these issues. We need to control this dreadful epidemic poised to threaten the social fabric.

Rural adolescent have limited privacy, lack of transportation to health care, poverty and farming accidents. Nurses working in the community must adopt culturally sensitive intervention to meet their needs. The changes in the youth are universally same only each one is different in copping the change according to social cultural values learnt and the guidance and health education received in time makes a difference.

Health promotion during the adolescent period can help them to escape the unintentional injuries. They need advice to take drivers education course and to wear seat belts. We need to inform them with a risk associated with drinking and driving fast and recklessly, avoid use of drugs.

Encourage them to swim with a friend, teach them basic rules of water safety, so that they can select safe and supervised places to swim, before that helps them to check sufficient water depth for diving swim with a companion. Use on approval flotation device in water or boat. Encourage them to play in safe places, caution against engaging in hazardous sports. Teach stranger safety, never to go with stranger.

Avoid personalized clothing in public places. Always listen to child's concern regarding others behavior, if any one makes him feel uncomfortable in any way, teach child to say no when confront with uncomfortable situation. Teach conflict resolution skills, screen for tobacco, alcohol, drug use and inform of the risks. Prevention information will provide them with information regarding diseases mode and transmission and related symptoms. Encourage abstinence from sexual activity and provide accurate information about the consequences of sexual activity. Foster positive skills that enhances successful coping. Demand privacy when in the bathroom or dressing.

Sexuality is God given gift. Body is Holy and is a temple of God where He lives. Therefore, we have to respect our bodies and keep it always clean and pure.

What are the changes found in growing up girls?

Do you find your cloths becoming every now and then tight? Do you feel bad when your parents scold or correct you?

This and many other change takes place due to hormonal changes in life.

During menstruation, the breast becomes larger and tender to touch. Be careful to protect breast from injury. They will get curly hairs which beginning to grow under her arms, keep clean. Menstruation last about 4-5 days and happens every month until a women is 45 to 50 years old. Some girls begin it before they are 12 years old and others may not start until they are older then 12.

Every 28 days the whole process of it is repeated. You can keep tract of your menstrual dates and be prepared for it. If you begin counting 28 days from the first day of menstruation, you can find out the date when your next menstruation will begin.

Follow menstrual hygiene such as -Fold clean cloth and make pads for you to wear so the blood would not soil your clothes, change the pads often when they become soiled to prevent bad odors, which come from wearing soiled napkins. Keep at least 6 clean pads ready. You can use pieces of old saris or other soft cloth. If the cloth is thin use, three layer about 18 inches square. Ready-made disposable pads too worn in the same way.

Some girls have pain, especially in the beginning when their bodies are not used to the experience yet. Some of them may have backache, crams, and bloated full feeling in the abdomen for few days before it begins. It is a sign that an egg has been made in her body, which can possibly grow into a baby. When the egg is fully developed, it bursts through the sac and come out, uterus with a soft lining. Take daily bath and comb your hair dress in clean clothes as usual. Do your usual work at home and take rest when you feel tired. You can eat any food you feel like eating.

Remember, menstruation is not sickness. It is a part of God's wonderful plan in preparing a girl to be a mother.

Adolescent is a period that extends from the onset of puberty until the time of sexual maturation, this period varies widely depending upon genetic and environmental factors. These are the formative years, the years of preparation for undertaking greater responsibilities, a time of exploration and widening horizons to ensure all round development. This development depends on his socioeconomic circumstances, the environment in which they live, grow, the quality of relationship with their family, community, and peer group and the opportunity for education.

Sex plays an important part in any intimate loving relationship. Sex is the sensual and sensory manifestation of the attraction between two people. However, it can also cause disappointment, frustration and unhappiness. To tackle problems such as these it helps if we are equipped with a knowledge and understanding of our sexuality and sexual behavior.

Sexuality is not just matter of inner drives- it is shaped by the customs and practices of the society we live in. sexual restrictions have been always existed; sex is not just sexual act. To understand fully we need to take holistic approach a whole person. We are not sexual machines, but an individual, Sex is a natural part of life, and a broad understanding of it can only serve to empower people in their relationships. Misinformation, ignorance or embarrassment, inhibitions, fears, anxiety develop as a results of influence of parents, society. Try to make sure that children have plenty of chances to play with other children. Do not be overprotective or possessive. Allow the child to grow up believing they are the center of the universe. Do not put too much pressure on child to succeed.

We have to understand this concept; what the human sex drive is and how it is controlled. What part of body responds best to stimulation? What makes one person sexually attractive to another? How does the human body work sexually? What determines the nature of sexuality? What controllers the way in which we form relationships and where does this feeling of sex come from? In addition, why do some people achieve longer lasting and happier relationships than others are all-important questions?

The brain as a sex organ—This powerful organ comprising billions of interconnecting nerve cells, which controls and coordinates all our bodily activities, also controls our sex lives. In fact, the brain is the control center for our sexual desire and sex drives.

The secret of success is often nothing more complicated than getting the timing right. When both of you are ready for commitment, is all that required for a successful relationship.

Some find it difficult to express feelings, reason the way you were brought up, from very early age where they were discouraged from expressing emotions.

Abnormal sexual development, genital abnormalities may be evident to parents and doctors when a child is born, or may become clear, as a child gets older. In the case of testicular feminization, the fetus is genetically male and the testes develop normally. However, the male baby's sex organs are indistinguishable from a female. She may be born with an enlarged clitoris or, in more severe cases; she can develop a penis and an empty scrotum, and look like a male externally. Individuals whose primary sex organs do not match their external genitals are known as pseudo-hermaphrodites. Some seek gender-reassignment/sex change operations in later life in order to match their external genitalia to their sexual identity.

- The *influence* of society, relatives and television-media-net, will probably influenced, however, parents in helping to provide their child with a strong sense of self worth, and strive to ensure that their children have equality of opportunity and support, regardless of *gender*.

  Sex by 18 for 50% women in state loses their virginity by the time they reach 18 years of age. About 39% of women get married before the legal minimum of 18 that force them into teenage pregnancy. Early marriage system leads the early sex.

- *Sexual images* on TV in videos and in film influence children, and may get negative and confusing messages that may not be acceptable. The importance of parents giving truthful, thoughtful and developmentally appropriate answers to their children's questions about sex, and parents need to supervise what actually children watch.

- *Talking about sex to children*, name of their genitals, how the baby's are made etc., is of important in today's fast forward life.

  Protecting children from sexual abuse—Parents can advice about possible dangers in the outside world, but what action can parents take to help their children avoid the various dangers? Parents should make sure children tell their parents immediately if anyone touches them in a way they do not like.

- *Puberty timeline*—Change causes great confusion and distress. Puberty is normal part of growing up. Despite sex education, some girls are still taken by surprise by their first menstrual period and boys by their first ejaculation. Parents can help by talking to their children about growing up and developing. Adolescent may have doubts about what is happening to them, and may need parental reassurance at some point.

- Keeping the skin clean and free from excess oil and dirt by regular washing with an antibacterial soap can help to reduce the incidence of skin problems such as *acne, body odors* that are very common among adolescents.

- *The hymen*—In some societies, women who are deemed not to have intact hymens are taken not to be virgins and are banished or even killed. In other societies, the bedsheets are displayed after the wedding night to sow off the bloodstains that indicate the bride was a virgin. This is unfair and may cause suffering, as in many girls, the hymen is already sufficiently stretched and it has little functional value and has only cultural value.

- Some boys experience a small degree of *breast development* during puberty. Do not be shock; breast swelling generally last for between 2 and 18 months.

- *Peer pressure*—One of the enjoyable features of adolescence is the formation of strong friendships that enable boys and girls to develop a separate identity outside the family. Yet pressure from friends of the same age can be irresistible. The urge to conform to a certain image during a time of change and uncertainty is very strong. Friends may try to convince an adolescent to skip school, take drugs or have sex, when he/she may not want to do these things. Saying no to peer pressure means that those friends drop you, be assertive and say no if you feel pressurized doing something you feel wrong rather then response to peer pressure. Adolescence generally needs help and advice about all kinds of matter from parents.

- *Parents as role models* they watch and are influenced by what their parents do and say. It is easy to tell a child that he/she should not smoke or drink but parents should bear this in mind themselves for the message they are trying to convey. Every father believes that when he was at the age of his child he was hard working, outgoing. This is like a sparrow packing in the mirror for seeing its own reflections. The father sees his own youthful days in his child. In addition, the mistakes that he has done he does not want his child to repeat. If the parents become friends to children and take them into confidence the children, will not hide anything from them; at this age the child needs guidance and prepare them for responsible behavior.

- *Being assertive* means saying what you feel without being aggressive, without compromising your position and, hopefully, without hurting someone else. Be honest and say you are not really interested when someone you do not like asks for a date. When your boyfriend/girlfriend wants to do something that, you do no want to do.

- *Sexual fantasies*—Fantasies are daydreams or imaginings experienced by most people. A person might fantasies that they are a famous singer or great football players. They are not real and are purely in the realms of the imagination. Sexual fantasies are the same. It has nothing to do with real life.

- *TV-Media* children get addicted and lose creativity and critical thinking. They watch horror films, nude scene and watch multi channel programmes which gives them drug effect, glamorous world, over night becoming rich, watch violence, rape scene this gets influences the mind and sometimes get transplanted into practical life. Watch TV by selecting educative programmes, sports, jocks and comedy, entertainment that gives you relaxation with knowledge.

- Talking about being *homosexual*—A difficult choice is where to hide their feelings or admit them openly and hope that friends and family will accept the way they are. Telling the parents can be greatest barrier, initially parents will get upset, angered to know their child is gay, later will accept because of the love they have for the children. For the adolescent to do this move usually takes a great deal of courage, anguish. So support them, as nothing will change the situation.

- Some parents worry that giving their young *teenager information about sex* will make them more likely to indulge in sex. Researchers say that if children are equipped with knowledge about sex in their teen, they are more likely to wait until they are older before starting their sex lives. When parents talk and discuss the different options available, young people are likely to take a responsible attitude of their actions.

- A new study has found that young girls who are sexually active are far more likely suffer from depression than those who remain virgins. Researchers found that teenage sex leaves many girls with feelings of guilt and low self-esteem. Portrayal young women as sex objects in media is harming there mental and physical health.

- *Unwed mothers*—If you think you are *pregnant*, confiding in anyone can be difficult. Telling parents would be insurmountable obstacle, as you may feel ashamed and guilty about what has happened, and you will be terrified that they will be angered or even reject you. Your parents will probably feel shacked and incapable accepting the situation. As the dust settles, you may find they are more helpful and supportive in a crisis, whatever the cause and will talk what could be done. If you cannot tell, your parents get counseling and seek advice of family clinic. If your partner builds up the courage to tell his parents, and if he wants to stand by you fine. The only answer is to talk about things, and own the responsibility of your action by handling well. Nothing is more precious then life. Respect and care for life.

Abortion—Think twice seriously before going for abortion. If you are a teenage girl, you need to know what abortion means, it is killing of human being. It is not like tonsil operation. One out of three teenage abortions has complications that might prevent girl from having children again. Abortion more than twice is as dangerous as childbirth; more than one third of mothers of aborted babies have mental problems later. So if you find yourself in trouble over pregnancy, never think that abortion is an easy way out. How are the babies in their mothers womb murdered? There are four ways; all are cruel and in- human. The vacuum suction, it works as a vacuum cleanser, cleaning up dirt, the baby comes out in little pieces. The cutting up method, the doctor just slices the baby to pieces inside the mother's womb. The surgical method, the doctor takes the baby out by surgical opening in the abdomen, the babies' then are generally used for experiments or else they are burned or drowned in water. The salt method, a salt solution is injected into amniotic sac and the baby is burned to death. God gives us the gift of freedom, some choose though abuse this freedom by destroy in the gift of human life by aborting their unborn babies.

• *Suicide* has become second leading cause of death after accidents in teenage group. Reckless driving and drug overdose. Anxiety, emotional fluxes, search for identity, frustration, defective coping, lack of affection and acceptance from their parents and peers, feeling of despair and hopelessness experience. The teen may feel responsible for parents divorce, or find himself simple lost in a new family situation, severe anxiety due to competition and pressures of getting good job. For the young people whose hopes have been raised only to be aborted, sense of failure may be overwhelming leaving to despair.

A suicide attempt is a desperate cry for help. Some of the signs and symptoms of potential suicidal behavior of adolescence is extreme fatigue, loss of sleep with nightmares, restlessness and early morning awakening, sudden loss of appetite, inactivity an boredom, tearfulness, withdrawal from previous enjoyed activities, writing many letters to friends, consumption of alcohol, giving away prized possession.

The cause may be long grief reaction to loss and significant other than death/separation, chronic illness, and family history of suicide.

Suicide attempts are often an impulsive act. Find out how long the young person been feeling bad and does he know what caused to feeling? It is important to explore possible reasons for wanting to die. Does he have a support system? Does he feel alone or is there someone with whom he can talk?

Methods used- jumping, hanging, poisoning, wrist slashing, inhalation of gas, ingestion of analgesic.

The teen should be encouraged to and show the alternative ways that could change the feelings. To provide sense of hope, do family therapy during this difficult period of change.

- *Substance abuse* in teenagers—Increasingly, young people turn towards smoking, drinking, or drug. How to help them to break this habit? Best ways to help their children is to set a good example.
- If there is a heavy *menstrual* flow that last for more then seven days.
  Irregularity in the menstrual cycle that cannot be attributed to long distance travel, excessive weight loss or illness
  Intervals between periods of fewer than 21 days or more then 60;
  Bleeding at any other times during the menstrual cycle other then at the start of a period or, briefly, around ovulation. It is important to get a medical opinion so that the serious disorder, if present, can be treated.
- *Breast tenderness*—Alleviates pain and tenderness wears a supportive, properly fitting bra. Take mild painkiller and take vitamin B_6.
- Many teens are *reluctant to see the doctor* when the experience symptoms- especially symptoms that affect their reproductive systems. Early detection means more option for treatment and higher survival rates. Be aware of what your body is telling you, when something appears to be wrong; in order to assess and monitor all the various aspects of health.

Losing that loving feelings due to many factors such as excessive alcohol intake leads to loss of desire. Depression tends to lower a persons sex drive. If overworked or exhaustion which leave little room for sex. Feeling of guilt because the way you are brought up to believe sex is not quiet nice may reduce desire. Mental stress tends to cause to loose the desire also worrying about money or business matters can diminish interest in sex.

Never take each other for granted. Talk to each other openly, honestly. Listen to the others point of view. Treat each other with respect. Show your appreciation of each other and do not end the day in anger. Make time for each other; do not be too serious, it is important to laugh together sometimes. Make joint plans or discuss your joint plans.

Every culture controls the sexual activities of its citizens. People who break the rules are regarded as criminals. Many forms of sexual activity are still prohibited by law. Sexual harassment is a different form of inappropriate behavior, action or words are abusive and offensive type. Unwelcome physical contact; groping, pinching, patting, or unnecessary touching. Unwelcome invitations and comments, pressure for dates, sexually suggestive jokes, remarks, pornographic pictures and calendars in the workplace. Some people derive sexual gratification from making obscure telephone calls. The caller attempts to engage the woman victim in intimate conversation. Various approaches are used to help the victim, and the approach will depend upon the specific problem presented.

Miracle of life—God created a man and a woman. God created human beings according to his own image and likeness, resembling them like him. He created male and female. He blessed them and looked at his creation the crown of his created work in man and God was very pleased. Nothing is more precious than human life. Respect and care for God given life.

Making motherhood safe and to have healthy mother and bouncing baby let us go through the process of fertilization how new life is formed.

Pregnancy and childbirth are special events in women's lives and the lives of their families. This can be a time of great hope and joyful anticipation. It can also a time of fear, suffering and even death.

Although pregnancy is not a diseases but a normal physiological/biological process.

It is associated with certain risks; each pregnancy represents a journey into the unknown from which too many women never return. Access to health care particularly at the critical time of birth, can help ensure that childbirth is a joyful event.

It takes many years for a girl to become a healthy mature woman. The first days of life or the miracle of life is a mystery. The miracle of life is when the ovum encounters the sperm, the new life is infused, and stats growing, it is already someone. Let us understand the biological process of this.

A new life begins when an egg cell from the mother is fertilized by the sperm cell from the father. The egg is one of the many thousands that develop in the sex glands called ovaries of the mother. The mother has two ovaries one on each side of the womb. In the lower part of the abdomen. After a girl comes of age, the egg cells begin to ripen one at a time. Once every 28-30 days one of the ripe eggs is released from the ovary sac into a nearby passage called the fallopian tube. The egg at the time is smaller than the head of the pin.

The sperm cell of the man develops in the man's sex gland called the "testes". Like the mother, the sperm cells of the father begin to mature or ripen after puberty. The sperm cell is so small that it cannot be seen by the naked eye. Nearly 5,00,000,000 of them could fit into a space the size of a thimble. They can be seen under a microscope and look like tiny tadpoles with oval shaped heads and long tail.

When they are released into the woman's body, they swim along into the womb and then on into the tubes projecting outward from the womb. If there is an egg cell in producing a fertilized egg.

As soon as egg becomes fertilized it begins to grow and passes down the tube into the womb. The original egg cell divides into two. The two cells divide to make four and the four divide to make sight and so on. The lining of the womb has been prepared for the arrival of the fertilized egg (ovum). A rich blood supply makes the lining thick, soft and spongy. About 10 days after the egg has left the sex gland (ovary), it becomes fixed (implanted) with the help of hairy growth (vittin) covering the ovum in the lining of the womb where it continues to grow.

After the fertilized egg is planted in the lining of upper part of the womb, it begins to increase in size. The hairy growth which attached itself to the womb for blood supply changes into a tube with placenta. The fertilized egg gets its nourishment from the mother through the tube, which passes into the umbilicus of the fetus. The egg continues to grow for 280 days or 9 months and one week until it becomes a full size baby. During this period, the mother does not have her usual menstrual periods. By the end of 2 weeks the cluster of cells are still barely large enough to be seen by naked eye. At the end of 3 weeks, the ovum is the size of a small grape. The hairy growth covers the ovum. By the end of 4 weeks, the sac with the embryo is the size of a pigeon's egg. The embryo is curved to resemble a bean the eyes and limbs are not yet developed. At the end of 4 weeks, the baby is still only about a quarter of an inch long. Now the inside parts like the heart and the stomach, the brain and the lungs begin to develop. The heart begins to beat although no one will be able to hear it for many weeks. At five weeks, the baby is the shape of a tiny quarter moon.

His head grows faster than any other part of the body. The backbone begins to form. By 1½ months, the baby is almost half an inch long and small short arms and legs have formed. By the 7th week, the ears and eyelids can be seen. The baby now floats in a sac of fluid, which is sometimes called 'bags of waters. Perhaps you are wondering why he does not drown. The answer is simple. He cannot drown because he does not use his lungs until after he is born and comes out into the air. He gets all that he needs from the mother's blood even the oxygen, which we get from the air. As the baby grows, the sac stretches like a rubber balloon. The fluid in the sac keeps the baby warm and acts like a cushion to protect him from any sudden bumps, which may happen from the mother's daily activities.

At the end of eight weeks, the sac with the embryo resembles a hen's egg. By now, the mother begins to suspect that she is pregnant. She has not had her regular menses for two months and her abdomen begins to enlarge. She may feel slightly nauseated early in the morning and does not feel like eating. By having, her urine examined at this time she can know for sure if she is pregnant or not.

At 12 weeks, the sac is the size of a duck's egg. The placenta is formed. By the 3rd month the baby is bout 2 ½ inches long and weight about one ounce. Tiny fingers and toes are already well formed and even tiny nails begin to show. The back is still curved but the head begins to straighten. Teeth are beginning to form deep inside the gums. The hair is beginning to grow on the head. By now the external sex organs of the baby have appeared. At four months, the baby is 4-5 inches long and weighs about 4 ounces. By the 5th month, the mother can feel the movement of the baby. For a while, the baby looks like a wrinkled old person but fat eventually fills out the spaces under the skin and makes it smooth. The doctor may now hear the faint beating of the baby's heart for the first time. The baby is bout 3 inches long weighing 10-11 ounces. The size of the womb increases up to the level of the mother's naval (umbilicus), and really begins to show. From this time onward, the size of the abdomen increases rapidly. By six months, the baby is quite active. He kicks and moves from one side to another. Sometimes the head is down and sometimes it is up.

After seven months, the baby usually stays in one position. He sleeps for long intervals and has active periods before he is born just as he has after birth. From the sixth month, onward fine soft fuzzy (hair) grows on the baby's body and at about seven months a soft creamy substance covers and protects his skin. The seven-month baby looks full-grown but he weighs less than 5 pounds (5 Kgs.) If he were to be born at this time his chances of survival are small. He would be too small and weak to nurse. His resistance to infection is low and his body temperature is unsteady. During the 8th and 9th months baby attains his full growth. The nose and ears take firm shape and the nails grow longer. The bones of the head become harder and close together. The hair on the head grows as longer. By now, the baby weighs 5 pounds or more and he is likely to live if born at the time and given proper care.

Now the baby is ready to begin his journey into the world. The mother has to work very hard. That is why the whole process is called labour. The muscles of the womb begin to tighten/contract and draw back/retract causing the baby to be pressed against the inside opening of the womb. This helps to widen the opening to the baby can pass through. The baby's head faces the right side of the mother and has dropped low down between the bladder and the rectum. It takes several hours, especially with the first baby, for opening to stretch large enough to allow the baby to come out. The doctor may put on rubber gloves and feel inside to find out how fast the womb is opening. Throughout the period, the mother has a feeling of crams in the abdomen and the back may ache. The baby is still inside the "bag of water" and some of the water collected at the bottom of the bag, which acts as a cushion to the baby's head.

The baby's position gradually rotates until the faces the mothers back. The mothers bladder and rectum are compressed which gives the mother the feelings that she needs to pass urine and motion. During this time, the muscles of the womb continue to tighten and relax attentively. Usually the bag of waters breaks by this time, due to the pressure, allowing the fluid to escape.

Finally, the outlet has opened completely. It will take about almost two hours for the baby to be born. At this time, the mother can help by bending down as though having a bowel movement. The nurse will stay with the mother and instruct when to bear down. Bearing down too soon may tire the mother needlessly. If the baby is very large and the opening is small the nurse may enlarge it by making a small out which latter is closed with a few stitches. This is better than having the opening torn by the force of the baby's coming out. The cut heals better than a tear. The mother does not feel the pressure already numbs the cut or putting in the stitches as the part.

Most babies are born head first with the face down, which is the easiest way. Sometimes, babies are born feet or buttocks first, or with the face turned upward. When this happens, the doctor may use special instruments to help the baby come out. If the doctor had a chance to examine the mother earlier, he will know the position of the baby. A doctor may be able to turn the baby before he is born so that the head will come first and the birth will be easier.

The baby is born but he is still attached to the mother by a long shiny cord. Inside the cord are the blood vessels through which the baby has been fed and through which the baby's waste materials have been transported from the body. The cord is cut between the two ties to prevent necessary loss of blood. Now the baby is taken to be cleaned and dressed while the mother waits for the final stage of labour. A few minutes later the mother again feels the muscles of her womb contract and out comes the bag, which had enclosed the baby during the nine months of growth, and the spongy pad, which was the source of nourishment for the baby. Labour is over and the mother is ready for a well-earned rest.

Not only the baby but also a family is born. The young husband feels a new tenderness towards his wife who has undergone the stress and discomforts of labour. Both view the baby with a sense of wonder and feel happy. Perhaps they love the baby and each other more because it cost them something.

Adolescent Health/Sex Education-II

Growing up is never easy, when high-spirited young boy/girl reach the age of 12-13 years a dramatic change takes place. Something unknown strange feeling a new unexplainable feelings come and the world is perceived differently. Up to this point, someone else has always made most of the decisions for him or her. Nevertheless, suddenly the whole situation changes at this point of time. Change raise serious problems for parents and teenagers alike they are often confuse and uncertain what to do. The young person feels quiet able to handle things for him. If there is an atmosphere of love and confidence in the home, even the most difficult young person will eventually pass through these years without permanent harm.

Therefore, parents must consider that each person deserves a fair chance to develop his/her own way. Expect some mistakes; this is how they learn to stand on their own feet as adults. However, parents must provide sensible rules for them to follow as they grow up with friendly guidance and counsel. Wise parents will avoid unfair comparison.

This is the clumsy age, which brings many changes into youth some quiet amazing. Boys who never could keep their hair tidy to their faced, washed, suddenly begin to comb their hair many times a day. Teenage girls are forever in front of the mirror, working out new hairstyles. Teenagers are very anxious to be accepted by those of their own age, and most of all by those of the opposite sex.

Every individual should acquire basic scientific knowledge about the human body including sex organs. On the horizon of adulthood- Everything you always wanted to know about human sexuality, but do not know whom to ask.

When did you begin your menses period? How often do you menstruate? Do you have premenstrual symptoms? How heavy is your menses flow? Do you experience any spotting between menses? Do you experience pain or discomfort during menses? (type, intensity, location, duration of your pain and onset, amount, character, duration of bleeding to be noted.) When was your last menses? Do you have unusual vaginal discharge? Have you had any STDs? Do you perform monthly BSE (breast self examination)? Have you noticed any abnormality? What is the most effective nursing intervention to help client overcome their anxiety related to the discussion of reproductive health problems? What are the psychological changes in sexuality that occur when a person ages?

So many factors lead to normal growth and development of child in to adulthood. It takes many years to mature child into adulthood and many questions that get crowed the minds of young ones. There is a primary and secondary development takes place.

The age at which secondary sex characteristics develop in the child are compared with the established normal ranges for male or female culture influences gender related and sexual identity.

A child's attitudes and behaviour about his meaning and use of the genitals begin in infancy and are mounded on the behaviour of significant adults.

Religions dictates often parallel those of a specific culture and strongly affect sexual activity. Person's religious beliefs often influence specific sexual particles the acceptable number of partners contraceptives use, specific treatments to terminate a pregnancy end fertility and remove barriers to infertility.

Male reproductive organs—brief information- the penis is the sexual organ, which is also used for emptying urine outside the body. During sexual intercourse, the semen is ejaculated through the penis. Normally, either urine or semen is discharged through it, at any given moment. Hence, urine and semen are not emptied together.

Describe anatomy of male sexual organs-scrotum, testes, seminal vesicle, vas deferens, prostrate gland, Cowper's glands, and urethra with the help of charts or slide, video with explanation.

In the same way, describe female reproductive organs- Labia majora, Labia minora, clitoris, hymen, vagina, uterus, fallopian tube, and ovary. Moreover, their functions.

What is puberty? The physical and psychological changes talking place due to hormonal changes. The signs of puberty in girls are the development of a breast bud, hair growth around the genital area. There is increase in height and she is likely to have the first menstrual period that shows the transition of childhood to adulthood talking place.

What is menstruation? When does it begin and when does it stop permanently? Why do women develop pain in the abdomen during menses? What is safe period?

Signs of *puberty in boys* seen are increase in the size of the testes, and penis, hair at the pubic area and later on face. The voice becomes hoarse and the Adams apple starts becoming prominent, sudden increase in height, gain weight.

Individual variation exists in the length, size and shape of the penis. In addition, the ability to reproduce does not depend on the length of the penis. The size of the penis depends on certain heredity and hormonal factors. Penile erection during sleep is a normal harmless phenomenon. The erection of the penis can occur even in childhood and the capability is observed even in old age. The failure to get penile erection may be due to certain organic diseases and psychological disorders. Premature ejaculation is generally caused by certain psychological disturbances. One must also remember that alcohol stimulates desire but takes away the action. In addition, lack of confidence, marital disharmony very high blood pressure, and uncontrolled diabetes can affect.

During adolescence, developing sexual attraction towards the opposite sex is common. This *attraction* and curiosity towards sex related issues and inability to get information may facilitate this further. This is a passing phase in ones life and it is normal to think about sex. This will disappear ones own; one should keep oneself busy and concentrate on study and activities, which will divert attention.

The influence of *peer pressure* is dominant, if every body in-group smokes the other even do not like will stars smoking due to peer pressure. Therefore the choice of peer who can influence ones own attitudes and behavior is crucial.

Peer pressure can lead to negative and positive outcome. It is a process of development of their own identity separate from their parents. Socially unaccepted behaviour one should not do it, which is also unacceptable to self. One can say no. If the group ask you consume alcohol, you should be mentally prepared about what you say when the issue arises; so that you are not caught unaware. Be mentally prepared to take opinion of elder's parents, teacher in case of dilemma. Never think obligated to pay back with sexual favors as shortcut.

There are ways in which one can *express love* and affection. Love is an emotion a feeling. It does not necessarily mean sex. One should plan before hand just how far one would want to go, and stick to your limits. In addition, say no to sex if the other partner says it is a way of expressing love.

Auto-Erotic: The adolescent takes interest in his own body. He craves for self-relief from tension, which implies him to handle his own sexual organs. This usually culminates in masturbation.

Masturbation is when an individual stimulates ones own sexual organs manually. Sexual satisfaction is sought without any direct contact. Either hands or mechanical devices do it. Masturbation is common amongst teenagers and becomes rare after marriage.

However, excessive masturbation develops mental arrogance and should be discouraged.

It also has bad effects, if it continues well into adulthood, even when the natural object of satisfying sexual desire is present.

Impotence is the inability to have penile erection even after sexual stimulation. It is associated with certain illness like long standing, uncontrolled diabetes, hypertension and certain spinal cord diseases. Psychological problems can also lead to impotency; it is managed with the help of medical specialists and psychotherapy and good counseling.

When the penis is introduced in the vagina, the *sex* is called penovaginal sex. When it is introduced in the anal cavity, it is called penoanal sex. If it is introduced in the oral cavity, it is called peno-oral sex.

During adolescence, individual may be impulsive and take decisions without realizing its consequences. Individuals are easily attracted to each other at the physical level. Infatuation is common in this group. One needs to understand the consequences like unwanted pregnancy and the risk of contracting SID/HIV infection. *Premarital sex* can lead to HIV infection. HIV infection can be acquired by having unprotected sex with an HIV infected person. Unsafe sex especially with an unknown person can lead to this infection. Performing a sexual act is a major decision. Careful analysis of the associated responsibilities is necessary before undertaking such a step.

Completion of education, setting into a *career* and obtaining financial stability are generally considered as the prerequisites for marriage. Social acceptance for sex in our society is mostly after marriage. Adolescence is not the right age for sex, as girls are not able to bear the burden of pregnancy physically, mentally or emotionally. Boys cannot shoulder the responsibility of parenthood.

There is a tendency to satisfy ones *curiosity* by sexual experimentation, disregarding the risks and social norms. Additionally peer pressure and other addictions lead a helping hand to foster risky behaviour. This is a passing phase in adolescence and disappears with time and emotional maturity.

Heterosexuality: In this phase, the object of attachment is a member of the opposite sex. This develops during late adolescence. This enables the boys and girls to develop a healthy attitude towards one another so that they may lead good social life.

Homosexuality is the sexual relationship between persons of the same sex that is man with man or woman with woman that is called *lesbian*. They tend to derive sexual pleasure through penoanal, peno-oral or mutual masturbation. They may also use certain mechanical devices to satisfy each other's sexual urge. Anal canal, unlike vagina is not elastic and does not have natural lubricants. This factor increases the chance of tears or micro-injuries, which facilitate transmission of HIV infection.

Sexual desire control lies in the brain this center in the *brain* when get stimulated one has sexual arousal.

Conception depends not on the frequency of sexual acts but the timing. If it has taken place during the unsafe periods, the risk of pregnancy is higher. Therefore, pregnancy is possible even due to the first sexual experience.

Good *personal hygiene* should be ensured all through especially when girl menstruates.

The sexual urge continues to exist even in old age.

Abstinence is a state of not performing an activity that is a person does not have sex with anybody.

All these changes are perfectly normal and are just part of growing. However, rapidly growing bodies are often awkward and hard to manage. Here they need sympathy and understanding, not harsh criticism during this stressful time. Striking changes are now talking place within the body, producing new reactions that are followed by deep feelings of guilt. Bad company and a lack of proper guidance may lead to a life of sorrow and tragedy.

The *nurses/teachers* understanding of development provides a unique perspective for helping *teenagers* and parents anticipate and cope with the stresses. Nurse/teacher must identify teenager's needs and desires. Any deviation in the timing of the physical changes can be extremely difficult for adolescent to accept. Nurse's/parents/teachers needs to support who undergo delay puberty.

In early *adolescent* secondary sex characteristics appear. They compare their normality with peer of the same sex. They are somewhat preoccupied with rapid body changes. They try out various roles. They start doing the measurement of attractiveness by acceptance or reject of peer. Conformity to group norms becomes vital and of importance. They have strong desire to remain dependent, there are a wide mood swings, intense daydreaming, and anger outwardly expressed with moodiness, temper outburst and verbal insults and name-calling are some of the common features found at this age.

As they grow into late adolescence starts to view problem, and are able to be comfortable with physical growth. Popularity is a major concern for teenagers. Accidents remain the leading cause of death in adolescence. Mostly motor vehicle accidents that are most common cause of death. Depression and social institution commonly precede a suicide attempts.

In such youth, there are some Warning signs such as decrease in school performance, withdrawal loss of initiatives, loneliness, and sadness and crying, appetite and sleep disturbances leads them towards low self-esteem results in tendency of suicide, guidance can help them focus on the positive aspects of life and strengthen coping abilities.

He has deep down craving and desire to be more like an admired idol. There is continues need of praise and approval from peer group and parents, the child wants to be first or best. Many find it difficult to sit still for a longer periods, may become interested, yet shy, around members of the opposite sex. They continuously do hero-worshiping.

Keep only cheerful friends. The grouches pull you down. Keep learning, learn more about the computer, crafts, gardening and never let the brain idle. An idle mind is the devil's workshop. Enjoy the simple things. Laugh often, long and loud. Laugh until you gasp for breath. Cherish your health and preserve it. Life is not a race, do take it slower, and hear the music before the song is over.

Adolescent Health/Sex Education-III

Adolescent health has always been over-shadowed by children's health. However, adolescence is a crucial bridge between childhood and adulthood. Any holistic approach to improving the health status of India's children must therefore, address adolescent health.

Due to low levels of educational achievement and persistent gender disparity; high unemployment rate in urban-rural setup; they have early sex, early marriage and child bearing. This is due to poor knowledge and use of contraceptives, unwanted pregnancies and abortions, short birth intervals and unplanned births. Above and over they have poor nutrition and antenatal care, lack of information and adequate access to health services are some of the major reasons in rural setting up where youthfulness ends.

Diseases such as diabetes and anorexia are becoming increasingly common among adolescents in urban areas and are a major public health challenge. Moreover, the stress faced by adolescents these days surfaces in disastrous and often, unthinkable ways, including suicides, murders, deviant behaviour and substance abuse.

Consequences of early marriage and early sex: India has a population of more than 200 million adolescents, of whom 36 percent in the 13 to 16 year age group are married.

As many as 64 percent of those in the age group of 17 to 19 years are already mothers

Early marriage has significant health repercussions; and while the problems faced by adolescent girls have received some attention, those encountered by male adolescents tend to go unrecognized. Sexual active by the time they are 18. Most adolescents reach sexual maturity before they are ready to handle or grapple with their own social, emotional and psychological development. Moreover, there is widespread lack of information among adolescents on reproductive and sexual health issue.

Be aware—The pursuit of happiness today that it was we are living longer than we have ever lived before but our lives are becoming unhealthy, our wants are more, our fears are more, our angers are more. Happiness is way of life. It depends on the thought process one engages himself into it. Those who are optimistic live happier lives than pessimist does. Calm yourself down, you cannot change the circumstances, try to relax your muscles, let the anxiety drain out of your body with deep breath.

Worry only adds up to your current stress levels and leads to reduced concentration levels. Take action, it is the antidote to worry. As things we endlessly worry about never, materialize. You set for yourself basing your view on someone else view leads to low self-esteem and loss of energy. Stop making comparisons, stay in touch with the real you, set your own slandered, believe in yourself and boost your self-esteem. When you cannot forgive and crave for revenge, you actually end up punishing yourself.

The anger that is bottled up within you weighs you down without you even realizing it. If you spend too much time with someone who does nothing but complains, it is bound to rub off on you. The negative vibes will definitely get you feeling low. When we badmouth others, we focus our energies on negative traits and give rise to negative emotions, mind your own business, will save you a lot of energy.

EATING DISORDER—OBESITY- GET RID OF AN UNHEALTHY LIFESTYLE

New food trends to make you smarter and younger consumer wants food that will give them sharper minds and tighten those wrinkles as well as help them shed a pound or two, better skin and digestion- now by some ancient culture and looking at food and some of the medicinal and wellness properties. Food industries to help develop new products, encouraged fruits and vegetables and eat verity of different colors food.

Imagine a car to be the human body. The radiator in a car can be compare to our water stores, while the fuel tank can be relate to our fat stores. When the radiator is low water, the car will stall on you. This has nothing to do with the fuel tank (burning fat in our case) so to compare our fuel tank (fat stores) with our radiator (water stores) would be absurd. To facilitate fat loss, one must drink water to remain well hydrated together with diet control and exercise.

More than half the world will be obese by 2030 with waistlines increasing rapidly around the world research study says. Be aware of those diet goodies, you might be stacking on more kilos than you deserve. The key areas that hold fat in your body needs to lose weight now. You must take roughly 10,000 steps a day, making a conscious effort those with desk jobs.

Make sure you smile everyday, a positive attitude can benefit you much being happy adds to your life either year, get the right nutrition. Shun diet foods, simplify your food choices, and choose foods that satisfy hunger they will make you feel fuller on few calories, which make it much easier to lose those unwanted kilos. Control your eating speed, eating slowly and relaxed state of mine will curb your desire to consume more than you need.

Cut food into smaller pieces, chew each mouthful thoroughly and do not reload your spoon before swallowing the previous mouthful. You will be able to savor the taste more. Try power walking or running around a local park. You only get out what you put in. Getting fit or toning your body is like running a business you need to put in the hard work and make sure that what you are doing works, be on a mission. Push your effort level up, and challenge your body.

Make time for exercise and prioritize it. Stop stress polluting your life, one worry can utterly spoil your happiness. Set aside time to do something pleasurable even if it is just for and hour, it gives you something to look forward to. Avoid energy drainers. Unlock your energy face up the issues, brisk walk will boost your energy, stimulate your brain to produce happy chemicals and exercise will lower your stress. Get your timing right, go to sleep before 11 PM, do not under estimate good night sleep, the body's repair system is at work in the night giving your body enough time to rejuvenate.

Stay healthy with morning walk- family play an integral part in maintains health. When parents are active and health conscious, children grow up to maintain their health.

However if families are careless about diet and health, illness like obesity lack of physical activity attribute to 1.9 million death globally.

Walk helps activates body cells, improves blood circulation, burns free fatty acids, to shed excess fat and fights obesity. Improves oxygen supply in the blood, relives blood pressure, joint pain and body aches. Our current lifestyles leave us feeling exhausted with tight muscles and an aching back along with a stressed state of mind.

Exercise helps lose weight and reduce body fat, increases muscular strength and appearance, increases stamina, de-stresses, improves sleep, fitness levels, and increases body immunity; reduces health risks and injuries.

Research-say obesity contributes to global warming. Obese and over weight people require more fuel to transport them to the food they eat and the problem ill worsen as population literally swells in size , where as thinner people eat less and are more likely to walk then rely on cars, a slimmer population would lower demand for fuel for transportation and for agriculture.

OBESE AT RISK OF PSYCHIATRIC DISORDERS, DEPRESSION AND ANXIETY

Child obesity is not only reaching epidemic proportions in our metros, but around the world, to make sure that the whole family eats healthy food. Never skip breakfast, research proves that breakfast eater have lower BMIS balance the meals- so not base any entire tiff in box on noodles, rice or bread. Avoid liquid calories-sweet filled mango shakes or other beverages that contains sugar. Liquid calories are digested much quickly than solid calories. Stock your fridge healthy foods.

They look into a fridge and eat whatever suits them. Limit snakes give juicy fruits and maximize actions. Over weight, children should be encouraged to eat healthy foods and cut calories consumption healthy lifelong change and diet stop eating junk foods. Adult over weight needs to shad extra kilos. About 60% overweight people have a heart related risk- what is worrying is more than 75% are unaware about it. Health is not the absence of illness. It is the presence of wellness. How prevalent are these health conditions? What health issues are related to being overweight or obese? What is necessary to lose weight? What should one do to get more benefits from weight loss? Early detection and action provides you an opportunity to reversal control and add more productivities years to their lives.

Being in shape helps to boost our professional image, self-esteem and raise or happiness quotient about looking good.

This is often expressed by dressing up self-confidence and redefining relationships and makes the difference in health, understanding why you eat what you eat, and the way you control your life. Once you lose your extra weight, make a commitment to sustain it.

Only when you change the behaviors and habits that cause weight gain will you have found the way to sustainable weight loss. Make weight loss bring you a life gain. Fitness tells you how to get belly fat out of your anatomy forever. Challenge you abdominal routine, strengthen the back muscles, evaluate your eating habits, incorporate cardiovascular exercise to burn calories and keep the check on your weight. Even when on a diet, ensure that your body does not miss basic nutrition. Starchy foods provide energizing carbohydrate, fibers, vitamins, minerals and antioxidants that keep immune systems healthy.

Tennis work all the major muscle groups, including the arms, legs, back and stomach and burns about 390 calories an hour, more if you keep missing the ball. Cycling works all the major muscles in your legs and it keeps your stomach in flat too because you work your abdominal muscles while trying to sit up straight and balance on the seat. It is good for all age groups. Jogging is a brilliant fat burner, 260 calories in 20 minutes and if targets your bottom, hips and thighs. Netball burns about 255 calories an hour and good for toning up wobbly thighs and bingo wings. It increases your fitness levels, which boosts fat burning more effectively. Start with warm-up to raise the body's core temperature and cool down gradually to lower body temperature. Right forms and technique protects joints and safeguards the body from exercise trauma. Focus on posture and keep your body properly aligned while exercising. Breathing is an important aspect. Good stretch after an exercise while body is still warm which prevents muscle soreness and increases flexibility. Drink plenty of water before, after and during to prevent dehydration. Progress gradually and systematically structured. Select exercise that is enjoyable and one that fits your personality, lifestyle and fitness goals.

Normal dieting and exercising is a way of life to get in shapes to improve physical health and appearance and attempt to control obesity. In eating disorder becoming thinner is what matters most, health is not the concern; that is not correct concept. It is not how fat or thin you are that matters but how healthy you are counts. In this highly cosmetic world everything from the color of our hair to toe nails is artificial the teenager feel that only when they have the perfect body their lives will be perfect.

Dieting sometimes results in their lack of energy and weakness, restlessness and insomnia. Very often it leads to Dizziness, fainting, and headaches. There could be an early loss of menstrual periods in girls. Thus, they develop depression, anxiety and sudden irritable mood. Hair begins to thin and brittle. They develop anemia and constant low blood pressure. They need medical treatment, nutritional therapy, counselling, behavioral therapy, family therapy.

Teenage years in our city mean going to junior college, having grilled sandwiches and fried foods for lunch every day, constantly munching on chips or snacks and bringing on a pizza when a cracker football match is on TV. A system of low fat snacks and fresh meals needs to be in corporate. Talk of staying healthy and keeping fit. Develop active lifestyle and good eating habits. You do not actually need a diet plan- what you need is an eating behavior insight. The eating behavior that is the way we relate to food. Have you ever noticed that the older you get the easier it is to gain weight and harder it is to lose?

Are you an emotional eater? Deal with your emotions, if tend to numb your problem with food, you eat because you have nothing else to do. You eat when you are sad, lonely, worried, you crave for certain foods when you are depressed to stress. Eating makes you feel better when you are burdened with problem, get to know weather you are physically hungry or emotionally hungry, let the craving pass, distract yourself from food. Talk a walk, watch a movie, play a sport, exercise, listen to music, read, call friend. Choose low calorie food, eat at regular time and eat a balance diet. Stress cause increased levels of cortisol which creates craving for sweet foods. Unfortunately, your worries return as you realize that you have been overeating and you become loaded with guilt. The key is moderation; learn to control your urges. Life events such as unemployment, health problem, family hassle, stressed out work, home etc. can trigger emotions that result overeating.

Exercise slow and steady as every one gets excited about a workout at the beginning. Most of us have our share of over eating triggers but understanding them can make tackling problem a lot easier. When you are feeling low, indulging in that dark chocolate cake can be a temporary solution because it raises the body's blood sugar level. However, uncontrolled eating can further make you feel miserable because you begin to loathe yourself for not having enough self-control. Tackle the issue that is causing the problem. Boredom drives many of us to overeating during the evening or the end of the day. Try to keep yourself stimulated activities other than eating.

Adolescent health—Health nurse/teachers/parents in modern times have a significant responsibility in effectively carry out sex education guiding the youth especially in rural areas. Health nurse can be of immense help in guiding to handle younger ones, when problem faced she can use services of experts such as psychologist, counselor. To work with the youth is a challenging and difficult area yet it is necessity in modern times if the youths are to be given proper direction for the benefit of the nation. They have to be physically and mentally fit.

Healthy development of adolescents is dependent on several complex factors; there socio-economic circumstances, the environment in which they live and grow, the quality of relationship with their families, communities and peer groups and the opportunities for education and employment among others.

The health of the youth is the outcome of all this and in addition nutrition and family, affection they receive as children. The health problems of adolescent and youth are different from younger children and older adults.

The physical growth, which occurs in adolescence, places extra demand and nutritional requirements. During this period additional requirements of nutritious food is needed nutrition is important and inadequate of it can lead to serious consequences throughout reproductive years and beyond.

Along with nutritional diet, a good amount of exercise increases the body's level of endorphins/natural sedatives; improves circulation, promotes cardiovascular health pent-up anxiety.

Skin infection and acne occur in quiet a few teenagers, causing many psychological strains, for they cannot bear anything marring in their appearance. There can be many disorders in the development of breast. All they need is reassurance for the size depends largely on the genetic and family history.

Genitourinary and gynecological infections occur in adolescence. This includes fungal and trichomonal infections which lead to leucorrhea which may cause intense itching.

Problems associated with development— problems can occur in the sexual development of a teenager. If the female, they can take the form of such rare conditions like imperforated hymen, absence or separate vagina or hypertrophied clitoris. Males could have undescended testes with an empty scrotal sac. They could have a micropenis or a feminine distribution of body hair and fat.

Boys usually go through intense psychological stress because of the size of penis compared with that of other boys.

It is the duty of responsible parents to give free and frank sex education. To avoid unwanted pregnancies and single parenthood, the accompanied social stigma and psychological stress are also not infrequent accidents of adolescent. Abortions, usually under unhygienic conditions, can lead to severe morbidity and even death.

Those turbulent teen years growing up are not easy. Changes always raise serious problems. Together with it brings confusion and uncertainties, what to do? Expect some mistakes; unfair competition. Rapid growth brings many changes and under friendly guidance, they are willing to accept suggestions. We are able to help them in their troubled minds. In addition, show them the brighter side of life by doing something constructive. The youths are the future of the country and we need to pay closer attention to them.

Have you noticed how you, as a person, constantly live with fear and anxiety? You have accepted it as a part of life. TV news is an overdose of violence, cruelty, hate crimes, bomb blasts, terrorist threats, communal riots, domestic brutality, border conflicts, wars, murder, dacoit TV brings all this our home, make it part of our life and conversation, extortion, kidnapping, road rage, casts, crimes, something horrible happening somewhere.

Same for the press, net- How do you take it all this and react to it? All this will have the positive and negative impact on your health and personality. Stop and touch deeply the present movement. All of us have the power to change the situation if we care to practice mindful walking, mindful breathing to encourage the energy of mind. Why do you continue to run? The present moment contains all the wonders of life including blue sky, sunshine.

Nurse and Counseling - I

You live in a complex, busy changing world. You are too embarrassed or ashamed to tell teacher or parents what is bothering you or just do not have an appropriate person to turn for counseling. The counselors do not diagnose or label you, he is the best person to listen to you, to find the best ways to understand and resolve your problem. These can be precious hours.

Counseling is also a satisfying and rewarding work role. You know that you have made a profound difference to the life of another human being. It is always a great privilege to be allowed to be a companion to someone who is facing his or her own worst fears and dilemmas. The role is challenging, e.g. coming to terms with trauma, depressed person feels a sense of being accepted and to believe that he is powerful, worthwhile person. Everything is getting one top of me.

What is counseling? It is not just something that happens between two people. In addition, a social institution is embedded in the culture of modern industrialized societies. It is an occupation, discipline of relatively recent origins.

Work with individual with relationships, which may be developmental, crisis support, psychotherapeutic, guiding or problem solving. The task of counseling is to give you an opportunity to explore, discover and clarify ways of living more satisfyingly and resourcefully.

It denotes a professional relationship between a trained counselors and you. Person to person relationship designed to help and understand, clarify your views of your life space and to reach your self-determined goals through meaningful communication skills. Your intimate concerns, problems or aspirations. It is a service sought by people in distress or in some degree of confusion who wish to discuss and resolve these in a relationship, which is more disciplined and confidential than friendship, and perhaps less stigmatizing.

A student may use a teacher as a person with whom it is safe to share worries and anxieties. A community nurse may visit a home to give medical care to a client who is terminally ill, but finds her giving emotional support to the spouse. That is role of the community counselors.

The aim of counseling therefore is insight- understanding of emotional difficulties leading to an increased capacity to take rational control over feelings and actions. Relating with others becoming better able to form and maintain meaningful and satisfying relationships with other people.

Self-awareness of thoughts and feelings that had been blocked off or denied. Self acceptance of a positive attitude towards self and ability to acknowledge areas of self criticism and rejection. Self-actualization, enlightenment assisting the person to arrive at a higher state of spiritual awakening. Problem solving person is not able to resolve alone.

Psychological education to understand and control behaviour. Acquisition of social skills maintenance of eye contact, anger control. Cognitive change the modification or replacement of irrational beliefs or maladaptive thought patterns associated with self-destructive behavior.

Empowerment skills, awareness and knowledge that will enable to take control of once own life. Social action by inspiring in the person a desire and capacity to care for others.

Some of the most important in counseling and psychotherapy have originated in philosophy. The field of moral philosophy also makes an input into counselling by offering a framework for making sense of ethical issues.

Counseling takes place when someone who is troubled invites and allows another person to enter into a particular kind of relationship with them, when they encounter a problem in living.

Confidentially, the counselor undertakes to refrain from passing on what they have learned from the person to any others in the person's life world. Affirmation the counselor enacts a relationship that is an expression of a set of core values, honesty, integrity, care, belief in the worth and value of individual persons, commitment to dialogue and collaboration, reflexivity, the interdependence of persons, a sense of the common good.

Resolution arriving at a personal acceptance of the problem or dilemma and taking action to change the situation in which the problem arose. Learning enable the person to acquire new understanding, skills and strategies that make them better able to handle similar problems in future. Counseling stimulates the energy and capacity of the person as someone who can contribute to the well-being of other and the social good.

In a mass urban society, counselling offers a way of being known and being heard. Someone in extreme need of emotional help and support.

Counseling for abuse done when some one takes advantage of ones power, position, unfair to treat person badly or violently, misuse, to speak in insulting offensive way, to or abuse, threatened, unfair, illegal practice, cruel treatment, rude remarks, insults, criticizing harshly, abusive language used can be referred to counseling.

Education given to a person who indulgence in constant thoughts of fear, anger, melancholy, remorse, envy, sorrow, hatred, worry. Help him for happy living by right food, proper exercise, fresh air, and sunshine and giving purpose in life. Counseling and helping skills can be voluntary professionals. Professional help is often a free-for-service nature. Furthermore, there is the assumption that professional helpers are suitably trained and qualified. It is a relationship. The emphasis here is on the quality of the relationship offered to the client. Characteristics of a good helping relationship are sometimes stated as non-possessive warmth, genuineness and a sensitive understanding of the client's thoughts and feelings.

It emphasizes self-help. Helping is a process with the overriding aim of helping clients to help themselves. Another way of stating this is that all clients, to a greater or lesser degree, have problems in taking effective responsibility for their lives. The notion of personal responsibility is at the heart of the processes of effective helping and self-help.

It is a process. The word 'process' denotes movement, flow and the interaction of at least tow people in which each is being influenced by the behaviour of the other. Both helpers and clients can be in the process of influencing each other. Furthermore, though some of this process transpires within session, much of it is likely to take place between sessions and even after the contact has ended. What begins as a process involving two people ideally ends as a self-help process.

Counseling and helping is a process whose aim is to help clients, who are mainly seen outside medical settings, to help themselves by making better choices and by becoming better choosers. The helper's repertoire of skills includes those of forming an understanding relationship, as well as interventions focused on helping clients change specific aspects of their feelings, thinking and acting, nurturing and healing, problem management, decision making, crisis management, support, life skills training.

What are skills? The meaning of the word skill includes proficiency, competence, and expertness in some activity. However, the essential elements of skill are the ability to make and implement an effective sequence of choices to achieve a desired objective. For instance, if you are to be a good listener, you have to make and implement the choices entailed in being a good listener. The fact that all skills involve choices does not mean that the activities have to be carried out in a mechanistic way. Rather the skills approach to helping may free you to be more spontaneous.

A distinction can be made in helping between a person orientation and a task orientation. With a person orientation, the major emphasis is on the quality of the human relationship offered by counselors and helpers. In an emotional climate of safety, freedom and being understood at a deeper level, technical skills become secondary. The client's own capacity for self-direction is released. Providing good relationships with clients is considered both 'necessary and sufficient' for change to occur. This is an underlying assumption of the client-centered or person-centered approach to helping.

Hearing involves the capacity to be aware of and to receive sounds.

Listening involves not only receiving sounds but, as much as possible, accurately understanding their meaning. As such, it entails hearing words, being sensitive to vocal cues, observing movements and taking into account the context of communications.

Social conversation is geared towards meeting the needs of both participants. In fact, social conversations have facetiously been described as 'two people, both of whom are taking turns to exercise their ego'. Though hearing may take place, listening may not.

A helping conversation emphasizes meeting the psychological needs of clients. As such, it places a high premium on listening to them.

Listening, however, does not just take place between people; it also takes place within each. Indeed your inner listening, or being appropriately sensitive to your own thoughts and feelings, may be vital to your outer listening involving understanding another. Furthermore, if you listen well to another, this may be very helpful to the quality of their inner listening.

Listening involves choices regarding both receiving and sending messages. Sometimes terms like 'active listening' and 'empathy' are used to describe this process.

Importance of Listening—Accurate listening, communicating and understanding is important in helping for a number of reasons.

1. *Creating Rapport:* You are more likely to develop an effective working relationship with your clients if they feel you have understood them.

2. *Creating an influence base:* The objective of helping is to help people to help themselves. To do this effectively, helpers may choose not always to be passive, but to influence their clients actively in developing self-help skills. Listening accurately to your clients is one way you can build your position as an influencer. It contributes to their perceiving you as competent, trustworthy and attractive.

   Furthermore, understanding clients from different cultural groups both as individuals and in terms of their culture contributes to your ascribed status and credibility. This may require special knowledge and cross-cultural sensitivity on your part.

3. *Creating a knowledge base:* If you listen well, most clients collaborate in providing relevant information about themselves. This helps you both in your initial assessment and in any later interventions, you make.

4. *Helping clients to talk:* All of us have some fears about revealing ourselves to others. Clients are often shy and anxious. They may have received much rejection in their pasts. Good listening helps them to feel affirmed, safe, accepted and understood. This in turn helps them to make the choices that allow them to share their world with you.

5. *Helping clients to experience and to express their feelings:* Accurate listening can help clients to acknowledge more of their inner flow of experiencing. The message some clients may need to receive is that it is OK to acknowledge, experience and express their feelings.

6. *Helping clients to own responsibility and to problem-solve:* Clients who are listened to sharply and accurately are more likely to assume responsibility for working on their problems than those who are not. One reason is that good listening may reduce defensiveness. This may increase their willingness to focus on their own behaviour rather than on what others do to them. Another reason is that good listening provides a base for the offering of well-timed confrontations and of different perceptions that encourage clients to assume rather that to avoid responsibility. Furthermore, good listening provides clients with psychological space and support for their self-exploration and problem solving.

   If your clients are to feel that you receive them loud and clear, you need to develop the ability to 'get inside their skins', 'walk in their moccasins' and 'see the world through their eyes'. The skill of listening to and understanding your clients is based on your choosing to get into their internal rather that to remain in your external frame of reference.

   The internal frame of reference involves you in understanding clients on their own terms. This involves choosing to listen carefully and to allow clients the psychological space to tell their own stories. It involves paying attention to vocal and bodily as well as to verbal messages.

Attending and Showing Receptiveness

How can you make good listening choices. Listening is very important in helping. Receiving information skills include attending and showing receptiveness, disciplined hearing and accurately observing body messages. Sending information skills include communicating your understanding and checking its accuracy.

Psychological Receptiveness

Being open to another person's experience of life is more difficult than it appears on the surface. Many carry round the illusion that they listen well, despite the pervasiveness of anxiety and of set ways of perceiving in most people's everyday communication.

As a helper, you need to be present to your clients. This entails an absence of defensiveness and a willingness to allow the expressions and experiencing of your clients to affect you. Ideally, you should be 'all there' – with your body, your thoughts, your senses and your emotions.

Process of presence has two chief aspects: Accessibility and expressiveness.

Accessibility entails a reduction of the usual social defenses against being influenced or affected by others. It implies a measure of trust and vulnerability.

Expressiveness entails making available some of the contents of one's subjective awareness without distortion or disguise. It implies a measure commitment and a willingness to put forward some effort.

Physical attending: Some of the main non-verbal ways you can demonstrate your interest and attention as listener are as follows:

Availability: It may seem obvious, but helpers may sometimes, be rightly or wrongly, perceived as unavailable to help. It may be that they are genuinely over worked. Some may be poor at letting their availability be known. Others may be giving out message, possibly without realizing it that creates distance.

You need to be clear about any formal and informal messages you convey about availability and access.

Relaxed body posture: A relaxed body posture, without slumping or slouching, contributes to conveying the message that you are receptive. If you sit in a tense and uptight fashion, your clients may either consciously think or intuitively feel that you are so bound up in your personal agendas and unfinished business that you are not fully aware of them. Crossed arms, crossed legs, a stiff body posture, finger drumming, leg bouncing and fidgeting may each indicate tension.

Physical openness: Physical openness means facing the speaker not only with your face but also with your body. To sit at a slight angle to your client, but still in a position where you can both receive all of each other's significant facial and bodily messages.

Slight forward lean: Leaning forward is a sign of your involvement. However, if you lean too far forward you look odd and your clients may consider that you invade their personal space. If you lean back, they may find this distancing. Especially at the start of relationships, a slight forward trunk lean can, without being threatening, encourage the talker.

Good eye contact: Good eye contact means looking in your client's direction so that you allow the possibility of your eyes meeting reasonably often. Staring threatens clients. They may feel dominated or seen through. Some clients even feel threatened at seeing their own reflections in shop windows. Looking down or away too often may indicate tension and boredom. Good eye contact also means that you see all the facial messages your clients send.

Appropriate facial expression: A friendly, relaxed facial expression, including a smile, usually demonstrates interest. However, if your client comes in agitated or weeping, a smile would be inappropriate. Your facial expression needs to show that you are tuned into their verbal, vocal and bodily messages.

Use of head nods: Each head nod can be viewed as a reward to the client giving the message that you are paying attention. Head nods need not signify that you agree with everything clients say, but rather that you are interested. As with all physical signals of attending, head nods can be used to control what clients say rather that to free them to communicate from their frame of reference. You need to become aware of whether, when and why you physically respond differently to your clients according to what they say for example, encouraging either their negative or positive comments about themselves.

Nurses provide counseling to help the patient accept actual or impending changes resulting from stress. It involves emotions, intellectual, spiritual and psychological support, patient who needs counselling have normal adjustment difficulties and are upset or frustrated. She encouraged individual to examine available alternatives and decide which choices are useful and appropriate. Help them adapt to changes in lifestyle or body image, during life threatening illness, patients and family need counseling to cope with the possibility of death. E.g. behavioral modification patient changes from smoking to meditation to cope with stress. Patient uses exercise as a health promotion activity, pain control, and anxiety assist children with coping with loss and grief.

Nurse and Counseling - II

Counseling is a process of assistance given to an individual in need with the aim of enabling him to learn and pursue realistic solutions to his difficulties. On going dialogue and relationship between client and Counselor for the provision of psychological support. Counseling differs from casual conversation since it is a focused, specific and purposeful discussion.

Human body made up of many tissues and organs, each having its own particular function to perform. The cell is the unit or the smallest element of the body of which all parts are comprised. Many parts of the body are symmetrically arranged. Human body is the nature's evolution. It is a machine unmatched in its design, unparalleled in the integrity of its functional systems and unfathomable in the depth of subtle and natural emotions. Human body keeps working day and night. The man has so far not devised such an efficient machine, which can work so effectively and for such a length of time.

Every organism in this universe is composed of cells. In human body there are numerous organs, each one has complex structure and carries out a definite functions. All organs are nourished with blood vessels and supplied with nerves. All the delicate internal organs are well protected by bony cage and muscles that provides a definite shape to the body. A bone consists of organic substance and inorganic matter, chiefly consisting of calcium salts. The spinal column is a backbone bears the entire weight of body and yet fully capable of bending and stretching for many years. Vertebrae acts as a cushion and softens and the impact of shocks and jerks through the spinal column. Spinal cord which is like a sot rope leaves the base of the brain and passes through this canal giving out small nerves, that pass out through the spaces provided in the vertebrae. These nerves serve different organs of the body.

All the bones of the skeleton are attached with the muscles, which help in the voluntary and involuntary movements of the body. The skin then covers the whole body to protect the internal organs. The skin also helps in the regulation of the body temperature. Human body is a perfect machine which can regulate itself, provided the natural rules of food, work and rest are observed. When we transgress natural rules, we create toxins in the body, which the body attempts to get rid of.

This attempt is considered as disease and is given different names according to different symptoms. It can be physical or psychological. Psychology is the science of the human mind and includes the different aspects of the mind, namely thought, emotion, behaviour and their accompaniments. A normal person should conform to the standards of thinking, feeling and behaviour of the culture, class, race, religion, age group to which he belongs. Failure to conform is abnormal and he is considered to be suffering from a psychiatric disorder.

Bogged down at work, de-motivated and have no one to rescue you from your duty woes? You need a counselor. There has been rise in job related stress, such as nursing and medical professions, constructions, IT, BPO. The hectic pre- and post-work life is causing employees stress. Let alone, late hours of work, even inter- and intra-traveling networking and hanging out lifestyle stress them.

With high salary come increasing job insecurities. You are as good as your last deal. Some stress is self created by peer pressure and the constant obsession to be better than the guy in the next cubicle owing to increasing work pressure, demanding job roles and a high pressure environment, many feel drained out. People are more open to counselors as they are mature and patient listeners. Factors like traveling, cost of living, relocation, languages and new cultures also induce stress among professionals. This has lead to growing need of counselors, alternative stress releasers such as yoga, exercises, socializing etc.

What are the psychological issues that employees face? Maintaining work life balance, domestic issues, not spending quality time with family, causes stress.

Ego manifests itself in different forms. We usually refer to ego as pride. We can have pride of knowledge, power and, wealth. We attribute all that we are and all that we have done to our own individual effort. We think we are superior to others in many ways. God is a creator and we are small specks in the entire scheme of creation. Some enlightened scientists begun questioning how much a perfectly diagnosed universe and such a complex well-planned organism as a human being could come about through chance.

The person sitting next to you is suffering. He is working away at problems. He has fears. He wonders how he is doing. He does not feel good about himself and he finds it difficult to love others. Deep within people, there is a great toughness for their own integrity, a great tenacity in the face of adversity. Human nature is the most indestructible thing that we know. It has an uninitiated ability to take whatever comes, to go on surviving in the midst of unbelievable difficulties and persecutions.

Sickness and pain have always been a heavy burden on humankind. Right attitude of the client towards sickness and openness to accept healing is an important aspect of life. Spiritual direction and counseling is a valuable practice .The problems are not only produced by illness but also by the stress and strains of today's lifestyle. These anxiety-producing stresses needs to be relived. This social interaction between a person requiring help and a helper who gives such help is called counseling. Counseling forms an important part of the nurse practitioners role, especially in the community where, the majority of problems occur.

Considering the unique role of the nurse in a hospital, the function of nursing is to assist the individual sick or well. The nurse provides, for the emotional and physical comfort and safety of the client. The client sees the nurse as bringing relief from pain or helping to allay his fears. The most significant factor is the nurse's ability to understand why, the client behaves as he does. The nurse must develop empathy that produces insight into the feelings and needs of the client. Clients are bewildered and afraid of what lies before them. Nurse should have within herself a deep spiritual experience, she will be able to cope with the overwhelming problems of suffering and sorrow, which will confront her nearly every day. The nurse is always with the client and, so she will be able to help them better.

First she has to take help in counseling for personal help herself, it helps her in their stress; stress due to the particular nature of her work and responsibility; stress due to the side of client, e.g. When her client dies, she feels it stress due to personal problems.

In the hospital, client is the most important person. Her responsibility is to assist the client in the hospital. Often the family feels the need to talk when, their relatives are ill, when the dear one dies, they need help, to build this inter personal relationship in which the counselor helps the other person to understand and cope his problems. Counselor provides sensitive understanding and skillful response, enters into his personal confusion and conflicts, and at the same time recognizes his emotional reactions so that he not only chooses better ways to reach his reasonable goals, but also has sufficient confidence, courage and moderation to act as this choice.

Nurse counselor needs deep communication, which gradually becomes an intense sense of sharing on understanding and being understood. Through her helping process, enabling him to utilize the resources he has now for coping with life. Where the client learns a new and more satisfying way of adjusting himself to his real environment. She creates an atmosphere through acceptance, reflection and clarification of feeling expressed. She assists client to discover himself and to find a more satisfying way to adjust himself. Become strong enough with self-confidence to act on his own choice.

In direct counseling, counselor is likely to lead the conversation and try to persuade the person to behave in certain prescribed ways.

In non-directive way counselor merely lends a friendly ear reflecting her thoughts and feelings and detailing the alternative forms of behavior. It is a client center counseling. The mutual frankness and honesty of Counselor and client as expected. Good of the person is the goal, the change in the person is part of the process, echoing his sentiments gains his confidence.

She does psychological counseling for clients personal growth. By fostering freedom within the client, improving his encounter with others, discovering meaning for his existence, finding personal meaning in the world of reality.

Aims of counseling is not to solve one particular problem, but to assist the individual to grow so that he can cope with the present problem and with later problem in a better integrated fashion. Thus, client becomes better organize to handle new problem in best manner. Counselor helps him to grow from a feeling of no worth to a feeling of worth, insecurity to security, inadequacy to adequacy, incompleteness to completeness, irresponsibility to responsibility, closeness to openness, and counselor removes the blocks that hinder the need satisfying ways and aims at personality growth.

Counselor helps to develop new skills, new approaches and new motives. The purpose may be to work through a problem, to make a decision, to bring about a change in behavior, to instill self-confidence, or to increase autonomy, efficiency. Through the intermediary and personal loving encounter client is helped to discover himself.

Characteristic of counseling- relationship as the core of the counseling process together with counselors technique and attitudes where, client begins to trust and have emotional security in the counselor. Every one wants to feel worth and mutual respect encourages growth. Spontaneity, authenticity, acceptance, reciprocal openness, mutual listening is very vital for client to lead to discovery that he is responsible for himself in this relationship.

Counseling is person centered and not problem centered. It stresses the emotional element, the feeling aspect of the situation than the intellectual aspect. It stresses the immediate situation, rather than the individuals past. It is a growth experience rather than the solution of the problem, where the client can work out his own understanding, which leads to voluntary choice.

Be a good listener; avoid questions as far as possible. Do not be judgmental; accept the client and his reactions, recognize the value of the period of silence. Avoid personal involvement, avoiding unnecessary reference to you, e.g. I would do in this way. Avoid client dependency, have your limits for the interview, you should not expect to obtain a total picture in one interview, you should not appear hurried, even though you are, allow him to formulate his own plan of action. End your interview in some such way as now, how would you summarize what we have been saying? On the other hand, what do you think is best for you? A comfortable room that will afford privacy and comfort must be given.

A client freely comes to the counselor for help in his own inner struggle. He is sick and he needs help. Total honesty from the part of the client is absolute, a disposition to be open and to discover oneself. Courage to own oneself with defects if any. Ability to trust and confine, he will get what he puts into it. An ability to accept anything meaningful change to take place.

There is a tendency for a client for unhealthy dispositions by seeking sympathy and support, rather than searching for a way out to solve his problem. Defending himself against a sense of weakness; and feels a strong need to lean on others. A feeling that his case is unique and that nobody will understand him properly. He has a strong fear of being condemned. His basic needs are affection, attention, security, achievement, and independence. Five major aspects of a person's life are, incomplete, unfinished, unresolved.

The counselor is called upon to enter into the feelings of the other man, her calling to entering into the confusion of tortured souls, empty herself; she must be given over to others. She should be intellectually able, professionally motivated, and emotionally mature. That is intellectual ability and judgment, resourceful, self-learner, interested in persons as individuals, regards the integrity of other person. Insight into his own personality and has a sense of humor. Sensitivity to the complexities of motivation. Ability to adopt a therapeutic attitude, ability to establish warm and effective relationship with others. Self-control and stability, discriminating sense of ethical values. Deep interest in clinical psychology.

As a surgeon carefully scrubs before an operation, the counselor should enter the counseling relationship scrubbed of her own self-concern and urges. She must keep herself fit like a sharpened sword. She must cultivate positive attitude. Beside she is expected to be a well-balanced personality. Value and respect different cultures, customs. She should shed his mask.

Factors that favor understanding is empathy that, is understanding with heart. Understanding takes place where there is rapport, confidence and trust in other person. Rapport is regarded as an indispensable characteristic for successful counseling.

Communication is the essence of counseling. It is more than talking; it is a conveying of experience in terms of their meaning. Facial expression, gestures, postures, verbal, non-verbal and emotional expression in dialogue.

The word communication comes from the Latin word *communicare* which means to share, to impart, to partake, etc. It means transmitting and sharing of ideas, opinions, facts and information between persons or groups in such a way that the meaning received is equivalent to those that is perceived and understood by the sender. Effective communication is indispensable.

It can be classified on the basis of relationship—formal and informal, on the basis of flow downwards, upward and horizontal, on the basis of expression—verbal, nonverbal, oral and written.

To understand the personal meaning of events we need listening. Be a good listener, follow LADDER pattern:

Look at the other person, maintain good eye contact

Ask appropriate questions

Don't interrupt

Don't change subject

Express emotions with control

Responsive listen.

Listening is truly an art, it comes from inner attitude of mind on the part of the listener and not just a well perfected verbal technique. We hear not only the words but we pick up the feeling tones, the personal meanings, even the meaning that might be below the conscious intent of the speaker. Can we sense the shape of this person's inner world; can we put ourselves in his shoes and appreciate, what it is like to be him? Hearing another person deeply, walk around, and see the world through the eyes of the other. It means that behind the aggression of the person we are able to sense the uncertainty and insecurity.

To listen means to welcome another into yourself, through welcoming presence, inviting look, smile and recognition. Listen to the whole person. Listen with your mind and heart. To listen is to accept, welcome the other into your life. To have to see to it that there is always a room in your inn, that the door is always open. A moment of complete attentiveness is quiet sufficient to welcome the other. There must be plenty of room. Let him come and go as he wills without having to commit himself. Feeling and relating- being with the person bridge connecting the islands of awareness of two human beings. Reflective listening, feeling between the lines. The confidences of the counselee must be respected.

For good listening, stop talking—You cannot listen if you are talking. Put the talker at ease, show that you want to listen, do not read your mail while he talks. Allow plenty of time, do not interrupt him, ask questions, this encourages him and shows you are listening. It helps to develop points further. Stop talking, nature has given two ears and one tongue. Be sensitive and be sober.

Disciplining your hearing—At its most basic level, good listening involves the capacity to hear and remember accurately what has been said. This may be easier said than done. For example, your clients may tell you more than you can easily remember, or they may not express themselves clearly, or may have distracting mannerisms. On your side, your own needs may get in the way of your hearing. You may be tired, angry or have unfinished business in your mind from a previous client.

Additionally, you may have made up your mind what the client's problem is and consequently selectively hear mainly what fits into your formulation.

Hearing vocal messages—As effective counselors, you should be skilled not only at picking up what clients say, but also how they say it. Frequently how clients communicate is much more revealing than what they actually say, as their words may be more concealing than revealing;

Volume	Loudness, quietness, audibility
Pace	Fast, slow
Stress	Monotonous, melodramatic
Pitch	High-pitched, low-pitched, shrill, deep

Observing body messages—Good listening involves choosing to see as well as to hear. Both you and your clients are always sending body messages, some dimensions of which are listed as follows:

- Eye contact staring, looking down or away
- Facial expression expressive of thoughts and feelings, vacant, smiling, hostile
- Gesture amount, variety, e.g. arm movements
- Physical distance near, far, ability to touch.

As age grows with other organs, the capacity hearing and visual of ears and eyes reduces, elderly will not be able to hear properly or see properly hence, it is important that you seat such a way that he can hear and see you properly, e.g. Abuse of elderly person let us take. Abuse of elderly persons can occur in their own homes, hospitals, home for aged etc. the abuses may be by family members, caregiver, neighbors etc. there are different forms of abuse, and sometimes-intentional harm may be done to the elderly.

Elder abuse is defined as the willful infliction (impose) of injury, unreasonable confinement, intimation, or punishment by an individual including a caretaker of goods or services that are necessary to attain or maintain physical, mental and psychological well-being.

Types of Abuse-Physical—Use of force resulting in bodily injury, physical pain or physical impairment, such act of violence as striking, pushing, slapping, kicking, pinching and burning. Inappropriate use of medication, restraints, force feeding, and physical punishment of any kind.

Psychological abuse—Emotional – infliction of pain or distress through verbal or nonverbal acts, verbal assaults, insults, threats, intimidation, humiliation, and harassment, abusing language, silence or isolation.

Abandonment—It is the desertion of person by individual who has assumed responsibility for providing care.

Financial or material exploitation includes the illegal or improper use of an elder's funds, property or assets. This may involve the use of funds without permission, forging a signature, misusing or stealing possessions, deceiving the elder into signing any document and improper use of power of attorney or guardianship.

Self neglect—It is the behavior of an elderly which threatens his own health or safety, e.g. personal care, meal preparation, poor hygiene, bad body odor, sores, rashes, soiled clothing.

In crisis management, counselors are faced with making immediate choices that help clients get through their sense of being overwhelmed.

Crisis may be defined as situations of excessive stress. Stress tends to have a negative connotation in our culture. This is unjustified if one thinks of stress in terms of adjustive demands or, more colloquially, challenges in life.

In an acute state of crisis, clients may be experiencing heightened or maladaptive reactions in a number of different, though interrelated, areas. Therefore counseling is a vast field and there is different specialty of choice of a group that one is interested.

There are numerous books in the sky, a lot of wisdom in the stars, music in the bamboos, poem in the flower, knowledge in leaves, proverbs in seeds, fables in the dew, angels in marbles, formulas in atoms, ideas in grains of sands, humor in animals, art in shadow and life of god in everything. Those who look see it and those who see it translate.